6.04-19

Surgical Treatment of Haemorrhoids

Springer
London
Berlin
Heidelberg
New York
Barcelona
Hong Kong
Milan
Paris
Singapore
Tokyo

Charles Mann (Ed.)

Surgical Treatment of Haemorrhoids

Springer

British Library Cataloguing in Publication Data
Surgical treatment of haemorrhoids
1. Hemorrhoids – Surgery
I. Mann, Charles V. (Charles Victor)
617.5′55
ISBN 1852334967

Library of Congress Cataloging-in-Publication Data
Surgical treatment of haemorrhoids / Charles Mann, ed.
p. ; cm.
Includes bibliographical references and index.
ISBN 1-85233-496-7 (alk. paper)
1. Hemorrhoids – Surgery. 2. Hemorrhoids. I. Mann, Charles V.
[DNLM: 1. Hemorrhoids – surgery. 2. Hemorrhoids – diagnosis. 3. Hemorrhoids – therapy. WI 605 S961 2001]
RC865 .S87 2001
617.5′55 – dc21 2001034455

ISBN 1-85233-496-7 Springer-Verlag London Berlin Heidelberg
a member of BertelsmannSpringer Science+Business Media GmbH
http://www.springer.co.uk

Printed in Great Britain

Typeset by Best-set Typesetter Ltd., Hong Kong
Printed and bound at The Cromwell Press, Trowbridge, Wiltshire, England
28/3830-543210 Printed on acid-free paper SPIN 10836267

Preface

Despite its unglamorous reputation, surgical treatment of haemorrhoids is one of the most important coloproctological procedures. The justification for this assertion relies on the experience that if a surgeon or clinic achieves a reputation for kind and efficient management of this most tender area, patients will present themselves in large numbers, and not only with haemorrhoidal disease; conversely, if a surgeon is ignorant or clumsy in this area, patients will go elsewhere for treatment. Two famous clinics with international reputations in coloproctology (St. Marks Hospital, London and the Ferguson Clinic, Michigan) started with the aim of providing the highest quality of care to haemorrhoids, and other anal conditions such as fistula.

In many instances, poor surgical results in haemorrhoid surgery are caused not only by wrong choice of procedure but also by being badly carried out. In too many cases, these faults are compounded by the operation being delegated to an inexperienced junior. Only when the need for meticulous standards of surgery for the treatment of haemorrhoids is recognised will haemorrhoidectomy shed its evil reputation amongst the general public.

For this reason, and to fulfil the aim of the book to encourage high standards of craftsmanship, an international panel of distinguished contributors has been invited to provide detailed descriptions of their techniques for the treatment of haemorrhoids. The reader will be enabled to select the procedure of choice for each patient, and assimilate those small, but vital, details of care that make all the difference to the result. If this objective is attained, patients should be spared brutal and unsatisfactory haemorrhoid surgery.

If the book contains a large number of chapters to describe a wide variety of techniques, this is a requirement to present the many procedures available for the treatment of piles. Most proctologists employ only a limited number of techniques, but all of them have to be aware of what is available, so that they can make informed judgements regarding correct management.

Despite increased critical appraisal of the results of surgery, in the case of haemorrhoid surgery many treatments are applied without a background of controlled clinical trials. Many "old" procedures persist, and many "new" procedures are taken up because of the personal preferences of the surgeon. In future, it is hoped that all procedures will be properly validated. Until this occurs, many surgeons will be reluctant to change their management; worse still, socio-economic pressures will usurp undue prominence in the choice of operation, and give insurance companies and politicians too much power over treatment protocols.

If the object of this book is realised, the surgical reader should have his interest in haemorrhoid surgery reinforced and should be able to measure his practise against the best international standards. At the least, the best technique for each operation should be adopted by all surgeons, which should reduce patient suffering to the lowest possible level.

The Editor wishes to extend his gratitude to the experts contributing their wisdom and experience to this book.

C.V. Mann MA, MCh, FRCS (Editor)

Contents

Contributors

Professor Timothy G. Allen-Mersh
Professor of Gastrointestinal Surgery
Division of Surgery
Anaesthetic and Intensive Care
Imperial College School of Medicine
Chelsea & Westminster Hospital
369 Fulham Road
London, SW10 9NH
UK

Dr Stephen I. Allison
Fellow Colon & Rectal Surgery
Athol Place Surgery
Wickham Terrace
Brisbane, 4006
Queensland
Australia

Dr Mireille C. Berthoud
Department of Anaesthesia
Royal Hallamshire Hospital, CSUH Trust
Glossop Road
Sheffield, S10 2JF
UK

Dr Julius C. Bonello
Clinical Associate Professor of Surgery
U of I College of Medicine
7303 N. Knoxville Avenue
Peoria, IL 61614
USA

Dr Sridhar Chalasani
Chief General Surgical Resident
York Hospital
1001 South George Street
York, PA 17405-7198
USA

Professor Marvin L. Corman
University of Southern
California - Centre
for Colorectal Diseases
450 San Pablo Street, #4500
Los Angeles, CA 90033
USA

Dr Francesco Cortese
Department of Surgery
"Tor Vergata" University, Rome
St Eugenio's Hospital, Rome
Italy

Mr S. Ellesmore
Department of Surgery
St Marks Hospital
Watford Road
Harrow
Middsx, HA1 3UJ
UK

Mr L. Peter Fielding
Professor of Clinical Surgery
Pennsylvania State University School of Medicine
Medical Director, Surgical Service Line
Chairman, Department of Surgery
York Hospital
1001 South George Street
York, PA 17405-7198
USA

Dr K.S. Ho
Registrar
Department of Colorectal Surgery
Singapore General Hospital
Outram Road
Singapore 169 608
Singapore

Professor Indru T. Khubchandani
Division of Colon and Rectal Surgery
Department of Surgery
Lehigh Valley Hospital
Allentown, Pennsylvania
USA
Professor of Surgery
Pennsylvania State University College of Medicine
Hershey, Pennsylvania
USA

Chefarzt Dr Han C. Kuijpers
Koloproktologische Klinik
Prosper Hospital
Mühlenstrasse 27
45659 Recklinghausen
Germany

Professor Roger J. Leicester
Consultant in General and Colorectal Surgery
Colo-Rectal Surgery Unit
St George's Hospital
Blackshaw Road
London SW17 0QT
UK

Mr Peter H. Lord
Previously Chief of Surgery
Wycombe General Hospital
England
and Vice-President
Royal College of Surgeons (Eng).

Holly Tree House
39 Grove Road
Beaconsfield
Bucks, HP9 1PE
UK

Mr Peter J. Lunniss
Senior Lecturer
Honorary Consultant Surgeon
Academic Department of Surgery
Room 442, 4th Floor Alexandra Wing
The Royal London and Homerton Hospitals
Whitechapel
London, E1 1BB
UK

Mr Charles V. Mann
Emeritus Surgeon
St. Marks Hospital and
The Royal London Hospital.

The Cosy
Basingstoke Road
Old Alresford
Hants, SO24 9DL
UK

Professor Giovanni Milito
Unita Di Colonproctologia Ed
Endoscopia Digestiva
Casa Di Cura Villa Stuart
Via Trionfale 5952
00135 Roma
Italy

Dr Per-Olof Nyström
Consultant Colorectal Surgeon
Colorectal Surgery
Department of Surgery, University Hospital
SE-581 85 Linkoping,
Sweden

Dr Hitesh Patel
Department of Surgery
Chelsea & Westminster Hospital
369 Fulham Road
London, SW10 9NH
UK

Mr Albert Peters
Surgeon, Marienhospital Erwitte
Erwitte
Germany

Dr Francis Seow-Choen
Head and Clinical Associate Professor
Department of Colorectal Surgery
Singapore General Hospital
Outram Road
Singapore 169 608
Singapore

Professor Rune Sjödahl
Professor of Surgery
Consultant Colorectal Surgeon
Colorectal Surgery
Department of Surgery, University Hospital
SE-581 85 Linkoping,
Sweden

Mr Alastair C.J. Windsor
Consultant Surgeon
St Marks Hospital
Watford Road
Harrow
Middsx, HA1 3UJ
UK

1 Surgical History of Haemorrhoids

S. Ellesmore and A.C.J. Windsor

For as long as man has been blessed with an anus, it is fair to assume that he has also been doubly blessed with haemorrhoids. The word "haemorrhoid" is derived from the Greek *haema* (blood) and *rhoos* (flowing), and it was probably Hippocrates (460 BC) who was the first to apply the name to the flow of blood from the veins of the anus. The term "piles" is derived from the Latin *pila* (a ball) and was widely used by the public at the time of John of Arderne (born AD 1307), and in his treatise of 1370 he remarks that the "common people call them piles, the aristocracy call them haemorrhoids, the French call them figs (*figer*, to clot), what does it matter so long as you can cure them". If only it was that simple.

The Egyptians

Although Egyptian writings left no specific reference to haemorrhoids, there are several descriptions which are unlikely to be any other condition. The *Edwin Smith Papyrus* (1700 BC) (Breasted, 1930) and the Ebers Papyrus (1500 BC) (Ebbel, 1937) both contain references to anal pathology and the *Edwin Smith Papyrus* reports, "if thou inspecteth a man in his anus, whether standing or sitting, suffering very greatly with seizures in both his legs. Thou shouldst give a recipe, an ointment of great protection; Acacia leaves, ground, titurated and cooked together. Smear a strip of fine linen therewith and place in the anus, that he may recover immediately".

The Greeks

The Hippocratic Treatises (460 BC) (Adams, 1849) provide some of the earliest details of both clinical description and surgical treatment of haemorrhoids and in the following reference, Hippocrates is seen to favour an operation to simply ligate the pile: "And haemorrhoids in like manner you may treat by transfixing them with a needle and tying them with very thick and woollen thread; for thus the cure will be the more certain. When you have secured them, use a septic application, and do not foment until they drop off, and always leave one behind; and when the patient recovers let him be put on a course of Hellebore." Further writings "On Haemorrhoids" (Adams, 1849) attributed to Hippocrates deal with haemorrhoidal excision and give mention to an expanding speculum akin to one found in the ruins of Pompeii, and remarkable similar to the Eisenhammer retractor of today. There also appears an interesting description of the aetiology of haemorrhoids: "The disease of the haemorrhoids is formed in this way: if bile or phlegm be determined to the veins of the rectum, it heats the blood in the veins; and being gorged the inside of the gut swells outwardly, and the heads of the veins are raised up, and being at the same time bruised by the faeces passing out, and injured by the blood collected in them, they squirt out blood, most frequently along with the faeces". It is good to see that our understanding of the aetiology of haemorrhoids has improved, though some would question by how much.

The Romans

A Roman contribution to the history of the haemorrhoid is provided by Celsus (25 BC–AD 14). In *De Medicina* (Celsus & Cornelius, 1938), he gives a description of the surgery, mentioning both the ligature and ligature-excision technique, and also mentions the postoperative complication of urinary retention. Galen (AD 131–201) also gives a good clinical description of haemorrhoidal disease, and advocates ligation of haemorrhoids for two hours when surgery is indicated. The intermittent occlusion of the vascular pedicle was also used in the nineteenth century to reduce pain and to avoid spreading gangrene.

The Far East

The only reference of note from Indian medical history is in *The Susruta Samhita* (Bhishnagratna, 1907), the ancient Sanskrit text of Hindu medicine. Opinions are divided as to its date, from fourth century BC to fifth century AD. The work is the Aryan equivalent of the Hippocratic Treatise, but is more surgically advanced. Of note are its emphasis on wound cleanliness and advanced surgical technique.

Following the collapse of the Roman and Greek civilisations, medical knowledge was nurtured by the Arab Empire; Rhazes (AD 860–932), Ali Abbas (AD c.994) and Avicenna (AD 980–1036) (Adams, 1844) all describe the classical operations for piles. However, the Arab scholars held the baton of medical knowledge for only a short time before returning it to Europe.

The Master Surgeons

At this time Europe was to see one of its finest periods of surgical advancement in the hands of the Master Surgeons. Theodoric (AD 1205–1296) trained at the University of Salerno, discarded Galenical doctrine and advocated healing by primary intention. Lanfrank (died AD 1315) of Milan migrated to Paris in 1295 and became the first great teacher of French surgery. Henri de Mondeville, Guy de Chauliac and John of Arderne (one of the most celebrated early colorectal surgeons), all educated at Montpelier, greatly advanced surgery in a pre-Renaissance revival. Interestingly, master surgeons wrote little during this period, and even less about the management of haemorrhoids. Henri de Mondeville (1260–1320) mentioned haemorrhoids only to warn against operating on them. Unfortunately, the era of the Master Surgeon came to an end with the practise of surgery by the barber and not the scholar; a situation that would remain until the middle of the eighteenth century.

The Barber Surgeons

The era of the barber surgeon lasted for nearly 350 years, and what writings there were from true surgeons were sadly very traditional. The notable surgeons of the time, Ambrose Pare (1510–1590), Master Peter Lowe (1612), Dr Read (1650) and Richard Wiseman (1622–1676), added little to the medical knowledge of haemorrhoids. In polite society at this time, the condition was known as "le mal de St Phiacre", an attempt to confer respectability by the possession of a patron saint; however, there seems to be some doubt about the appropriateness of the chosen patron who was the patron saint of gardeners!

The Renaissance

The eighteenth century saw the end of the barber surgeon and a return of science to medicine. Lorenz Heister (1739) published a work on *Chirurgie*, one of the first textbooks to contain detailed illustrations. He states on haemorrhoids, "but the moderns judging the methods of the ancients too cruel, and often pernicious, generally leave the case to nature, except when the discharge is profuse . . .". He described ligature with excision, "he is then to tie up the bleeding tunercles with a needle and thread, cutting off those parts which are distended beyond the ligature, taking care at the same time to leave a few of the smallest veins open as before observed".

In the same period, Morgagni (1749) (Morgagni, 1769) published his theory on the aetiology of haemorrhoids, differing from the Hippocratic dogma held by the ancient and mediaeval writers. Morgagni stated, "without doubt, it was not very easy for the blood to pass through a liver of that kind [cirrhotic]. But why, then, you will say, did it not stagnate equally in the other veins which go to the trunk of the vena portarum? And for this very reason it was that I said you would immediately understand it, or at least in part. Add therefore, to omit other things, the very great length, which is peculiar to this one vein [the superior haemorrhoidal] among the others, so that it is much more difficult for the blood to be carried upwards, from this vein, than from the others, especially as the situation of the human body requires it, which without doubt is one of the reasons why other animals are not subject to piles. And if you ask why, in those bodies in which there is any impediment to the quick motion of the blood upwards, the veins of the legs in particular are dilated into varices, you will find the same thing to be the cause of them chiefly which we assign for the piles."

The Nineteenth Century

At the end of the eighteenth century and the beginning of the nineteenth century, men such as Percivall Pott, William Cheselden and John Hunter created an environment in which writing was encouraged, although interestingly none of these men wrote about haemorrhoids themselves. There was great debate about the relative values of ligation and of excision of haemorrhoids, neither without mortality, and ligation with the added morbidity of intense pain. It would appear that the surgeons of the time had not differentiated between the sensitive anal skin and the insensitive rectal mucosa.

Jean Louis Petit, who wrote a three-volume book on surgery in 1774 (Petit, 1774), rejected excision due to potentially fatal haemorrhage and anal stenosis, and ligation due to pain and gangrene. He noted that the skin of the anus was sensitive and therefore recommended excision ligation, and in 1835, Brodie (Brodie, 1836), in writing about the problems of ligation alone, stated: "The application of the ligature to internal piles in general causes but little pain, and only a slight degree of inflammation follows, for the mucous membrane has nothing like the sensibility of the skin, and does not resent an injury in like manner". In a *Dictionary of Practical Surgery*, Samuel Cooper (1809) both quoted and supported Petit's favour of excision/ligation and, although the technique was not universally accepted, one has to remember that this was before the advent of general anaesthesia and this technique took longer to perform than both excision and ligation alone. Sir Astley Cooper (1836) supported ligation, following the death of three of his patients on whom he had performed an excision – two from bleeding, one from peritonitis – and Copeland described many complications from the excision/ligation technique, including pain, retention of urine, stricture and tetanus. He recommended rectal bouginage, popular with the French schools, thought to treat the increased anal tone which was the cause of haemorrhoids.

The founder of St Marks Hospital, Frederick Salmon, in his short book of rectal surgery (1828), advised bouginage. But we learn later from Allingham (1888) that Salmon modified the excision/ligation operation, incising the perianal skin, dissecting between the haemorrhoidal plexus and the anal musculature as high as the rectal mucosa, then ligating the pedicle. Little has been added to the operation of haemorrhoidectomy since then, the exception being Whitehead's (1882) operation which involved removing the pile-bearing area of the anal canal and restoring mucosal continuity by the suturing of rectal mucosa to anal skin. It was not adopted in the UK due to the side-effects of stricture, incontinence due to loss of sensation, and soiling due to the presence of rectal mucosa in the anal canal, although it enjoyed greater popularity in America.

The Twentieth Century

The success and safety of Salmon's operation sounded the death knell of the ligation alone technique. Many surgeons have modified this operation since, but none has altered the technique to any great extent. Those worthy of mention are Smith (1876), Alfred Cooper (1887), Quain (1854), Bryant (1861), Goodsall (Goodsall & Miles, 1900), Wallis (1907), Cripps (1884), Ball (1908), Miles (1919), Lockhart-Mummery (1923), Gabriel (1948), Devine (Devine &

Devine, 1948), and, of course, the modification described by Milligan, Morgan, et al. (Milligan et al., 1937).

The end of the twentieth century saw two further developments; the diathermy haemorrhoidectomy, as described by Alexander-Williams (Sharif et al., 1991), and the stapled haemorrhoidectomy, using either a linear or a circular stapling device (Longo, 1998). All the various techniques are presently practised and supported by different surgeons, and, as yet, no one technique has proved superior to the others or been universally adopted. The debate as to the aetiology of haemorrhoids continues, with currently accepted theories including varicosity of the anal submucosal veins, vascular hyperplasia and downward displacement of the anal canal lining. It seems logical that a better understanding of aetiology may allow a more appropriate and effective surgical approach.

Conservative Management

The history of haemorrhoids would not be complete without mention of the more conservative treatments we all practise on a daily basis. In 1657, Riverius (Riviere, 1657) was supposed to have used the topical application of nitric acid, a technique reintroduced by Houston (1843). In 1860, quacks were injecting phenol solution into piles, a technique later adopted by the medical profession, after Andrews (1879) thought it to be too dangerous to be used by the quacks.

Cauterisation was revised by Cusack, using a special clamp. This clamp was later modified by Smith, Allingham and von Langenbeck, among others.

Banding was introduced by Barron (1963), and, in many outpatient departments, has found favour over injection.

That the haemorrhoid should be featured in the medical literature of the past four thousand years, that patients in the past were prepared to risk death as a complication of surgery, and that present treatments are still far from perfect, implies that there is more to the humble pile than one first imagines.

The authors would like to acknowledge the late Sir Alan Parks, whose seminal article on the surgical history of haemorrhoids has formed the core research material for this chapter (Parks, 1955).

References and Further Reading

Adams F (1844–1847) The seven books of Paulus Aegineta, Book 6, Sec 79, London, 2, p 403
Adams F (1849) The Genuine Works of Hippocrates, London, 1, pp 333, 825
Allingham W (1888) Diagnosis and Treatment of Disease of the Rectum, Fifth edition, London. Revised by Allingham HW, p 143
Andrews E (1879) Med Rec N Y 15:451
Ball CB (1908) The Rectum, its Diseases and Developmental Defects, London, p 210
Barron J (1963) Office ligation for internal haemorrhoids. Am J Surg 105:563–70
Bhishnagratna KKL (1907) An English Translation of the Susruta Samhita, Calcutta, 2, p 316
Breasted JH (1930) The Edwin Smith Surgical Papyrus, Chicago, 1, p 507
Brodie B (1836) Thirty-six lectures on disease of the rectum. Lond Med Gaz 18:182
Bryant T (1861) Guy's Hosp Rep, 3s 7:91
Celsus AC (trans 1938) De Medicina, Book 7, Ch 30, Para 3, Spencer WG (trans), London, 3, p 465
Cooper AP (1836) The Principles and Practice of Surgery, London, p 426
Cooper S (1809) A Dictionary of Practical Surgery, London, p 367
Cooper, A (1887) A Practical Treatise on the Diseases of the Rectum, London
Cripps H (1884) On Diseases of the Rectum and Anus, London, p 52
Devine HB, Devine J (1948) The Surgery of the Colon and Rectum, Bristol, p 323
Ebbel B (1937) The Papyrus Ebers, Stockholm, pp 43–4
Gabriel WB (1948) The Principles and Practice of Rectal Surgery, Fourth Edition, London
Galen Galeni Opera ex Octava luntarum. Editone Venetiis apud luntas, MDCIX
Goodsall DH, Miles WE (1900) Diseases of the Anus and Rectum, London
Heister L (1739) A General System of Surgery. Book 5, p 249
Houston J (1843) Dublin J Med Sci 23:95
Lockhart-Mummery JP (1923) Diseases of the Rectum and Colon, London
Longo A (1998) Mundozzi Editore, p 777
Miles WE (1919) Surg Gynecol Obstet 29:497
Milligan ETC, Morgan CN, Jones LE, Officer R (1937) Lancet 2:1119
Morgagni JB (trans 1769) Seats and Causes of Disease, Letter 32, Article 10, Alexander B (trans), London, 2, p 105
Parks AG (1955) De Haemorrhois, a study in surgical history. Guy's Hosp Rep 104:135–56
Petit JL (1774) Traite de Maladies Chirurgicales et des Operations, Paris, 2, p 137
Quain R (1854) The Diseases of the Rectum, London
Riviere L (1657) Praxis Medica cum Theoria Lugduni, Ninth Edition, Book 10, Ch 10, p 184
Salmon F (1828) A Practical Essay on Strictures of the Rectum, Third edition, London, p 205
Sharif HI, Ling Lee, Alexander-Williams (1991) Int J Colorect Dis 6:217–19
Smith H (1876) The Surgery of the Rectum, Fourth Edition, London
Wallis FC (1907) Surgery of the Rectum, London, p 47
Whitehead W (1882) Br Med J 1:148

2 Anatomy and Development of Haemorrhoids (Including Classification)

Peter J. Lunniss

Introduction

It is, at first sight, somewhat surprising that, in this age of rapid technological advances and medical achievements, our understanding of one of the commonest afflictions of the human race is, at best, limited. Literature relating to haemorrhoids spans many centuries, but the scientific basis of most of these contributions may be justly disputed. Theories relating to aetiology abound, and conversations with colleagues and lay people alike reveal an astounding spectrum of concepts. It is prudent, therefore, to return to an appreciation of the relevant anatomy, from which appropriate criticisms concerning theories of the development of haemorrhoids may be made.

Anatomy

Examination of the anal canal of foetuses clearly shows the mucosa and submucosa above the dentate line to be uneven and thrown into folds; the so-called anal cushions (Fig. 2.1). There are variations in the numbers and positions of these cushions, but there are usually three, corresponding to those seen in later life. These are described classically as occupying the left lateral, right posterior and right anterior positions, and which continue proximally as the primary rectal foldings, described in detail by Johnson in 1914. Slightly later in foetal development, secondary foldings are seen (the rectal columns of Morgagni), both over and between the primary folds, and between the bases of which lie the rectal sinuses. This area is the caudal limit of the so-called epithelial transitional zone, below which the anal canal is lined by stratified squamous epithelium, and which is richly innervated by sensory nerve endings serving several modalities including touch, pain and temperature. The bulk of the anal cushions themselves, situated in the upper part of the anal canal, are lined by rectal-type mucosa with only visceral afferent innervation, and although there is perception of stretching, sensitivity to noxious stimuli is much more blunted than distally.

Between the epithelial layer and the internal sphincter lies the submucosa consisting of vascular, muscular and connective tissue supportive elements. The key to the understanding of this layer (and indeed the anal sphincter complex itself) is the conjoined longitudinal muscle of the anal canal (Lunniss and Phillips, 1992; Fig. 2.2). The longitudinal muscle is a direct continuation of the smooth muscle of the outer muscle coat of the rectum, augmented in its upper part by striated muscle fibres originating from the medial components of the pelvic floor. In the foetus, this layer is very prominent as it descends between internal and external sphincters, and, indeed, is a thicker muscle layer than the internal sphincter. With age, however, there is a gradual replacement of muscle fibres by fibrous and connective tissue, such that in late adult life, very few muscle fibres are seen in the distal part of the sphincter complex, and the layer itself is relatively much thinner.

As it descends, the longitudinal muscle layer gives off ramifying extensions that pass medially and

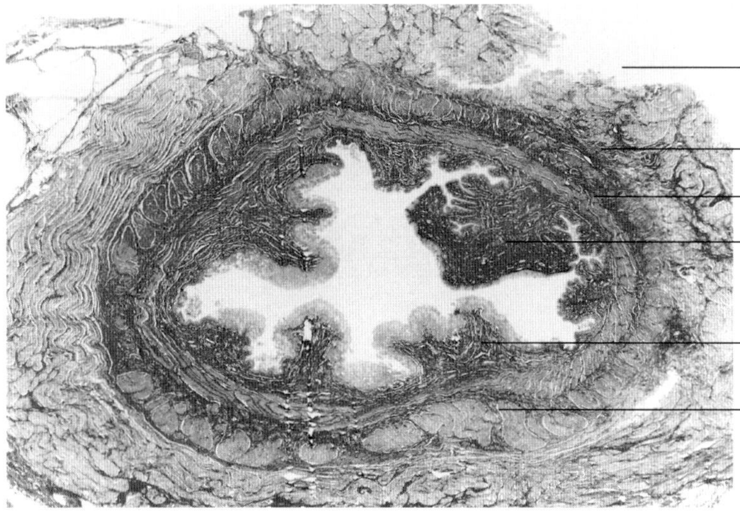

Figure 2.1. Transverse section of a foetal anal canal just above the dentate line. The mucosa and submucosa are thrown into 3 primary foldings (the anal cushions) and several much smaller secondary foldings. The longitudinal muscle layer, at this age, is wider than the internal sphincter, and the muscle bundles are well seen. From this layer, muscle and connective tissue fibres pass outwards between the fibres of the external sphincter and inwards across the internal anal sphincter to enter the submucosa. With age the muscle:connective tissue ratio falls, and few muscle fibres are seen in the anal canal of the elderly.

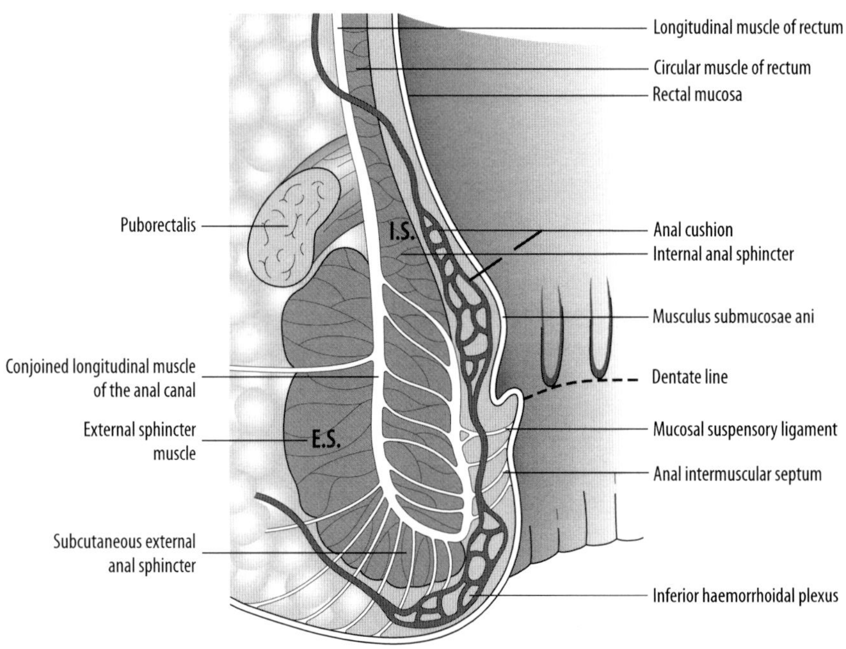

Figure 2.2. Line drawing to show the relevant anatomy of the anal canal. The longitudinal muscle layer of the rectum, augmented by fibres from the medial part of the pelvic diaphragm, descends as the conjoined longitudinal muscle layer of the anal canal. As it descends, fibres pass medially across the internal anal sphincter and blend with the smooth muscle fibres of the submucosa (Treitz's muscle, musculus submucosae ani). The orientation of fibres crossing the internal sphincter changes from inferomedially above the dentate line to superomedially below it. The inferior terminal ramifications of the conjoined longitudinal muscle layer, inserting into the skin of the anal verge, define the subcutaneous component of the external anal sphincter. The most medial of these fibres, looping around the inferior border of the internal anal sphincter to insert into the anoderm below the dentate line is known as the anal intermuscular septum (its site seen on examination as the intermuscular groove). The condensation of fibres at the level of the dentate line is known as the mucosal suspensory ligament (of Parks).

laterally across the sphincter components. Most of the muscle continues down the intersphincteric space before splitting into multiple terminal septa, which surround the muscle bundles of the subcutaneous portion of the external sphincter to insert into the skin of the lowermost part of the anal canal and adjacent perianal skin. Milligan and Morgan (1934) named the most medial of these septa, passing around the inferior border of the internal sphincter, the "anal intermuscular septum". Above this level, medial extensions cross the internal anal sphincter and form part of the supporting meshwork of the submucosa, blending with the submucosal smooth muscle layer and thereby supporting the mucosa itself. Some authorities consider that those fibres crossing the internal sphincter to enter the submucosa originate from the internal sphincter itself rather than the longitudinal muscle layer (Kerremans, 1969; Lawson, 1974), but my own observations, especially when foetal anatomy is considered, are consistent with those of the anatomists of the last century (Rudinger, 1878; Roux, 1881) in that fibres traverse the width of the internal sphincter from longitudinal layer to submucosa. These fibres cross the internal sphincter in an inferomedial direction above the dentate line, and in a supramedial direction below the dentate line. Sir Alan Parks (1954) described the increased density of fibres that are inserted into the mucosa of the anal crypts at the level of the dentate line the "mucosal suspensory ligament" (although he considered this to be derived from the sheath surrounding the internal anal sphincter). One feature of this structure is that it separates the superior and inferior haemorrhoidal plexuses, another is that the mucosa is more firmly tethered to underlying tissues at this level than above. Fibres that cross the internal sphincter at a higher level to reach the subepithelial space interlace with those that have crossed more distally as well as with the true submucosal smooth muscle, first described by Treitz in 1853, and variously named since.

The exact origin of the smooth muscle fibres in the submucosa of the anal canal is perhaps not crucial in a discussion on the anatomy of haemorrhoids. What is of paramount importance, however, is an appreciation that there is a meshwork of supporting tissues (muscle fibres and connective tissue) within the subepithelial space that is intimately linked to deeper structures within the anal sphincter complex, including the internal sphincter, longitudinal muscle layer, external anal sphincter, and, indeed, extending beyond the sphincter complex (Courtney, 1950). With age, the smooth muscle component of this mesh is reduced, and muscle fibres are gradually replaced with fibroelastic connective tissue, which in turn becomes fragmented.

In addition to the meshwork support to the lining of the anal canal, the subepithelial space contains venous dilatations supported by the same fibroelastic, connective tissue and smooth muscle scaffolding. Debate has centred on the nature of the vascular component of haemorrhoids, but the seminal anatomical studies of Thomson (1975) have clarified this issue. Although the vascular component of the subepithelial space in the unborn is not prominent, venous dilatations, similar to those seen in adults, have been observed histologically in infant specimens. These vascular dilatations are seen in the submucosa both above and below the level of the dentate line, but are much more numerous above, although tending to be larger below. The description of the blood supply to the upper anal canal by Miles, constant with bifurcation of the main trunk of the superior rectal artery into right and left branches, and with subsequent division of the former into anterior and posterior divisions thereby determining the sites of haemorrhoids around the anal circumference, was questioned by Thomson. He demonstrated that, in fact, the divisions of the superior rectal artery were not constant, and that furthermore, the anal submucosa in a proportion of his specimens received a blood supply from the middle and inferior rectal arteries. He was also able to show the presence of free communications between tributaries of the superior, middle and inferior rectal veins, as well as tiny direct arteriovenous communications with the submucosal venous dilatations. These communications have been shown both histologically and radiologically, and the oxygen tension of the blood contained within the venous dilatations (as well as the colour) is more arterial than venous.

Function of the Anal Cushions

To some extent, ideas as to why anal cushions exist must be teleological. No circular muscular structure alone can contract to the extent that its lumen is obliterated and irregularity of mucosal contour and distensibility are seen in other situations where luminal occlusion occurs. Thus, it is very attractive to suppose that the anal cushions, by their triradiate disposition and potential to vary in volume secondary to their vascular components, exist to effect an effective seal to prevent leakage of any rectal contents to the outside. Of course, at the time of defaecation, the anal canal must open up to allow passage of stool, which may be of considerable and surprising diameter. Simple compression of the vascular spaces and flattening of the cushions may be sufficient, but the presence of smooth muscle fibres and connective tissue mesh within the subepithelial space, linked intimately with internal sphincter, longitudinal muscle and external sphincter, begs a more active role. Recently, pharmacological studies in vitro have demonstrated fundamental differences in the responses of the longitudinal anal and internal anal muscle components to various agents. Thus, stimulation of cholinergic muscarinic receptors causes longitudinal anal-muscle and rectal smooth-muscle contraction, but internal anal-sphincter relaxation; alpha-adrenergic receptor stimulation results in rectal smooth-muscle relaxation but internal sphincter- and longitudinal anal-muscle contraction (O'Kelly et al., 1993). Subsequently, the role of nitric oxide as the neurotransmitter of intrinsic non-adrenergic, non-cholinergic inhibitory neurones involved in rectal smooth muscle and internal anal sphincter relaxation and the recto–anal inhibitory reflex has been substantiated (O'Kelly, 1996; Stebbing et al., 1997). The differing orientation of the fibres entering the subepithelial space suggests that if contraction of the longitudinal muscle layer were to occur at the time of defaecation, then the anal cushions would be pulled in a craniad direction in the proximal anal canal, and the distal anal canal would be everted (Shafik, 1976). Similarly, the orientation of the fibres crossing the internal sphincter would result, upon their contraction, in the shortening of that muscle.

Changes in the Anal Cushions with Ageing

The arrangement of the muscle and connective tissue elements in the internal and external anal sphincters does not alter with age. However, in addition to the gradual replacement of smooth muscle by connective tissue in the longitudinal muscle layer itself, a similar change occurs in those extensions ramifying inwards across the internal sphincter to the submucosa (and outwards across the external sphincter). With age, the submucosa becomes relatively thicker when compared to the internal sphincter, and the connective tissue fibres are less organised, becoming thicker, looser and fragmented, and contain relatively more elastin (Haas and Fox, 1980). The consequences of these changes are presumably a generalised loss of support to the sphincter complex as a whole, and a specific loss of support to the mucosa and submucosa of the anal canal, rendering them and the vascular structures contained within them more susceptible to those stresses imposed upon them. Thus, with reduced support, and over time, one may imagine the anal cushions becoming stretched in a caudal direction. As a consequence of physical prolapse, the cushions may become more prone to surface trauma, and loss of the muscle elements of the submucosa may reduce the contractility and strength of the walls of the vascular components, rendering them more likely to bleed or thrombose.

Anatomy of Haemorrhoids

The prevalence of haemorrhoids seen at proctoscopy far outweighs the prevalence of symptoms arising from them. If we accept that anal cushions, seen in the foetus, are normal structures that have a function, the term haemorrhoids should be applied only if there is change in morphology, loss of function, or development of symptoms associated with them. The anatomical changes that occur with ageing have been described. Anatomical assessment of haemorrhoidal tissue compared with tissue from age-matched asymptomatic controls is, of course, extremely difficult. There is a spectrum of symptoms that may originate from different patho-anatomical causes; surgical haemorrhoidectomy is usually reserved for patients with marked symptoms associated with significant pile masses; haemorrhoidectomy specimens may not reflect anatomical arrangements in vivo since only the mucosa and some of the submucosa is excised, with division of any supporting structures on the deep surface; and tissue examined ex corpora cannot reflect completely that which occurs in a dynamic situation in vivo.

Histologically, haemorrhoidectomy specimens often reveal squamous metaplasia (usually visible to the naked eye) secondary to recurrent or permanent prolapse of the pile mass. Immediately beneath the mucosa a dense capillary network may be seen (which may in some cases be the site of some haemorrhoidal bleeding, rather than the deeper vascular structures). The bulk of the haemorrhoid is formed by the muscular and connective tissue stroma in which lie the vascular structures (predominantly venous dilatations). In contrast to the anal cushion of early life, the supporting structures show a higher proportion of collagen than muscle fibres, and are fragmented and disorganised (Haas et al., 1984). Apart from the squamous metaplasia, these changes are seen equally in sections taken at post-mortem, and would seem to begin in about the third decade as a normal effect of ageing. However, some have emphasised in addition to the above findings, a severe chronic inflammatory process in haemorrhoidectomy specimens involving the connective tissue stroma and blood vessel walls themselves, with associated thrombosis, ischaemia and mucosal ulceration.

As Thomson (1975) noted, venous dilatations exist in the subepithelium below the level of the dentate line. These may be seen on clinical examination of normal subjects to form a circumferential ring at the anal margin if the subject is asked to raise intra-abdominal pressure, and are part of the external or inferior haemorrhoidal plexus. In some patients, these dilatations and the overlying skin are prominent at the same site around the circumference as the primary internal haemorrhoidal pathology (suggestive of similar aetiology). In others, the vascular component is less distinct and the skin is redundant, forming tags. These latter may represent the aftermath of previous haemorrhoidal prolapse which caused oedema, stretching of the skin, and fragmentation of the tissues supporting the anoderm, but may also relate to previous external haemorrhoidal plexus congestion. Such tags may create difficulties in anal hygiene, as well as causing social embarrassment.

Prevalence of Haemorrhoids

Problems of definition, sociocultural attitudes and availability of medical services all contribute to ignorance about the prevalence of haemorrhoids in man. For instance, the claims by Burkitt (1972) that haemorrhoids were rare throughout rural Africa, but more common in those African communities exposed to western influences (especially dietary) and in American Negroes may simply be explained by differences in availability and acceptance of medical practices. In the West, reported incidences of haemorrhoids depend upon the method of enquiry; hospital-based studies reflect the degree to which patients are referred by their primary physician; and population studies (made on the basis of symptoms rather than signs) risk overestimation since most anal symptoms, whatever the true aetiology, are ascribed to piles. Estimates based on proctoscopic studies similarly overestimate prevalence because of the issue of definition, that being when does an anal cushion become a haemorrhoid? Certainly, there is often little correlation between what is seen at proctoscopy and the presence, nature and severity of any symptoms.

Although men seek medical help for symptoms relating to haemorrhoids more commonly than women, the prevalence is probably equal between the sexes (Johanson and Sonnenberg, 1990; 1991). Women, of course, are often symptomatic during and after pregnancy, as well as at certain times during the menstrual cycle, and although oestrogen receptors are found in haemorrhoidal tissue, nonhormonal mechanical influences such as raised intrapelvic pressure would seem more important in aetiology. A positive family history is common, but whether this relates to genetic predisposition or other factors such as increased awareness, dietary and behavioural similarities, is unclear.

Theories of Development

Portal Hypertension and Varicose Veins

Misconceptions concerning the vascular anatomy of the anal canal (specifically the lack of appreciation of communications between portal and systemic systems and the "normality" of venous dilatations) led to theories that lasted several centuries. Man's upright posture (we know little about haemorrhoidal problems in animals), lack of valves in the portal veins and raised abdominal pressure were thought to contribute to the development of anal varicosities. If raised portal venous pressure were indeed the cause, one would expect a high incidence in subjects suffering from portal hypertension. Although such patients have a higher incidence of ano-rectal varices, these are a separate anatomical and clinical entity from haemorrhoids, which are seen no more frequently than in those without cirrhosis, portal hypertension and oesophageal varices.

Other Vascular Causes

Virchow and Allingham (quoted by Thomson, 1975) considered haemorrhoids to be haemangiomatous. Others of the same era thought them to result from changes in the erectile tissue that formed part of the continence mechanism, and Stelzner, as recently as 1963, postulated that they might result from hyperplasia of the "corpus cavernosum recti".

Infection

Repeated infection of the anal lining, secondary to trauma at defaecation, has been postulated as a cause of weakening and erosion of the walls of the veins of the submucosa (Quenu and Hartmann, 1895 [quoted by Thomson, 1975]; McGivney, 1967). This hypothesis is difficult to accept, as one of the truly incredible properties of the anal canal is its resistance to infection, as well as the ability of its mucosa to heal after surgical intervention despite the torrent of micro-organisms passing over it. Similarly, there is little histological evidence to support the role of infection as a *primary* aetiological factor.

Diet and Stool Consistency

Much emphasis has been placed on the role of constipation in the development of haemorrhoids, and, indeed, attempts at "normalising" bowel habit comprise much of the management of sufferers. Burkitt (Burkitt, 1972; Burkitt and Graham-Stewart, 1975), comparing the incidence of haemorrhoids and varicose veins in rural versus developed communities, put the blame firmly on lack of dietary fibre. A fibre-deficient diet results in prolonged gut transit times which is associated with the passage of smaller, harder stools which require more straining to expel. Parks (1956) proposed that the presence of a hard faecal mass in the rectum could obstruct venous return resulting in engorgement of the anal veins (the ampullary pump); some emphasise the act of straining at stool itself to be the cause of the disturbance of vascular flow; and others blame sitting for prolonged periods on the lavatory with a relaxed perineum.

A large-scale study, however, has shown the epidemiological pattern of constipation to be different from that of haemorrhoidal disease (Johanson and Sonnenberg, 1990). Most haemorrhoidal sufferers have a bowel habit that falls into the spectrum of normality, and, indeed, an association has been demonstrated between haemorrhoids and diarrhoeal disorders (Johanson, 1997). It can also be argued that if there is an association between haemorrhoids and constipation, then it is the former causing the latter.

Defaecatory Position

If straining at stool, or just protracted sitting with an unsupported perineum and impairment of venous return, are implicated in the development of haemorrhoids, one might expect differences in incidence according to the position adopted during the act of defaecation; i.e., squatting defaecation as opposed to pan defaecation. To my knowledge, however, there is no information in the literature addressing this issue, although observational evidence by the editor suggests that in those assuming the squatting position, although still prone to haemorrhoidal symptoms, the pile masses are more commonly seen in the antero-posterior axis rather than laterally.

Anal Hypertonia

The association between raised anal canal resting pressure and haemorrhoids in sufferers as a whole compared to normal controls is well known (Gibbons et al., 1988; Sun et al., 1992; Ho et al., 1995). Whether anal hypertonia causes symptoms attributable to haemorrhoids or whether anal cushion hypertrophy causes anal hypertonia is the subject of debate. The fact that surgical haemorrhoidectomy restores resting pressures to the normal range is not absolute evidence that the pile masses themselves are the cause of the hypertonia, as it is possible that simply their presence raises internal sphincter tone, and lateral sphincterotomy alone in patients with haemorrhoids restores resting pressures (Schouten and Blankensteijn, 1992). These, and other physiological findings, are discussed in much greater detail in the following chapter. It should be remembered, however, that there is a significant proportion of patients who suffer haemorrhoidal symptoms in whom the anal canal is relatively patulous, and perhaps associated with perineal descent and pudendal neuropathy. One study has indeed found that patients with prolapse as their main symptom had lower basal anal canal pressures than those with bleeding haemorrhoids (Hiltunen and Matikainen, 1985).

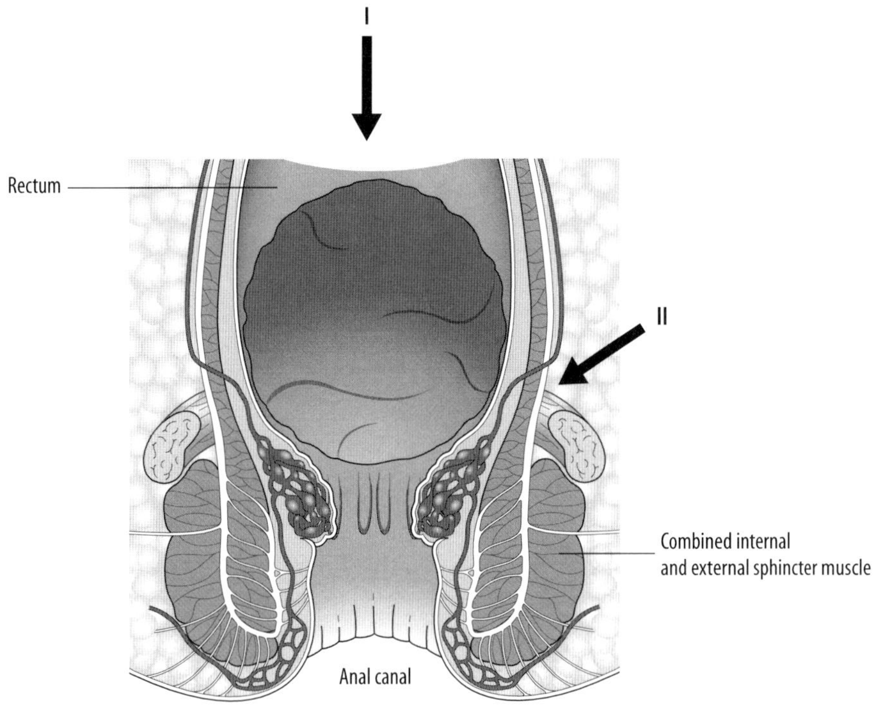

Figure 2.3. A theory for the transformation of anal cushions into haemorrhoids. Two mechanisms are possible, each superimposed upon the changes seen in the anal canal as a consequence of ageing.
Mechanism I. Forcing a large hard bolus of stool across the ano-rectal junction and through the upper anal canal displaces the anal cushions, which are forced downwards, stretching their submucosal attachments to the deeper structures of the sphincter complex. At the same time, the veins of the ano-rectal junction are compressed, and despite the existence of a collateral circulation, venous return is impeded, causing venous engorgement of the anal cushions.
Mechanism II. Abdominal straining or an increase in intrapelvic pressure impedes venous return from the anal cushions proximally, causing engorgement and stretching of the submucosal attachments.
Results. The cycle of recurrent forced descent of the anal cushions coupled with engorgement of their vasculature makes them not only larger by degrees but also less securely tethered to the wall of the anal canal. Increased size makes the resulting haemorrhoids more susceptible to surface trauma, causing bleeding and inflammatory changes. Both mechanisms may be involved in many patients with piles.

Ageing

The effects of ageing upon the anatomy of the anal cushions have already been described. Presumably, they arise with continued use of the anal canal for defaecation over time, although we do not know what changes might occur as a result of ageing alone (no studies having addressed changes over time in the defunctioned anus). If we accept the findings of Thomson that there are few differences in anatomy between symptomatic piles retrieved at operation and the anal cushions of cadavers who had no evidence of piles, then there must be other reasons why some people are symptomatic and others not.

The Author's Opinion

The fact that haemorrhoidal and ageing anal cushion anatomies are similar is fundamental to any theory of development. The major questions that must be answered are: why should some people become symptomatic and others not, and what determines which symptom should predominate. It is logical to suppose that size of pile mass must have an influence. However, the two major haemorrhoidal symptoms, bleeding and prolapse, may or may not coexist (the character of the bleeding may itself fall into one of several types). It is therefore reasonable to suppose (as evidenced by the number of theories aforementioned) that there is more than just one factor involved. Further evidence to this effect is provided by the spectrum of findings on clinical examination, both between individuals with symptoms, and within individuals over time who have not been specifically treated. One subgroup of patients includes those, in relative youth, possibly with stressed lifestyles, who complain of anal discomfort worsened at the time of defaecation or after prolonged exercise and with the occasional passage of blood with the motion. In such patients, digital examination and proctoscopy are difficult due to discomfort; digital examination reveals heightened sphincter tone and at proctoscopy, the submucosa at the dentate line is congested circumferentially with blood vessels. No gross prolapsing is evident, and although at the time of examination under anaesthesia a previously unseen fissure may be revealed in a proportion of these subjects, this finding is by no means invariable. Local interventions may have a higher complication rate of pain. Another group, in whom discomfort is less dominant, but bleeding more so, may have less spasm on examination, but significantly larger and engorged pile masses, which are more easily describable as lying in the primary positions of anal cushions, and which are associated with a greater degree of prolapse on straining. In others, prolapse itself may be the dominant symptom, to such an extent that the mucosa above the dentate line at the site of the pile masses appears to have descended beyond the distal limit of the internal sphincter and is apparent at or beyond the anal verge. Such patients may bleed spontaneously into their underwear, completely unrelated to defaecation. In these patients, there is often a significant associated cutaneous or subcutaneous component, secondary to either synchronous involvement of the inferior haemorrhoidal plexus or through skin stretching as previously described. Finally, there are those subjects, often elderly, in whom the anal canal is patulous, and in whom the distinction between haemorrhoidal pathology and mucosal prolapse is difficult.

In addition to the main symptoms of bleeding and prolapse, patients may also complain of perianal irritation. This may arise from mucus secretion from the caudally displaced rectal mucosa, from minor leakage through a now imperfect anal seal, or because of difficulties in cleaning after defaecation because of irregularity of the anal verge.

The spectrum of descriptions above does not support the view that one aetiology is solely responsible, and the main symptoms, bleeding and prolapse, should be considered in turn. Prolapse is more easily explicable if the effects seen with ageing are considered. Thickening of the submucosa, combined with weakness of those structures supporting the mucosa and submucosa render the anal cushions susceptible to the effects of forces imposed both at defaecation and whilst sitting with an unsupported perineum. Initially, there may be some "elasticity" to the masses, such that they retract to their original positions once the forces are withdrawn, but, with time, overstretching and fragmentation make the prolapse more constant and pronounced. Such changes may also occur in the anoderm below the dentate line as well as the skin and structures deep to the skin of the anal verge, resulting in the cutaneous components observed. Whether the anal linings of patients with prolapsing piles have greater shearing forces acting upon them, or whether the ageing process is simply accelerated, perhaps as a consequence of some unknown disorder of connective tissue, is unclear. Similarly, the influence of underlying anal tone in predisposition to prolapse has yet to be determined. In those with anal hypertonia, discomfort on defaecation may be explained by increased stimulation of the rich sensory network around the dentate line, and more severe pain may be caused by inability of any prolapsing tissue to reduce back up into the zone of lower pressure. Perhaps shearing forces on the upper anal canal lining are greater when attempts are made to evacuate through a relatively hypertonic muscle complex. In a patient already with some degree of prolapsing of the anal cushions, the development of weakness of the anal sphincter complex itself or as part of generalised perineal weakness would allow the degree of prolapse to worsen, perhaps from an asymptomatic to a symptomatic state.

For anal bleeding to occur, there must be some disruption of the mucosa and underlying vascular structure. In view of the intermittent nature of the bleeding, most often associated with defaecation, traumatic forces must be implicated in aetiology. Thomson suggested that the fault lay at the rich capillary bed immediately deep to the mucosa, and in those patients with general congestion at the level of the dentate line rather than the much more prominent vascular structures seen in others; this seems reasonable. Although by no means inevitable, the bleeding from these bigger structures, so striking at proctoscopy, and often described by patients as dripping into the pan, may be much more than might emanate from ruptured capillaries, and the venous dilatations, must be the likely source. We know that the amount of blood contained within the cushions is variable, and either increased inflow (unlikely) or decreased outflow must cause the distension. One can see pile distension in the clinic simply by asking the patient to bear down, and the combination of relative obstruction to outflow, traumatic forces acting on the surface of the pile, and degeneration of the structures supporting the submucosa and its contained blood vessels make bleeding from haemorrhoids quite understandable. The contribution of a possible inflammatory process within the pile leading to thrombosis, ischaemia and bleeding is unclear, but is suggestive of a previous or ongoing secondary event.

In addition to those changes which may occur in the main anal cushions (the primary foldings), similar changes may be seen also in the anal lining between the main cushions (the secondary foldings). In order to avoid confusion in terminology, haemorrhoids should be described as occupying either the primary or secondary *positions*, rather than simply primary or secondary; the latter description having implications in aetiology.

Classification of Haemorrhoids

No single classification of haemorrhoids can be described as perfect. Any classification is only as useful as the ease with which it can be implemented and the information that may be gained from it. Presumably, such classifications have developed so that the effects of intervention may be compared. However, the disparity between symptoms (and their severity) and physical signs in a condition where symptomatic relief is the goal, but in which management is influenced by anatomical and physiological considerations, makes construction of a useful classification that is not unwieldy difficult. Problems of classification occur elsewhere in surgery; for example, the staging of colorectal malignancy where Dukes' staging (the simplest) may be appropriate for discussions concerning prog-nosis in populations, but is probably insufficient for application to individuals or research; or Parks' classification of anal fistula, which does not embrace all those seen in surgical practice.

The classification most commonly adopted attempts to combine appearance with symptoms; i.e., first-degree piles being those which bleed, second-degree those which bleed and prolapse but reduce spontaneously, third-degree those which need to be reduced manually, and fourth-degree those which cannot be reduced. This classification fails on several points. Not all symptomatic haemorrhoids bleed; anal discomfort, soiling and other symptoms are not specifically addressed; and the cutaneous components (which may also be symptomatic) are not incorporated into the classification. These failings do not necessarily invalidate this classification, but indicate potential for refinement for greater applicability.

A symptom-based classification, attractive in the sense of comparative studies of the efficacy of treatment modalities, needs to be sufficiently comprehensive to incorporate all symptoms which may be attributable to haemorrhoids, in nature, frequency, and even interference with lifestyle. Such a classification would be unwieldy. It would also suffer from the fact that some symptoms may not, in fact, be due to the presence of haemorrhoids, and that bleeding, for instance, often a marked feature of "early" haemorrhoids, may be an unimportant symptom in "late" haemorrhoids.

Classification based upon clinical findings on examination is attractive in the sense that such findings have an influence on management strategy, but suffers the drawbacks that appearances in an individual may change without any specific intervention (especially when prolapse is not a feature), and that treatment efficacy is based upon symptom amelioration rather than restoration of normal anatomy. Anatomically, haemorrhoidal *position* may be described as primary (at the sites of the anal cushions), secondary (between the anal cushions), or circumferential. The degree of *prolapse* may be recorded as absent, below the level of the dentate line at rest or on straining, or visible at the anal margin at rest or on straining. There may or may not be associated mucosal (non-haemorrhoidal) prolapse. The state of the *anal verge* (presence or absence of skin tags, external haemorrhoidal plexus congestion) may be described. In addition, the state of the *anal tone*, and degree of *perineal descent* should be ascertained.

Classification of Primary Internal Haemorrhoids

If we accept the evidence that haemorrhoidal development is to a large degree an accelerated process of normal ageing, involving caudal displacement and increase in size of the anal cushions together with changes in the structures contained within them, a classification based on morphology (size and degree of prolapse) is logical. The principles of such a classification (Table 2.1) are as follows:

Table 2.1. Classification of Internal Haemorrhoids

	Stage	Morphology	Principal Presentations	Possible Additional Features	Visual Confirmation Related to Size	Expected Presentation in Age Group (Years)†	Conventional Management
Non-prolapsing	0	Anal cushions	1. Bleed very rarely 2. No prolapse	None	No definite increase	All ages; <20 if symptomatic	Dietary/lifestyle advice; medications; *Consider sclerotherapy or IRC for non-responders*
	1	Small haemorrhoids	1. Bleed intermittently 2. No prolapse	None*	Minor definite increase seen on proctoscopy	20–45	Sclerotherapy/IRC *Consider banding or stapling for non-responders*
Prolapsing	2	Intermediate haemorrhoids	1. Prolapse but return spontaneously 2. Bleed frequently and sometimes profusely	Pruritus Skin tags rare	Moderate increased size of individual pile masses which prolapse on straining	>30	Banding/Stapling *Consider surgery for non-responders*
	3	Large haemorrhoids	1. Prolapse, and need aid to reduce 2. Bleed frequently and often profusely	Pruritus Discomfort Some skin tags common	Major increase in size, including circumferentially. Prolapse easily and require replacement	>40	Operation by usual techniques
	4	Very large haemorrhoids +/– additional features (interno-external haemorrhoids)	1. Prolapse which is permanent and irreducible 2. Bleed profusely which can soil underwear#	Pain + pruritus, soiling Many skin tags usual Complications, e.g., thrombosis	Extreme increase in size with haemorrhoids also in secondary positions and skin tags	>50	May require operation, but by modified technique, e.g., anoplasty

IRC – infrared coagulation.
* – some patients complain of pain, for which a clearly recognisable cause cannot be demonstrated. A fissure may be responsible.
\+ – pain, if severe, is usually caused by complications, e.g., thrombosis, fissure-in-ano.
\# – occasionally, permanently prolapsed haemorrhoids cease to bleed because of mucosal thickening and squamous metaplasia.
† – there is considerable variation in the relationship between age and size (degree) of haemorrhoids.

1. Primary internal haemorrhoids are those unrelated to a specific condition (vide infra).
2. Grading and treatment can be related, and treatments compared accordingly.
3. Symptoms develop when anal cushions (normal structures) progress into abnormal haemorrhoids, usually by increased size.
4. The major abnormality in haemorrhoids is a change in size rather than a complete change in make-up.
5. Although the increase in size cannot be accurately measured, recognizable effects that are associated sufficiently closely with size provide an appropriate way of dividing haemorrhoids into separate groups.
6. The most accurate reflection of size is prolapse, which is either not present (small), intermittent (intermediate), permanent unless reduced (large), or irreducible (very large).
7. If one follows the expected natural progression, i.e., anal cushions do not become very large haemorrhoids without passing through intermediate stages, categorization by size as estimated visually and confirmed by the degree of prolapse is an excellent guide to "best treatment".
8. There must be included an initial stage (Stage 0), in which patients (young) may bleed but have no prolapse evident. Normal anal cushions may bleed.
9. Once prolapse has developed (Stage 2), changes are irreversible without treatment.
10. Age is a useful additional feature in staging, but the degree of overlap is so wide that it should not be relied upon in individual cases.

11. Other symptoms are secondary effects that are too variable to be incorporated in the primary classification, but are important as supporting evidence.
12. Any inflammation seen in haemorrhoids is as a consequence of mechanical irritation rather than a primary event.
13. Pain in most instances should *not* be attributable to primary internal haemorrhoids, and another cause sought. The discomfort associated with Stage 1 haemorrhoids is usually associated with anal hypertonicity. The discomfort associated with Stage 3 haemorrhoids is variable, ranging from a dragging sensation to severe proctalgia, probably arising from sources in the wall of the anal canal or pelvic floor. Pain suffered by patients with Stage 4 haemorrhoids usually relates to a secondary complication (thrombosis, ulceration, etc.).

No useable classification can be applied to every individual case. Perhaps one solution would be the design of a computerised comprehensive database incorporating all anatomical, physiological and symptom variables, from which natural history, and the effects of interventions (including unwanted effects) could be more accurately determined. Nevertheless, an attempt at a simpler classification can be made that accounts for most of the known facts, and which assists in choosing and comparing the interventions usually employed for the categories defined by the grading criteria. The classification described is simple enough to be practical, is based on accepted evidence of aetiology, and reflects appropriate management. At present, it is impossible to make valid analyses of the results of specific treatments because case selection is variable and ill defined. It is to be hoped that if a standardised classification were to be adopted worldwide, properly conducted clinical trials of treatment could be carried out that would reveal their true results.

Secondary Internal Haemorrhoids

Secondary internal haemorrhoids are those which have arisen from a specific condition, although the mechanisms may be the same as those involved in the formation of primary internal haemorrhoids (increased intrapelvic pressure and interruption of normal venous circulation, shearing forces acting on the anal lining, weakening of mucosal and submucosal support, etc.). The most important cause, albeit relatively uncommon, is carcinoma of the ano-rectum, but there are many others which may be categorised as follows:

1. Local, e.g., ano-rectal deformity, hypotonic anal sphincter.
2. Abdominal, e.g., ascites.
3. Pelvic, e.g., gravid uterus, uterine neoplasm (fibroid, carcinoma of uterus or cervix), ovarian neoplasm, bladder carcinoma.
4. Neurological, e.g., paraplegia, multiple sclerosis.

External Haemorrhoids

These are "haemorrhoids" which are situated in the venous channels of the inferior haemorrhoidal plexus deep to the skin surrounding the anal verge. They are not true haemorrhoids at all, and are usually only recognised as a result of a complication, which is most typically a painful solitary acute thrombosis. There is a subgroup of young patients, however, who have little in the way of internal haemorrhoids, but who suffer pain and minor bleeding (noticed on the paper) on wiping after defaecation, and in whom the mechanical trauma of over-zealous cleaning is probably responsible. External haemorrhoids associated with internal haemorrhoids ("interno-external piles") result from progression of the latter to involve both haemorrhoidal plexuses, and are best thought of as being an external extension of internal haemorrhoids (Stage 4).

EDITORIAL COMMENT

Over the last fifty years, there have been extensive revisions of the structure of the anal muscles, the arterial supply to the anus and the organisation and functions of the anal mucosa. Most recently, the dissections of the anal sphincter muscles by Professor Shafik (Cairo) and the researches of the anal cushions by W.H.F. Thomson (Gloucester, UK) have been very influential for our understanding of the anal organ. Thomson's demonstration of the relationship between the anal cushions and haemorrhoids greatly advanced perception of haemorrhoidal disease and its presentations and treatment. Although there is no proof that the realisation that haemorrhoids are essentially normal structures has been directly responsible for any particular treatment, is has been coincidental with accelerated progress towards non-operative treatments.

References and Further Reading

Burkitt DP (1972) Varicose veins, deep vein thrombosis, and haemorrhoids: epidemiology and suggested aetiology. BMJ ii:556–61

Burkitt DP, Graham-Stewart CW (1975) Haemorrhoids – postulated pathogenesis and proposed prevention. Postgrad Med J 51:631–6

Courtney H (1950) Anatomy of the pelvic diaphragm and anorectal musculature as related to sphincter preservation in anorectal surgery. Am J Surg 79:155–73

Gibbons CP, Bannister JJ, Read NW (1988) Role of constipation and anal hypertonia in the pathogenesis of haemorrhoids. Br J Surg 75:656–60

Haas PA, Fox TA (1980) Age-related changes and scar formations of perianal connective tissue. Dis Colon Rectum 23:160–9

Haas PA, Fox TA, Haas GP (1984) The pathogenesis of haemorrhoids. Dis Colon Rectum 27:442–50

Johanson JF (1997) Association of haemorrhoidal disease with diarrhoeal disorders. Dis Colon Rectum 40:215–21

Johanson JF, Sonnenberg A (1990) The prevalence of haemorrhoids and chronic constipation. An epidemiologic study. Gastroenterology 98:380–6

Johanson JF, Sonnenberg A (1991)Temporal changes in the occurrence of haemorrhoids in the United States and England. Dis Colon Rectum 34:585–91

Johnson FP (1914) The development of the rectum in the human embryo. Am J Anat 16:1–57

Hiltunen KM, Matikainen M (1985) Anal manometric findings in symptomatic haemorrhoids. Dis Colon Rectum 28:807–9

Ho YH, Seow-Choen F, Goh HS (1995) Haemorrhoidectomy and disordered rectal and anal physiology in patients with prolapsed haemorrhoids. Br J Surg 82:596–8

Kerremans R (1969) Morphological and Physiological Aspects of Anal Continence and Defaecation. Arscia Uitgaven, Brussels. pp 57–67

Lawson JON (1974) Pelvic Anatomy II. Anal canal and associated sphincters. Ann R Coll Surg Engl 54:288–300

McGivney J (1967) A re-evaluation of etiologic factors of haemorrhoidal disease. Arizona Medicine 24:333–6

Milligan ETC, Morgan CN (1934) Surgical anatomy of the anal canal with special reference to anorectal fistulae. Lancet ii:1150–6, 1213–17

O'Kelly TJ (1996) Nerves that say NO: a new perspective on the human rectoanal inhibitory reflex. Ann R Coll Surg Engl 78:31–8

O'Kelly TJ, Brading A, Mortensen NJ (1993) In vitro response of the human anal longitudinal muscle layer to cholinergic and adrenergic stimulation: evidence of sphincter specialization. Br J Surg 80:1337–441

Parks AG (1954) A note on the anatomy of the anal canal. Proc R Soc Med 47:997–8

Parks AG (1956) The surgical treatment of haemorrhoids. Br J Surg 43:337–51

Roux C (1881) Contribution to the knowledge of the anal muscles in man. Arch Mikr Anat 19:721–3

Rudinger N (1878) Topographisch chirurgische Anatomie des Menschen. Cotta JG, Stuttgart, pp 111–12

Schouten WR, Blankensteijn JD (1992) Ultra slow wave pressure variations in the anal canal before and after lateral internal sphincterotomy. Int J Colorect Dis 7:115–18

Shafik A (1976) A new concept of the anatomy of the anal sphincter mechanism and the physiology of defaecation III. The longitudinal anal muscle: anatomy and role in sphincter mechanism. Invest Urol 13:271–7

Stebbing JF, Brading AF, Mortensen NJ (1997) Role of nitric oxide in relaxation of the longitudinal layer of rectal smooth muscle. Dis Colon Rectum 40:706–10

Stelzner F (1963) Haemorrhoids and other diseases of the corpus cavernosum recti and the anal canal. Deutsch Med Wochenschr 88:177–82

Sun WM, Peck RJ, Shorthouse AJ, Read NW (1992) Haemorrhoids are associated not with hypertrophy of the internal anal sphincter but with hypertension of the anal cushions. Br J Surg 79:592–4

Thomson WHF (1975) The nature of haemorrhoids. Br J Surg 62:542–52

Treitz W (1853) Uber Einen Muskel am Duodenum des Menschen, uber elastische Sehnen, und einege andere anatomische Verhaltuisse. Viertal-Jahrschrift fur die praktische. Heilkunde 37:113–44

3 Pathophysiology of Haemorrhoids and the Consequences for Surgical Treatment

Han C. Kuijpers and Albert Peters

The anal canal is the terminal portion of the intestinal tract. It plays an important role in maintaining faecal continence. It is surrounded by strong sphincters and, due to the tonic contraction of these muscles, it is completely collapsed at rest and represents an antero-posterior slit. The proximal anal canal is covered with anal mucosa that contains an abundance of nerve endings responsible for fine sensory discrimination. This is called the anal sensation. The so-called rectal sensation is located in the pelvic floor muscle. The rectal mucosa itself does not contain receptors and is insensitive to stimuli. Rectal sensation is important to give awareness of the arrival of material in the rectum, whereas anal canal sensation may contribute to the discrimination of the nature of the material.

A perfectly smooth anal canal is seldom found on proctoscopy. Longitudinal columns are seen ending below at the linea dentata and, above, converting into vascular structures called the anal cushions. These are normal specialised highly vascular structures that lie in the left lateral, right posterior and right anterior aspects of the anal canal. Anal cushions are normal parts of the human body, demonstrable in children, foetuses, and even in embryos.

The anal submucosa receives arterial blood from the superior, middle, and inferior rectal arteries through a variety of branches. There are rich plexus' of vascular tissue beneath the epithelial lining of the anal canal called the corpus cavernosus recti. These plexus connect arteries to veins without intervening capillaries thus creating the vascular component of the anal cushions. These arteriovenous channels control the size of the anal cushions by regulating the blood volume flowing through them. Rapid filling of the cushions can be observed during anoscopy by asking the person to strain during examination. This observation is clinically supported by the finding of bright red arterial bleeding at the time of operation.

The cushions consist of mucosa, submucosal fibroelastic connective tissues, smooth muscle, and blood vessels. A network of connective tissue is formed around the haemorrhoidal venous plexus to anchor the cushions to the anal sphincters within the upper half of the anal canal. It is built up from fibres from the submucosal smooth muscle, derived partly from the internal sphincter and partly from fibres from the longitudinal muscle, with some elastic tissue. It also supports the anal lining during defecation. The vascular cushions and the muscularis are normally only loosely attached to the underlying circular muscle.

The role of the vascular cushions in the process of normal rectal evacuation is incompletely understood but it is likely that anal cushions complement anal sphincter function by providing the fine control over the continence of liquids and gases. They seal off the entrance to the anal canal and prevent the loss of small amounts of mucus and gas through the longitudinal mucosal folds in the anal canal. When the anal canal is inspected from above by inserting a colonoscope through the distal limb of a double-loop sigmoidostomy, the three cushions can be seen closing off the anal canal proximally, lying against each other as three fluid-filled malleable bags. Some patients have minor alterations in continence after haemorrhoidectomy which may arise due to the excision of the vascular cushions. During the act of defecation, when they become engorged and tense with blood, they cushion the anal canal lining. Because they are separate structures, rather than a continuous ring of vascular tissue, they allow the anal canal to dilate during defecation without tearing.

Haemorrhoids are engorgements of the anal cushions that tend to bleed or to prolapse. Haemorrhoidal disease is among the commonest diseases in the western world. At least five per cent of the general population suffers from haemorrhoidal disease, and the incidence increases with age. Whites are affected more frequently than blacks and increased prevalence rates have been associated with higher socioeconomic status.

The mechanisms that contribute to the occurrence of haemorrhoids are still not well understood. Various theories have been proposed regarding the exact nature of haemorrhoids. Many factors have been implicated in the causation of haemorrhoidal disease such as the absence of valves in the haemorrhoidal plexus and draining veins, and obstruction of venous return due to raised intra-abdominal pressure. Historically, these swellings were considered varicosities of the haemorrhoidal plexus. An extension of this concept is that haemorrhoids are masses of dilated venules. Failure to empty rapidly during the act of defecation, abnormal mobility of the cushions, and entrapment by a tight internal anal sphincter are other suggested causes of congestion. There is no doubt that there is a familial incidence of haemorrhoids. Haemorrhoids and varicose veins often coexist suggesting a general defect of the walls of the veins.

Failure of the cushions to empty rapidly is an often-postulated but never proven hypothesis to explain the cause of haemorrhoidal disease. Anatomical vascular pathways of venous drainage through the rectal musculature have been demonstrated and it is suggested that a faecal mass impacted in the rectum may compress these veins. Furthermore, the act of straining constricts the intermuscular veins by raising intra-abdominal pressure and so impedes the rapid emptying of the cushions. Another cause of obstructed venous drainage is increased pressure in the portal system. Since the veins in the portal system have no valves, every obstruction in the portal system (cirrhosis, thrombosis) will reflect in a higher pressure in the haemorrhoidal system. No relationship, however, has been found between haemorrhoids and portal hypertension. The incidence of haemorrhoids in patients with portal hypertension is about similar to the 50 per cent prevalence claimed in the general population. On rare occasions, it will result in true varices in this area. This cause is not seen very frequently.

The erect position of man leads to the effect that the entire column of blood in the portal system presses on the haemorrhoidal plexus. This may be the cause of why haemorrhoids more frequently occur in professions involving prolonged standing or heavy lifting. Haemorrhoidal disease is not featured in veterinary medicine.

The pressure in the portal vein can also be increased by outside compression on the venous backflow. The most common cause of this type of haemorrhoid is pregnancy. The symptoms may be considerably aggravated during delivery. Such patients were commonly asymptomatic previously and usually will be so again after delivery. Recent work has suggested that certain hormones such as follicle stimulating hormone, prolactin, and glucocorticoids may be responsible for initiating this disorder in female patients. Haemorrhoids may also be due to pelvic tumours such as an ovarian cyst or fibromyomata of the uterus. The myth that rectal carcinoma predisposes to enlarged anal cushions by obstructing venous drainage has never been confirmed. It must be recognised, however, that in the majority of patients no explanation for the onset of symptoms can be found.

Another theory is that internal sphincter dysfunction may be the responsible factor in initiating the disease state. Patients with haemorrhoids usually have increased internal sphincter activity and ultraslow anal pressure waves. Ambulatory anorectal physiology recordings have shown that there are also more frequent episodes of the sampling reflex which is thought to result from efforts to pass out the irritating haemorrhoidal mass. The high internal sphincter tonus creates further venous obstruction and pain at defecation. This in turn will increase the hypertonus of the internal sphincter and cause more pain and more venous congestion. Some, therefore, suggest that an internal sphincter abnormality may be an aetiological factor in the pathogenesis of haemorrhoids. Others, however, believe that it is the presence of the haemorrhoidal masses that produces the increased sphincter activity. Direct needle puncture of anal cushions in haemorrhoidal patients has shown abnormally high pressures in the blood vessels, suggesting that the high resting pressure in patients with haemorrhoids is of vascular origin. When the anal cushions prolapse outside of the anal canal or have been resected, the anal pressure is not raised. The increased internal sphincter activity, therefore, is likely a secondary phenomenon of the presence of haemorrhoidal mass rather than the cause; the raised resting pressure being the result of abnormal engorgement of blood in the anal cushions.

There is some evidence that the external sphincter in patients with haemorrhoids is in a state of increased contraction. External sphincter fibre size was increased when compared with a control group. There was no clear relationship with age, degree of haemorrhoids, history of straining or constipation, or perineal descent. This muscle hypertrophy likely represents an increased workload as a result of an increased reflex stimulation due to the presence of the haemorrhoids. EMG recording has confirmed this increased activity by demonstrating a significantly greater electric activity in the external sphincter of patients than in controls. This external muscle hypertrophy might also contribute to the raised anal canal pressure.

The presently accepted concept is that their nature is likely due primarily to laxity of the elastic network and the anal canal epithelium, which, by sliding downwards, causes distal displacement of the anal cushions. The anchoring and supporting connective tissue above the vascular cushions disintegrates, thereby allowing these structures to slide distally. The fibres become attenuated with age and during pregnancy and may be fractured from undue stress related to straining to move constipated stool. The anal cushion, which is no longer restrained by its fixation to the submucosa, is able to engorge excessively with blood, and subsequently congests and hypertrophies. When congested, they are more likely to bleed and to become oedematous. The oedema causes swelling and stretching of the tissues and finally hypertrophy. There can be stasis in the veins with clot formations and swelling or erosions of the lining, resulting in bleeding and, later, prolapse. The haemorrhoid becomes symptomatic.

Straining at stool is an important risk factor. The prevalence of haemorrhoids is lowest among people living traditionally in developing countries and intermediate in countries with populations between socio-economic extremes. It is suggested that the low incidence of haemorrhoidal disease in rural societies is related to a high fibre intake. Fibre-depleted diets are the fundamental cause of constipation. Constipation results in straining during evacuation of solid faeces causing engorgement of the anal cushions. During repeated straining, the normal supportive fibres of the cushions are stretched and the cushions will progressively prolapse beyond the dentate line. The passage of hard stool has a shearing effect on the vascular mucosa and facilitates its prolapse from the anal canal. Prolonged straining keeps the cushions outside the lower edge of the internal sphincter, which in turn constricts and congests them.

When the primary haemorrhoids are large, secondary haemorrhoids will develop in between them in the left anterior, left posterior, and right lateral positions, and the ultimate appearance will be a circular prolapse. There are two components to each haemorrhoid, one above (internal) and one below (external), the dentate line corresponding to the two venous plexus.

Internal haemorrhoids are symptomatic exaggerated submucosal vascular cushions located above the dentate line and covered by transitional and columnar epithelium. At first, they bulge into the lumen of the anal canal and produce painless bleeding (first-degree haemorrhoids). When haemorrhoidal disease progresses, they protrude during defecation and reduce spontaneously (second-degree haemorrhoids). During the next stage, protrusion occurs spontaneously or at the time of a bowel movement, and requires manual replacement (third-degree). Finally, they are permanently prolapsed and irreducible despite attempts at manual replacement. The prolapsed haemorrhoids lying outside the anal canal may become strangulated by the internal sphincter activity with possible thrombosis of the venous plexus (fourth-degree haemorrhoids). This condition may result in gangrene with the risk of abscess formation.

External haemorrhoids are the dilated venules of the inferior haemorrhoidal plexus which is located below the dentate line and covered with squamous epithelium. A thrombosed external haemorrhoid or perianal haematoma is a 2–4 cm diameter dark-blue lump at the anal verge. *External skin tags* are discrete folds of skin arising from the anal verge. Such tags may be the end result of thrombosed external haemorrhoids, or may be a complication of some anal inflammation such as anal fissure, frequent injections for sclerosing haemorrhoids, or inflammatory bowel disease.

Haemorrhoids are nothing more than a sliding downwards – a prolapse – of the upper part of the anal canal lining. Often they are not a sign of disease but merely of aging of the supporting tissues. When seen in combination with a complete rectal prolapse, it is illustrative to see how they disappear after abdominal rectopexy. The presence of large cushions in the absence of symptoms is no indication for treatment. Haemorrhoids should be treated only to alleviate symptoms. The general principle of prolapse treatment is either to resect or to re-fixate the prolapsing tissue. Treatment of haemorrhoids, therefore, is based on either resection of the haemorrhoidal tissue or creation of scar tissue in the lower rectal or upper anal mucosa.

There is a wide variety of treatments for haemorrhoids, ranging from dietary precautions through a variety of non-operative methods of mucosa fixation and widening of the anal canal, to a host of different techniques of excision of the anal cushions. The choice of method depends on the type and classification of the haemorrhoids and the presence of anal tags, and on the expertise of the operator. There is no place for routine manometry in planning treatment. It is always imperative that other causes of blood loss than haemorrhoids be excluded.

The aim of dietary manipulation and education is to avoid straining on defecation. The bad routine of sitting in the squatting position on the toilet for long periods at a time reading the daily newspaper has to be avoided. Counselling should also include the suggestion of removing reading materials from the lavatory as a prophylactic measure. These measures will prevent further disintegration and fracture of the anchoring and supporting connective tissue above the vascular cushions. In the squatting position, the pelvic floor is relaxed with the result that the cushions hang by their connective tissues and are not supported by the relaxed pelvic floor.

Further conservative treatment consists of the production of submucosal scarring (sclerotherapy, infrared coagulation) in the upper anus or low rectum or by removal of redundant mucosa (banding) which results in fixation, retraction, and partial atrophy of the cushions, returning them to their normal anatomical sites. Any safe means of creating cell death and tissue disruption will suffice but inappropriate damage to the anal sphincters should be avoided.

Surgery should be reserved for those who fail conservative measures or who have third- or fourth-degree haemorrhoids with severe symptoms. Second-degree haemorrhoids with skin tags are another indication for surgery. Surgical intervention is necessary in only 10 per cent of patients with haemorrhoids. Many different techniques of haemorrhoidectomy have been described. In general, they consist of excision of the haemorrhoidal complex (internal and external haemorrhoids, redundant rectal mucosa and skin tags) and ligation of the arterial pedicle. The method of handling the mucosa and perianal skin differentiates various techniques. In some, the mucous membrane is closed down to the dentate line and the external wound left open whereas other techniques employ primary closure of the entire wound. The open method combines removal of the haemorrhoidal complex with excellent drainage of contaminated wounds, whereas closed haemorrhoidectomy claims to offer prompt healing of wounds, diminished drainage, and less postoperative haemorrhage by avoiding open wounds. Postoperative nursing is easier after closed haemorrhoidectomy and the fear of infection has proved to be groundless in a large number of reports. Circular excision of the proximal anal mucosa and haemorrhoidal tissue, and suturing the rectal mucosa to the dentate line or below should be avoided since this leads to a "wet" anus deformity if performed incorrectly (Whitehead deformity). Several "flap" techniques have been described to treat haemorrhoids in combination with anal tags. They are based on mobilising the anal tags and suturing them to the rectal mucosa after excision of most, if not all, anal mucosa. These procedures deal more with cosmetic than functional aspects; since anal mucosa is replaced by skin, intra-anal scarring is huge especially when flap fixation is inadequate, and wide anal dilatation is needed to gain adequate access to perform the procedure, which are serious criticisms.

Impaired continence is the dreaded complication of ano-rectal surgery. Major continence disorders hardly occur after haemorrhoid surgery but the incidence of minor disorders, mainly soiling, is considerable, varying from 10 to 50 per cent. This is understandable for sphincter-dividing procedures such as fistulotomy (30–50%) or sphincterotomy (10–30%), but it is quite surprising that the incidence is only slightly less after non-dividing procedures such as anal stretch (15–25%), advancement flaps (20%) and haemorrhoidectomy (10–20%). Local scarring is not the explanation. Resting pressure decreases after haemorrhoidectomy, which often results in the clinical phenomenon of soiling. The cause is potential internal sphincter damage due to over-dilatation by the anal retractor. When possible, the use of an anal retractor should be avoided to obtain better manometric and clinical results.

There is no advantage in adding resting pressure-reducing procedures such as sphincterotomy and anal dilatation to routine haemorrhoidectomy since haemorrhoids are not the result of an internal sphincter dysfunction. Moreover, they carry the added risk of incontinence.

With the role of the proximal anal mucosa in faecal continence in mind, a procedure that leaves as much anal mucosa as possible and creates an intra-anal scar as small as possible is to be preferred e.g. closed haemorrhoidectomy. This is another reason not to perform a Whitehead procedure with its large circular wound.

An interesting new surgical procedure is the circular stapler haemorrhoidectomy according to Longo. It is based on the principle of a circular rectal mucosectomy about three cm above the anal canal. As after rectopexy, the haemorrhoids are pulled up and will shrivel within minutes. The complete proximal anal mucosa is preserved after this procedure, intra-anal scars are not created and a retractor is needed only to create a low-rectal purse-string suture. The advantage of this procedure is that any intra-anal manipulation is avoided with considerably less postoperative pain as a result.

Haemorrhoids are a nuisance. The best treatment is the least intervention possible to achieve this goal with a minimal risk of postoperative-impaired continence. The surgeon should not only, therefore, have expertise in finding the most appropriate match of disease and therapy, but should also be aware of the cause of haemorrhoids and the function of the continence mechanism in order to avoid needless and harmful procedures.

EDITORIAL COMMENT

As can be appreciated from the historical survey in Chapter 1, haemorrhoids is not a disease that has appeared recently. Nevertheless, the lifestyle of modern urban populations is very conducive to their development. Increased appreciation by medical practitioners of the factors that cause the appearance and enlargement of piles give hope that their prevalence can be reduced by suitable responses on the part of both doctors and the public. The benefits that can be gained from such elements as increased exercise, more fibre, plentiful fluids and regular defecation need to be incorporated into surgical programmes for the management of haemorrhoidal disease.

Surgical interventions should be the least required to relieve symptoms and preserve normal tissues. Scarring should be minimised and anal mucosa conserved.

References and Further Reading

Goldberg SM, Gordon PH, Nivatvongs S (1980) Hemorrhoids. In: Essentials of Ano-rectal Surgery. Lippingcott, Philadelphia

Gravie JF (1999) Treatment of stage III and IV hemorrhoids by the Longo technique. Ann Chir 53:245–7

Ho YH, Seow-Choen F (1996) The role of impaired pelvic floor relaxation in the pathogenesis of haemorrhoids and fissure. Seminars in Colon & Rectal Surgery 7:186–91

Ho YO, Seow-Choen F (1997) Randomized controlled trial of open and closed haemorrhoidectomy. Br J Surg 84:1729–30

Keighley MRB, Williams, NS (1993) Haemorrhoidal disease. In: Keighley MRB, Williams NS (eds) Surgery of the Anus, Rectum and Colon. WB Saunders Ltd, London

Kuijpers JHC (1994) Iatrogenic fecal incontinence. In: Kuijpers JHC (ed) Colorectal Physiology: Fecal Incontinence. CRC Press Inc.4:65–7

Thomson JPS, Leicester RJ (1992) Haemorrhoids: pathophysiology and clinical features.. In: Henry MM, Swash M (eds) Coloproctology and the Pelvic Floor. 2nd Edition. Butterworth-Heinemann Ltd, Oxford

Thomson WHF (1975) The nature of haemorrhoids. Br J Surg 62:542

van Tets WF, Kuijpers JH, Tran K, Mollen R, van Goor H (1997) Influence of Parks' anal retractor on anal sphincter pressures. Dis Colon Rectum 40:1042–45

4 Diagnosis

Charles V. Mann

General Principles

It is frequently taken for granted that the diagnosis of haemorrhoids is easy. Two assumptions underlie this view – one, that a patient complaining of bleeding on defaecation, especially one below thirty years of age, is virtually certain to be suffering from haemorrhoids, and two, that the diagnosis does not need to be confirmed by a meticulous process of examination that is designed to exclude other (and often much more serious) conditions; both are wrong. The clinician must always keep the possibility of alternative causes of the bleeding in his mind, and only reach the diagnosis of haemorrhoids when all other causes have been excluded. This may require not only a trained specialist in coloproctological disorders, but backup with endoscopic, radiologic and haematological investigations. Most medical students at some stage are taught the well-known aphorism "if you do not put your finger in it [anus], you may put your foot in it". While this nostrum highlights the absolute requirement of a digital examination in any case presenting with bleeding per rectum, it also carries the unfortunate and misleading message that this is all that is required. As will be seen from later discussions, this is very far from the truth, regardless of the age of the patient. Not only does the diagnosis of haemorrhoids require examinations additional to the insertion of the index finger, it disregards the vital importance of a detailed history for making the diagnosis; medical students should be taught a second aphorism, viz., "that if you do not obtain a proper history, you will form part of medico-legal history".

Haemorrhoid Size ("Degree")

In addition to establishing the diagnosis, it is necessary to make an accurate assessment of the size and extent of the haemorrhoids (see Classification; Ch. 2, p. 14). Are they external, internal, or both? Are the internal haemorrhoids prolapsing or non-prolapsing? Are prolapsing haemorrhoids of second, third, or fourth degree? What is their circumferential extent? Accurate answers to these questions must be obtained before any management is decided. The circumferential extent of haemorrhoids and the difficulties this may cause for treatment is often ignored.

Other Considerations

Whilst it is tempting to rely exclusively on the size of haemorrhoids when recommending treatment, it is essential to be aware of the holistic background if problems are to be avoided. These considerations may be put best in the form of questions. Why has the patient presented himself (or herself) at this time when the symptoms may have been present long-term? Is the patient optimistic about some new treatment being advocated or nervous about the possibility of cancer? Is the patient unusually young, or is there a strong family history of piles? Is the patient pregnant, or planning further children? Is the patient elderly, or have a weak anal sphincter? Does the patient have a regular diet associated with diarrhoea (curries) or constipation (fast food). Is drug or alcohol abuse a possibility? Is there a history of sexual deviancy and/or the probability of HIV exposure? Does the patient present with hidden or overt personality features that suggest they may be "difficult" or litigious? Has the patient been persuaded to seek treatment because of the dominant influence of their partner or a friend? It should not require emphasising that the answers to these questions should influence the therapeutic advice that is given.

Concomitant Conditions

Further to the questions listed above, to which the answers are usually obvious and relevant, certain conditions need particular emphasis because of their importance.

- *Women of fertile age.* Pregnancy is a prime cause of haemorrhoids. It is a mistake to carry out a haemorrhoidectomy, not only if the patient is pregnant, but also if further children are planned.
- *Elderly patients.* Old patients often have weak sphincters. A haemorrhoidectomy may lead to partial (or even, complete) incontinence.
- *Concomitant diseases.* Colitis and Crohn's disease, especially when the ano-rectum is affected, can cause complications following almost any treatments for haemorrhoids, and special considerations apply which are considered in Ch. 23. Immune deficiency diseases, especially HIV infection, can cause healing difficulties and even death after haemorrhoid treatments (see Ch. 23).
- *Mental disturbance.* Patients often try to conceal a psychiatric history and direct questions may be necessary to reveal it; a present or past history of drug treatment, including regular resort to tranquillisers, should always be obtained. Unless this is done, a great deal of unpleasantness may result, which may include a prolonged medico-legal battle. It should always be remembered that haemorrhoids are not a life-threatening condition, and do not in themselves constitute an absolute imperative for treatment.

Despite the above admonitions, the diagnosis of haemorrhoids is one of immediate visual recognition. Their characteristic appearance as fleshy vascular cushions covered by reddish blue smooth mucosa is not easily confused with any other anal condition. However, it is also necessary to make sure that, even if haemorrhoids are the primary diagnosis, other diseases are not present. Some possible concomitant diseases are referred to above, but one requires special emphasis – *carcinoma*. Carcinoma of the ano-rectum may not only be associated with haemorrhoids it can also cause haemorrhoids (so-called "secondary haemorrhoids"). The exclusion of carcinoma, or other rarer malignant conditions, is an overriding consideration in patients presenting with haemorrhoids.

Providing the clinician always carries out a complete programme of evaluation, errors of diagnosis and management should not occur. If invasive treatments are required, and always before haemorrhoidectomy, a gynaecological history and examination is advisable. An enlarged uterus (fibromyomata, gravid uterus), ovarian tumour or pudendal neuropathy can cause or aggravate haemorrhoids. If the patient is taking oral contraceptive drugs, haemorrhoidectomy should not be carried out until they have been stopped for the appropriate period preoperatively, usually two to four weeks.

The History

Every haemorrhoid case history should include details regarding (i) age, (ii) gender, (iii) marital status, (iv) children, (v) family history, (vi) previous treatment, (vii) principal complaints, with their duration, (viii) additional symptoms, and (ix) social and work background. It is the author's experience that few hospital records of haemorrhoid cases contain more than half this information, and most of them much less.

During the course of eliciting this information, the clinician can form a clear opinion of what the patient expects from his treatment, and, equally important, whether he feels confident that he can offer that elusive result – a "complete cure". The specialist must distinguish between symptoms which are definitely due to the haemorrhoids (which he has a good chance of curing) from those arising from other causes which the patient ascribes to haemorrhoids; in many cases, the latter will not respond to the haemorrhoid treatment. The author has experience of cases in which, after a successful haemorrhoidectomy, the patient remains dissatisfied because of symptoms which arise from anxiety (proctalgia), depression (constipation), irritable bowel syndrome (frequent and/or irregular bowel actions), dietary indiscretion (flatus incontinence) persistent pruritus (mucus leakage) and even headache; in the latter example the patient was quite certain, and said so to his lawyers, that his migraine was definitely caused by his haemorrhoidectomy, as was his impotence. Although the author convinced the judge that his fellow surgeon was not responsible for this patient's problems, lawyers are adept at stoking patients' disappointments if they are convinced that haemorrhoid treatment will result in a cure of all their symptoms. The surgeon should never promise more than he can deliver.

Each major element of history taking will now be considered in turn.

(i) Age

If the patient presents at an unusually early age (say, less than 25 years old), extra care must be exercised to eliminate other diagnostic possibilities. Colitis, Crohn's disease, adenomatous conditions (including familial polyposis), and carcinoma can all present in young subjects with symptoms that can mimic haemorrhoids. Any additional symptoms to bleeding, such as pain-altered bowel habit or mucus discharge, should alert the clinician to the strong possibility of alternative or additional pathology.

If a young patient presents with prolapsing haemorrhoids, unless there is a history of childbirth(s), one has to consider the possibility of a predisposition for developing piles. In such cases, there is often a strong family history, although there is no evidence whether this is genetic or environmental (toilet habits, diet). However, its importance lies in its association with the enhanced likelihood of recurrent haemorrhoids following treatment. The author avoided recommending a haemorrhoidectomy in such patients until they reached forty years of age because of the high chance for early recurrence (unpublished data).

For young females, the likelihood of future pregnancies should also influence their treatment, and indicate caution before advising haemorrhoidectomy (see next).

(ii) Gender

Pregnancy is a prime cause of haemorrhoids, both primary and recurrent. Haemorrhoids, which may be large and troublesome during pregnancy and soon after delivery, tend to improve over the ensuing months. Both these factors should be taken into account before deciding on operative treatment.

Anal intercourse is not uncommon in females, as well as males. Anal symptoms (bleeding, pain, pruritus, mucus) may result which can be wrongly ascribed to any piles that are present. The clinician should have a high index of suspicion for anal intercourse when these symptoms are combined with an atonic sphincter or anal fissures.

A weak anal sphincter may result from obstetric injury (forceps delivery, prolonged second stage of labour) or age. Elderly females are particularly prone to have a weak anal sphincter. This must be taken into account when treatment is decided, which should be as conservative as possible, and should never include an anal stretch.

(iii) Marital Status

This should draw attention to the possibilities for haemorrhoid development associated with pregnancy and parturition (see above). Divorce may be associated with relevant personality and lifestyle changes, including drug and alcohol abuse as well as an unsatisfactory diet.

(iv) Child Birth

The importance of obtaining a detailed obstetric and gynaecological history has already been referred to in (ii) above.

(v) Family History

In addition to any family history which indicates an enhanced predisposition to haemorrhoids, it is important to enquire what the results of treatment were for other family members with haemorrhoids. If such members suffered a very painful operation, and/or developed any complications from treatment, it is advisable to discuss these when the patient is advised on his/her own management.

(vi) Previous Treatment

Following on from the above there are other important reasons for obtaining an accurate picture of any previous treatments that have been given to the patient.

- *Previous sclerotherapy.* This can leave residual areas of adherent mucosa that can make a subsequent haemorrhoidectomy more difficult, especially a closed-type operation.
- *Previous sphincterotomy or anal dilation.* In both cases, the anal sphincter is likely to have reduced tone; therefore, any subsequent procedure that may further reduce sphincter tone is to be avoided. The author has seen two patients where repeated attempts to heal an anal fissure by multiple sphincterotomies or dilatations resulted in an incontinent patient; in one of these, it is doubtful if a fissure was the cause of the patient's anal pain, which was probably nervous in origin.
- *Previous haemorrhoidectomy.* Unless the first operation had been obviously mismanaged, it is usually unnecessary to repeat a haemorrhoidectomy as any recurrent haemorrhoids are likely to be of limited extent, and isolated. They should respond to conservative management (e.g., banding).
- *Previous fistulectomy.* By almost any technique, an operation for a fistula-in-ano reduces both the anatomical and physiological integrity of the anal sphincters. In some cases, the bulk of the haemorrhoids may even aid continence by acting as a plug of tissue sealing the anal lumen. A haemorrhoidectomy should be avoided whenever possible and banding used instead.

(vii) Principal Complaints

These are 1) bleeding on defaecation and 2) prolapse, although there may be secondary complaints as well.

Bleeding on Defaecation

Bleeding occasioned by haemorrhoids is painless. If there is pain, another diagnosis (e.g., fissure-in-ano) is almost certainly the cause. The bleeding is usually at, and/or immediately after, defaecation. If the blood drips into the pan, this is highly suggestive of haemorrhoids. In some patients, large prolapsed haemorrhoids cause blood on the underwear between defaecation due to trauma to their exposed surfaces, but it should be noted that sometimes fourth-degree haemorrhoids do not bleed (or bleed very little) because their exposed mucosa becomes thick and calloused. Bleeding unrelated to defaecation almost always arises from another cause, e.g., carcinoma.

Prolapse

This is a feature of larger haemorrhoids. Alternative causes of this symptom are mucosal prolapse, full-thickness rectal prolapse, fibro-epithelial and adenomatous polyps, and anterior rectal wall prolapse, all of which must be excluded.

In most normal patients, a haemorrhoid history is lengthy – usually years. In some very nervous patients, a single episode of blood loss can precipitate attendance in the clinic (usually because of fear of cancer) but this is rare. A short history in a calm individual should heighten the clinician's suspicion of possible alternative diagnoses, which may be serious. The assumption by patients that anal bleeding is due to haemorrhoids can delay presentation with disastrous consequences. One young patient (24 years old) referred to the author with long-standing bleeding attributed to haemorrhoids was found to have an incurable rectal carcinoma.

(viii) Secondary Complaints

These are symptoms which may be associated with haemorrhoids, but often arise from other causes which are unrelated, or only indirectly related.

- Mucus discharge. Mucus derives from the secretory epithelium above the dentate line. It can cause symptoms from haemorrhoids only if these are associated with prolapsed mucosa, i.e., very large. In many cases, the symptom is not directly due to the haemorrhoids but comes from another source, e.g., a mucus-secreting rectal adenoma; "mucus colitis"; non-specific proctitis.
- Pain. Prolapsed haemorrhoids can cause a dragging pain until they are reduced. A thrombosed haemorrhoid often causes severe pain. As stated previously, apart from these two examples, pain usually arises from non-haemorrhoidal causes, e.g., fissure in-ano.
- Pruritus. Most cases of anal and perianal irritation arise from neurotic or dermal causes, but mucus discharge (see above) can cause this symptom.
- Anaemia. Anaemia of sufficient severity to cause symptoms rarely arises from haemorrhoids. The author has seen only two such cases – both

females, in whom menstruation may have been a critical factor. If a patient is found to be anaemic, another cause should be sought, which should always include a haematological profile, chest X-ray and gastro-intestinal surveys of the upper and lower tracts of the intestine.

- Altered bowel habit. A change in bowel habit should never be ascribed to haemorrhoids. Any patient with haemorrhoids whose bowel habit is abnormal, especially if it has changed, should be thoroughly investigated for alternative diagnoses which include proctocolitis and neoplastic diseases; tests should include a full colonoscopy. If the tests are negative, enquiry should be made into laxative usage (diarrhoea), analgesics and antidepressants (constipation) and the possibility of irritable bowel syndrome also should be considered (see below).

(ix) Social and Occupational Background

Reference has been made already to the influence of gender and sexual orientation on the development of haemorrhoids. Occupation can also be an important factor, either as a cause or for management. Some athletes (weightlifters, tennis players) exert themselves in extreme bursts of muscular activity, which can be associated with thrombosis of external haemorrhoids secondary to hyper spasm of the anal sphincters, whilst a professional cyclist may wish to avoid a haemorrhoidectomy! While these are extreme examples, a proper history should include enough information so that the proper context for treatment selection is made clear.

Examination

Like the history, the patient's examination can be divided into well-defined separate parts which will be described individually, as follows.

General Appraisal

This starts from the moment the patient presents himself, and is directed towards the answers to two questions: 1) is the patient's general appearance and fitness consistent with a simple diagnosis of haemorrhoids? and 2) is the patient's age and physique a contraindication to standard management.

The patients' age and physique are obvious factors to take into account, together with their personality and mental state. The patients' weight, blood pressure and urine (specific gravity; protein; sugar) should have been tested already and the results made available to the clinician. If a patient has a history of smoking or any chest disorders (chronic bronchitis, asthma, emphysema) or evidence of reduced respiratory sufficiency (wheezing, breathlessness, persistent cough, cyanosis), an expert appraisal is mandatory, which should include a chest X-ray. A history of cardiac problems, especially of myocardial infarction, requires preoperative workup by a cardiologist, as well as the anaesthetist, if operative treatment is contemplated; and if the infarct was recent (less than six months prior to his attendance) any surgical treatment should be postponed until cardiac revascularisation is maximised (which takes approximately six months). Some clinics have a policy of routine preoperative assessment in designated facilities, usually staffed by anaesthetists. While this may be an excellent additional precaution, it is unnecessary for most patients, and should not replace the surgeon's overall responsibility for assessment. In particular, there is still a requirement for a check-up at the time that operative treatment is being carried out, or preferably a short while beforehand, not least because the patient's health can change in the period between the outpatient (office) assessment and the carrying out of any operative procedure.

Since the majority of patients with haemorrhoids do not require an operation, not all of the advice obtained is relevant. However, if the clinician's initial assessment is unfavourable, it should be acted upon appropriately, which may indicate referral to another specialist, usually a physician. Willingness to engage the help of colleagues is not a diminution of a surgeon's status but confirmation of his wisdom. Overoptimistic advice on the safety, simplicity and results of invasive treatments is a prime source of patients' discontent, and can be damaging not only to a patient's life and health but also to the surgeon's reputation.

Abdominal Examination

This is carried out in all cases. It is most conveniently performed immediately prior to the special positioning required for a haemorrhoid examination. Like all abdominal examinations, it is carried out in the required way for each of the abdominal quadrants but should include special attention to the inguino-scrotal areas where enlarged lymph nodes may be a sign of anal malignancy.

Although an open mind should be retained, certain specific signs should be looked for. *Abdominal distention*. This may be due to ascites or obstructed bowel. *Hepatic enlargement*. This may denote cirrhosis or metastases. *Splenomegaly*. This may arise from portal hypertension or a haematological disorder, including sickle-cell disease. *Abdominal mass*. This may be caused by a gastrointestinal neoplasm or other lesions, such as Crohn's disease or an ovarian tumour. *Pelvic mass*. Uterine enlargement may indicate pregnancy, fibromyomata, or uterine or ovarian carcinoma, making an immediate vaginal examination mandatory, followed by referral to a gynaecologist or obstetrician. Many of the lesions uncovered by abdominal examination may be a cause of haemorrhoids, especially those which are associated with back pressure on the pelvic venous system.

Reference has been made already to the importance of examining for enlarged inguinal or femoral lymph nodes, which can be not only a pointer to an anal malignancy (sometimes misdiagnosed as haemorrhoids) but also to a disease of the blood-forming tissues. As it is known that leukaemia can cause thrombosis in the anal veins (as elsewhere) and the author has seen such a case, this finding may assist diagnosis is such a rare presentation.

Preparation

Ano-rectal diagnosis is more accurate if faeces are not present. In most patients, the degree of faecal presence in an unprepared ano-rectum is sufficiently small that an adequate examination is possible without special preparation, and preparation by suppositories or enemas may eliminate significant residues (blood, mucus, pus) or produce a false appearance of an "inflamed" mucosa. At present, the question of routine preparation versus no preparation is so evenly balanced that a definitive standpoint is not possible. However, two points may swing the policy of a colo-proctological clinic in one or other direction, viz., 1) if the clinic uses a flexible endoscope for examining their patients at their first attendance it is necessary for them to employ routine bowel preparation, and 2) if the clinic does not employ routine preparation, the means to achieve this must be readily available for those cases that require it. The threshold for employing distal bowel preparation should be low, as the penalties for wrong diagnosis are serious.

If bowel preparation is indicated, the author recommends the use of a mini-enema, which is easy to give in the clinic and acts promptly; suitable preparations are Micralax (Celltech) or Klean-Prep (Norgine). Stimulant suppositories (Bisacodyl; Dulcolax (Boehringer) are a possible alternative, but are often slow to work and sometimes do not achieve adequate faecal evacuation.

Position

One of two positions is generally chosen: either the left lateral knees-up position or the face-down, knee-elbow position (Fig. 4.1). Both positions have their advocates, and there is no evidence that proves that one is superior to the other. In some clinics, an on-back knees-up lithotomy position is preferred.

The left lateral position is probably the simplest, and does not require a special couch; putting a small cushion beneath the lower buttock and hip improves access. It is comfortable for patients and the least embarrassing; in frail or disabled patients, especially the elderly, it may be the only one that can be tolerated.

The knee-elbow position also has some favourable points. It separates the buttocks efficiently and enhances access; it diminishes problems from faecal or other intraluminal residues by causing them to run "downhill" away from the ano-rectum; and it assists in straightening out the recto-sigmoid angle, which facilitates the passage of examining instruments through this sometimes difficult zone.

The lithotomy position (Fig. 4.2) requires a special couch with leg supports. It can be embarrassing for patients, especially young females. In obese patients, the weight of the abdomen can cause engorgement of the anal veins. Because of the angle of vision, it imposes increased difficulty for examining the anterior aspects of the anal canal and rectum. On the other hand, it is easy to speak to the patient in this position, and it permits the best access for an assistant, if one is required. The lithotomy position may increase the ano-rectal angle, which can make instrumental perforation slightly more likely if any force is used to pass an endoscope through into the sigmoid colon.

Special couches have been manufactured for use in colo-proctological clinics. They are expensive and

1. The left lateral position

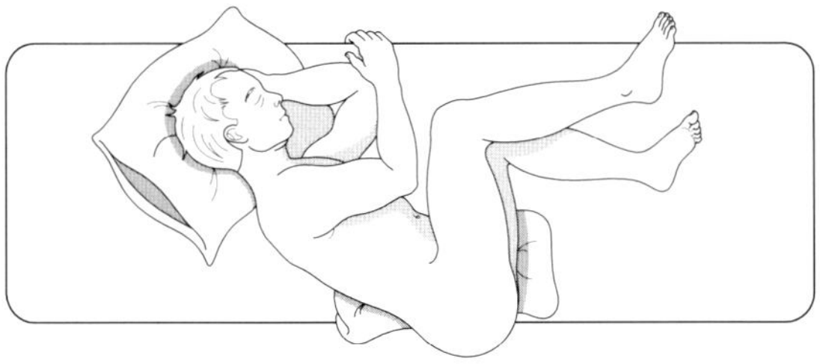

Advantages

1. Easy for the patient to adopt and maintain.
2. Minimises patients embarrassment.
3. Causes least physical problems for elderly or incapacitated subjects.
4. Facilitates verbal exchanges between surgeon and patient.
5. Allows a nurse or parent to sit near the patient's head to assist with reassurance and control.
6. Allows easy access to instrument trolley.

Disadvantages

1. Does not open out obese buttocks.
2. Does not reduce (straighten) the recto-sigmoid angle.

2. The knee-elbow position

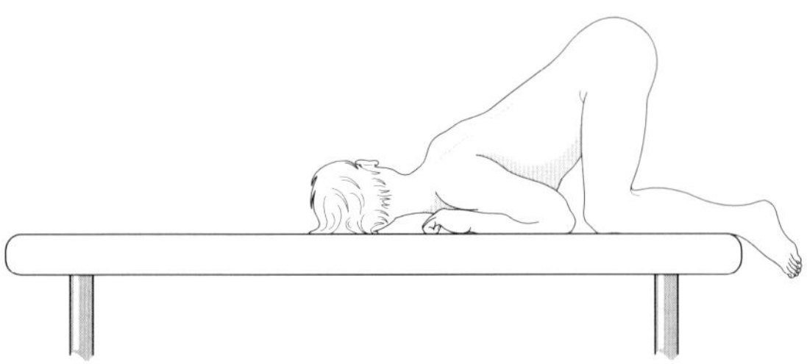

Advantages

1. Facilitates visual inspection by opening out the buttock.
2. Assists use of instruments (e.g., proctoscope, sigmoidoscope) by encouraging gravity flow of fluids away from their tips.
3. Reduces (straightens) the recto-sigmoid angle.

Disadvantages

1. Embarrassing, especially for females.
2. Difficult for elderly patients to adopt or maintain.
3. Often needs an assistant to steady the patient.
4. Interferes with verbal exchanges between surgeon and patient.
5. Prevents easy access to instrument trolley.

Figure 4.1. Positions for examination.

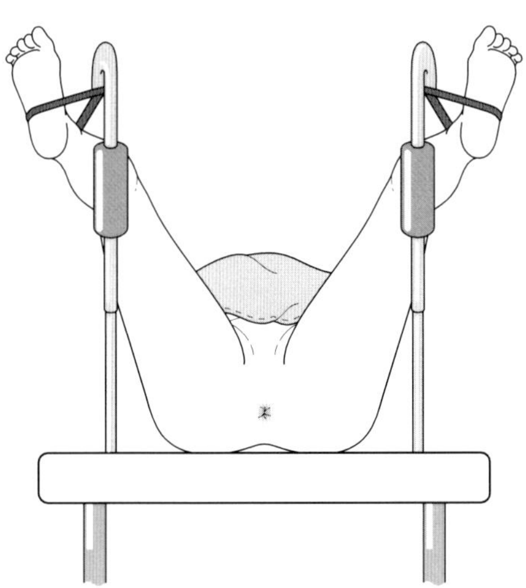

This is the position that is favoured also by gynaecologists, and should be used if a vaginal examination is a possibility. It is not commonly used in rectal clinics in the UK or North America, but is frequently used in European centres. It requires a table with leg supports. The position makes access to the anterior quadrants of the ano-rectum more difficult, as well as increasing the difficulty of negotiation of the recto-sigmoid junction.

Figure 4.2. The Lithotomy position.

require extra time for the patient to be properly positioned and secured. Their great advantage is that once the patient is settled in, they can tolerate a relatively prolonged examination and/or treatment session. This can be a definite advantage if endoscopy with either the short ("flexiscope") or long type of colonoscope is required. Most proctology departments do not use special tables for everyday use.

Whatever position is adopted for routine use in the clinic, it should be applied by an accurate, repeatable method which ensures optimum conditions for the examination. In particular, it should maximise patient confidence and comfort, allow excellent illumination of the perineum and anus, permit total visual and instrumental control to the examining clinician, and give access to an assistant if one is called for. Because the proctologist may need to spend considerable time conducting the necessary manoeuvres required for a complete examination (and possible treatment) of his haemorrhoid patients, if the examination position permits him to be seated, with his instruments within easy reach, he will be encouraged to carry out an unhurried and faultless treatment session.

Visual Inspection

When patients have been correctly positioned, they should be relaxed, comfortable, and able to respond to comments and instructions. Patients obtain comfort from a modicum of conversation with the proctologist or an assistant, which should include informing them about what is happening, and should include constant reassurance that they should not experience pain – only discomfort at worst. If any treatment is planned, the patient should be informed; this point is discussed in more detail elsewhere (see Sclerotherapy p. 57). If a patient's buttocks are bulky, they may obscure visualisation, in which case adhesive strapping should be applied to retract the overlying folds; in some extreme cases an assistant's fingers must also be employed to expose the area to be inspected. Good lighting is essential, which should be focussed on the anus without causing dazzle. Both lighting and table height should be adjustable so that the best elevation and angle is provided. Because visual inspection usually proceeds seamlessly to anoscopy, rectoscopy, and often treatment(s) as well, it is helpful if the most-often used instruments for these purposes are within easy reach.

Even when the patient is almost certainly a case of haemorrhoids, visual examination starts with the perianal skin and perineum. Thin rubber gloves are worn from this point onwards, which are changed as required, and always between each patient. Inspection is carried out with the patient relaxed, but also during a maximum straining effort, which brings prolapsing ano-rectal structures, including haemorrhoids, into view and gives information on the tone of the anal sphincters. Particular attention is paid to the presence of 1) dermatitis; 2) surface discharges (especially pus and mucus); 3) areas of abnormal skin (plaques, discolouration, infiltration, lichenification, increased or decreased pigmentation, blistering or ulceration); 4) skin tags; 5) haemorrhoids; 6) mucosa; 7) fissuring (both single and multiple); 8) sinuses and fistulas; and 9) tone of the anal sphincter (tight, patulous).

If non-specific or "inflammatory" skin changes are discovered, it should prompt enquiry regarding the use of skin preparations or suppositories as these may be irritant or sensitising; in the case of more specific lesions, these may be due to psoriasis, eczema or other dermatological conditions.

- *Dermatitis.* Common causes of this in haemorrhoid patients are local-anaesthetic-containing creams and suppositories (sensitising) and antiseptic ointments (both irritant and sensitising).
- *Surface discharges.* Both mucus and pus may appear on the perianal skin from internal causes such as inflammatory bowel diseases (Crohn's disease, colitis); venereal diseases (chlamydia, gonorrhoea, syphilis) or from a sinus track or fistulous opening; and more rarely from a deep chronic fissure-in-ano.
- *Abnormal skin.* This may be caused by psoriasis (characteristic plaques); eczema (areas of inflamed skin, usually with similar areas on other parts of the body, often with a history of atopy); sarcoid (bluish-red infiltration); lichen planus (white thickenings); Bowen's disease (hard intradermal plaque); leukaemia (discoloured thickening); melanoma (increased pigmentation); vitiligo and albinism (depigmentation); application of steroid creams (thinning, depigmentation); allergic reaction (blistering); Crohn's disease, tuberculosis, squamous carcinoma (characteristic ulcers, the latter with its typical heaped-up edge). The

presence of warts (condylomata) must be particularly noted.

- *Skin tags.* A single skin tag is of little significance, but multiple tags usually indicate underlying haemorrhoids, often large. Their presence may complicate treatment (see under Open haemorrhoidectomy, Ch. 11, p. 83).
- *Haemorrhoids.* The presence of visible haemorrhoids confirms their large size, especially if they are seen without the patient straining.
- *Mucosa.* This may be related to prolapsing haemorrhoids, but can also be due to an anterior rectocele or a true procidentia (mucosal or complete); both require confirmation by specific tests.
- *Fissuring.* The external end of a fissure-in-ano may be discovered, which can require gentle stretching of the anal verge. If the fissures are multiple or situated in the less common anterior or lateral aspects of the anal circumference or are unusually painless, this should raise suspicion of Crohn's disease.
- *Sinuses and fistulas.* These may be unassociated with specific pathological conditions but may be due to Crohn's disease, tuberculosis and, rarely, a neoplasm.
- *Sphincter tone.* A tightly closed anus may indicate spasm due to a fissure. A patulous anus may be caused by anal intercourse or be the consequence of age. Altered sphincter tone may have important consequences for treatment.

A haemorrhoid is a bluish-red cushion of tissue, covered by smooth mucosa which is usually reddest at its upper (internal) origin above the dentate line. A haemorrhoid usually has a narrowed base. First-degree haemorrhoids are visible only by anoscopy, but larger haemorrhoids protrude to a greater or lesser extent through the external anal orifice. They may be associated with skin tags and sometimes by a fissure-in-ano. Straining increases prolapse and vascular engorgement of haemorrhoids. In Caucasians, haemorrhoids occur most prominently in the left lateral ("three o'clock"), right posterior ("seven o'clock"), and right anterior ("eleven o'clock") positions, but the squatting defaecatory position, as commonly used by Muslims, encourages their development in the anterior quadrant predominantly. In most cases, the diagnosis of haemorrhoids is one of instant visual recognition. Haemorrhoids can be complicated by thrombosis, usually in the external anal venous network, causing a hard bluish-black swelling; if untreated, the blood clot may erode its covering epithelium and ulcerate through; this can cause confusion with a neoplastic ulcer, and occasionally an anal carcinoma has been disguised by thrombosis. Widespread thrombosis of prolapsed haemorrhoids ("strangulated piles") is associated with severe pain and requires emergency treatment; the appearance of the swollen black mass of tissue, usually involving the entire circumference of the anal orifice, is unmistakable, together with the stricken visage and straddled walk of the agonised patient, a source of frequent jokes.

If undue time appears to have been spent on the conditions that may be identified with, or substitute for, a diagnosis of haemorrhoids by their visual appearances, it is because these additional or alternative diagnoses may affect management in important ways; many will require preferential treatment in their own right; most will complicate any proposed treatment for haemorrhoids; some will prohibit haemorrhoid treatment and a few (e.g., skin tags, fissure-in-ano) can be treated alongside any treatment for the piles. Before leaving this aspect, certain additional points merit individual mention. Damaged or diseased skin should be cleaned up or cured before operative treatment of haemorrhoids is performed. Any ulcerating lesion should be biopsied if there is the slightest frisson of doubt about its nature. A common prolapsing anal lesion, especially in juveniles, is a stalked polyp, which may be fibro-epithelial or adenomatous; such a lesions should not be mistaken for a haemorrhoid and should be removed completely for full histological analysis.

In summary, at the end of visual inspection the proctologist should have identified not only the presence of any external or prolapsing internal haemorrhoids but have formed, taken together with the history, a shrewd assessment of the degree of haemorrhoidal mass that is present. Providing no other conditions are found to complicate management, it is usually possible at this stage to form a judgement on likely treatment for the haemorrhoids, and if office-based techniques are envisaged, it is a good principle to discuss these with the patient before any further procedures are undertaken. Another opportunity may arise after rectoscopy, but obtaining verbal consent to any instrumentation, and especially an invasive treatment, must take place before they are proceeded with.

Once visual examination is completed, the surgeon should proceed to anal and rectal examination, using the index finger and appropriate instruments (Fig. 4.3). Because anoscopy (proctoscopy) is frequently attended by treatment (e.g., sclerotherapy, banding) it is usually best to carry out rectoscopy (sigmoidoscopy) prior to proctoscopy, so that the proctoscope only needs to be inserted once. However, there is a final point that requires repeated emphasis; visual inspection needs to be done twice, once with the patient relaxed and again with the patient making a straining effort. During straining, lesions that are otherwise hidden in the anal canal descend into view (e.g., a polyp). In the case of haemorrhoids, they may prolapse, thus placing them in a different category (second-degree). Important differential diagnoses (e.g., mucosal or full-thickness rectal prolapse) may become evident, and any reduction in anal sphincter tone may become apparent, e.g., by a "gaping" response.

Digital Examination

This is not directly useful in the diagnosis of uncomplicated haemorrhoids. However, it is vital for lubricating the anal canal with a suitable clear jelly (e.g., KY jelly). The introduction of the index finger should be cautious and gentle, and it should be rotated so that all surfaces within reach are adequately greased.

Digital examination may reveal complications (e.g., thrombosis) or other diagnoses, and must be done with the intention to extract all the information possible.

With the finger fully inserted, the patient is asked to strain, which may bring pathology, such as a carcinoma, on to the end of the finger, even one sited in the upper rectum.

Before removing the finger, which must also be done gently, the patient should be asked to squeeze the finger (which is a further check on the muscle tone of the external sphincter muscle) and strain down (which can confirm that the anal sphincter is weak). If the straining effort is continued as the index finger is withdrawn, haemorrhoids (or other lesions) may follow it, and highlight that they are second-degree.

After removal, the finger is examined for any telltale evidence of blood, pus or mucus indicative of other pathology. The proctologist will also have learnt whether the rectum is loaded with faeces, which necessitates bowel preparation before proceeding further. Although lubrication should not have been lavish, any excess jelly is removed before subsequent instrumentation is carried out.

Rectoscopy, Sigmoidoscopy (Fig. 4.3)

The discussion that follows applies to the use of a rigid instrument.

Rigid rectoscopy does not necessitate routine bowel preparation for its employment. Most of the patients who are examined will have such sparse faecal contamination of their rectum that it does not interfere with a complete examination; of the remainder, many will have small solid boluses that can be manoeuvred out of the way, or liquid residues that can be sucked out with a large-bore sucker; only in a few cases will faecal quantities be sufficient to require bowel preparation for the examination. As discussed previously, bowel preparation not only imposes delay, with additional pressures on staff and toilet facilities, but can result in loss of diagnostic evidence (e.g., blood in the rectal lumen). In some patients, the preparation can work too vigorously and can cause such volumes of liquid stool that it is impossible to proceed; in many patients the preparation can cause irritation and reddening of the rectal mucosa which can be mistaken by the observer for inflammatory changes ("colitis").

Rigid endoscopy requires that the instrument is passed through the recto-sigmoid junction into the lower sigmoid colon, i.e., to a full 25 cm from the anal verge. Unless this is done, the examination is diagnostically incomplete. This is most easily achieved with a small-bore (20 mm diameter) instrument. Proximal lighting is essential. Since the advent of HIV infection, suitable disposable instruments have been developed. Surprisingly, it is not only true that small-bore rigid rectoscopes do not impede diagnosis, but facilitate it, it is also a fact that most diagnostic manoeuvres (e.g., biopsy, polypectomy) are also easily carried out through them. Small-bore rectoscopes also make it easy to get past small faecal boluses and to negotiate any narrowing to the lumen. Most importantly, they are much more comfortable for the patient.

Although the diagnosis of haemorrhoids is not made by the use of a rectoscope, every case of haemorrhoids requires at least a complete examination of the rectum and distal sigmoid as an integral part of their workup. One has only to become aware of one

1. Rigid instruments

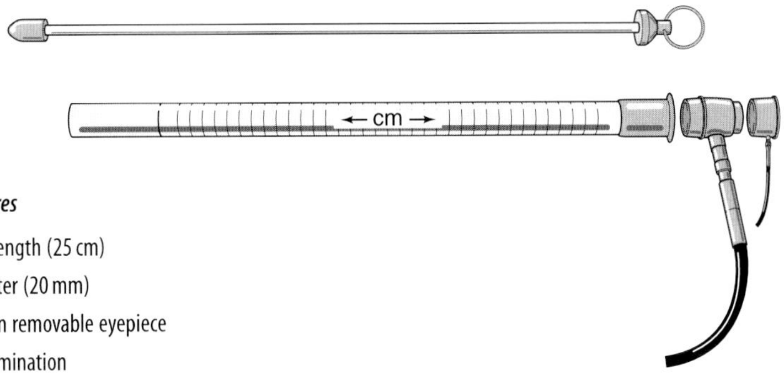

Desirable features

1. Convenient length (25 cm)
2. Small diameter (20 mm)
3. Magnification removable eyepiece
4. Proximal illumination
5. Disposable

Note: A small diameter instrument of sufficient (but not excessive) length is very manoeuvrable without impairing visual appreciation or passage of biopsy instruments.

2. Flexible instruments

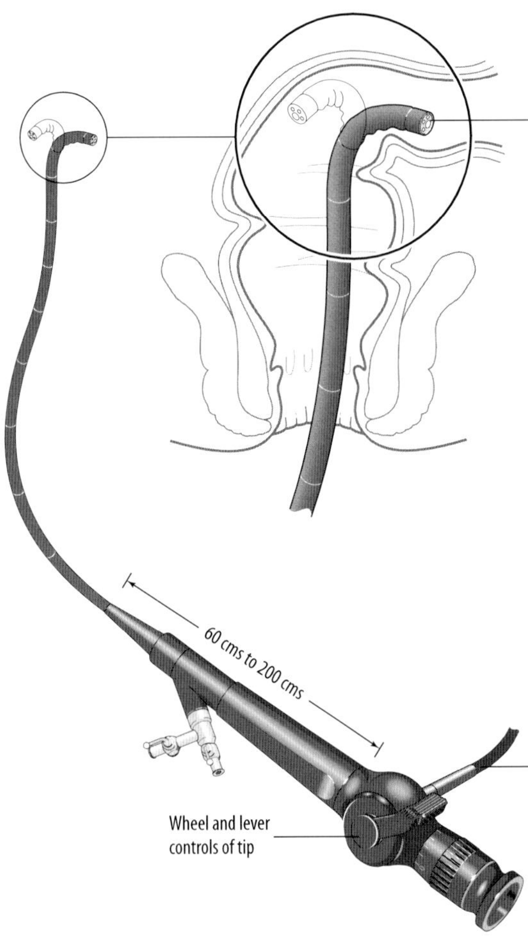

Desirable features

1. Robust design and cost-effective maintenance
2. Variable length
   i) 60 cms ("flexiscope")
   ii) 105–200 cms ("colonoscope")
3. Fibreglass optics
4. Mobile tip (320° arc)
5. Special instruments for:- biopsy, snaring, cutting, etc
6. Easy irrigation
7. Secure cleansing process

Figure 4.3. Diagnostic sigmoidoscopy (rectoscopy).

case of haemorrhoids that has been treated when a carcinoma is lurking in the more proximal bowel to ensure that such complete examination is carried out in every case. In the example cited, of a haemorrhoidectomy performed distal to a proximal carcinoma, the danger is not only delay in treatment of the colon cancer, but of malignant implantation in the open receptive surfaces of the haemorrhoidectomy wounds – truly a disaster of the utmost gravity.

Certain precautions can be taken to increase the chances of a complete rectoscopy. An increase of head-down tilt helps to straighten out the recto-sigmoid junction. In obese patients, use of the knee-elbow position can also ease passage through the recto-sigmoid junction. If required, patients can be additionally relaxed by a small dose of a tranquilliser (Valium), which can be administered intravenously. Minimal use of air-insufflation or force prevents pain, and reduces any slight chance of accidental perforation of the bowel.

If a co-morbid condition is discovered by rectoscopy, it is usually necessary to modify treatment for any haemorrhoids that may be present.

Flexible Recto-Colonoscopy

This has become the routine method of examination in some clinics; in others it is used to supplement rigid rectoscopy. In most cases, the flexible instrument of choice is the short version of the colonoscope, 60 cm in length. For maximum efficiency, its use implies bowel preparation, whose disadvantages have been described earlier.

The advantages of a flexible instrument are 1) it is less painful than rigid scopes, 2) it is longer than the standard rigid sigmoidoscope, so increasing diagnostic potential, and 3) it is easier to pass through the recto-sigmoid junction.

The disadvantages of routinely employing a "flexiscope" are 1) bowel preparation is advisable, 2) the instrument is expensive, 3) extra training is required in its use, 4) operative procedures are more limited, 5) special cleaning methods are required, often by expensive machines, and 5) examination of the proximal rectum, especially just above the ano-rectal junction, is often unsatisfactory.

The individual proctologist must weigh the advantages and disadvantages of flexible rectoscopy against each other with regard to the demands of his individual practise requirements. Whatever the decision regarding its routine application, he must be skilled in its use, so that he can resort to it without hesitation when indicated.

If there is any suspicion of malignancy above the rectosigmoid junction, total colonoscopy (195 cm) is necessary.

Anoscopy, Proctoscopy (Fig. 4.4)

As for rectoscopes, disposable proctoscopes are now available, and their use is recommended.

Before embarking on proctoscopy, forceps, small swabs, suction facilities and the common instruments used for the treatment of haemorrhoids in the clinic should be immediately to hand. It is a great advantage to have an assistant within call who can calm a nervous patient, provide an extra pair of hands, and fetch any instruments or preparations that are not already set out for the surgeon's use.

The anoscope should have a wide bore (20–30 mm) and is inserted on an introducer. Generous lubrication is advantageous. Insertion of the proctoscope should be gradual and gentle, allowing the anus to adjust to its presence; it should be put in to its fullest extent before the introducer is removed, also very gently. When the introducer comes out, there may be sudden release of flatus, fluid or faeces, and the surgeon's eyes and face should be protected at this moment; some surgeons wear goggles and a mask, but most do not. Any pain caused by introducing the proctoscope is noted, and if it is more than mild, the examination is discontinued until an explanation is found. In the author's experience, pain is usually an indication of another condition (fissure-in-ano, perianal abscess) or a complication (thrombosis). If pain is more than slight, further persistence with examination for, or treatment of, haemorrhoids without a thorough examination under anaesthesia is both useless and potentially harmful.

Many proctoscopes are marketed, with varied designs. Disposable proctoscopes are now available. Designs with an angled end or a longitudinal groove are very useful for isolating individual haemorrhoids, which can be invaluable for many office treatments (e.g., sclerotherapy, banding), and are recommended (Fig. 4.4).

Using the proctoscope, every aspect of the entire length of the anal canal is inspected. Normal as well as abnormal structures are noted; the identification of the dentate line (a pale wavy line halfway up the anal canal, which denotes the junction between

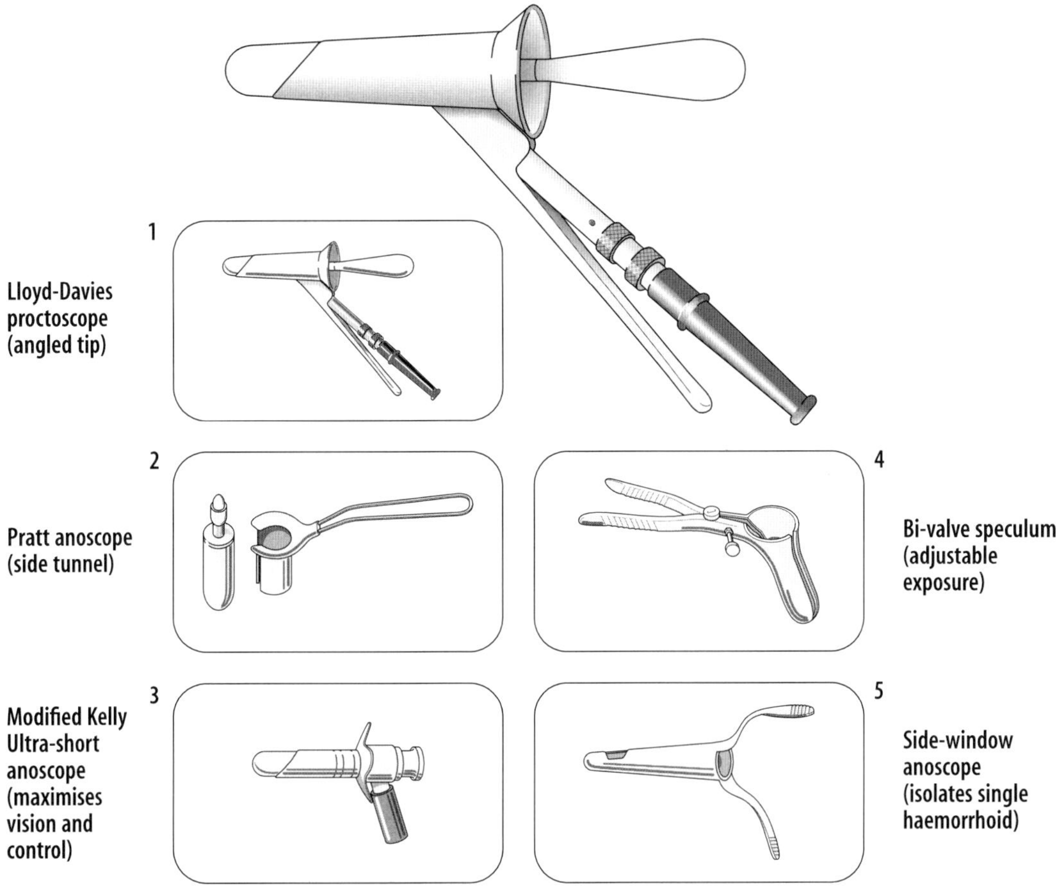

Desirable features

1. Relatively short length (7–10 cms)
2. Relatively wide bore (20–30 mm)
3. Angled or split tip (see inserts)
4. Proximal illumination
5. Close-fitting obturator
6. Short broad handle
7. Disposable

Inserts 1–5

These show the many varieties of anoscopes for the diagnosis and treatment of haemorrhoids. Most incorporate some, but not all, of the most desirable features. A wide bore, proximal illumination and an angled tip are the most important features.

Figure 4.4. Proctoscopy (Anoscopy).

squamoid and cubical epithelial linings) is especially important because the mucosa above the line is relatively insensitive – a vital point for many office treatments.

Certain conditions encountered on proctoscopy and which commonly accompany haemorrhoids, should be mentioned as they frequently modify treatment options. *Fissure-in-ano*. If not already discovered as a result of the history, visual and/or digital examinations, proctoscopy may reveal or confirm the presence of a fissure, and it contraindicates treatment of the piles by sclerotherapy or banding. Admission for combined treatment of both lesions under anaesthetic should be arranged. *Fistula-in-ano.* The presence of a fistula may be revealed by a purulent discharge from its internal opening. Treatment for the fistula takes precedence over that for haemorrhoids *Warts/condylomata.* Occasionally a single (or just a few) wart(s) is found by proctoscopy, without any peri-anal involvement. They can be fulgurated alongside treatment for the haemorrhoids. *Fibrotic or oedematous (crypt) tag.* A fibrotic tag at the entrance to an anal crypt can be snipped away at the same time as the piles are treated. An oedematous tag may be evidence of cryptitis, which should be treated before the haemorrhoids are touched. *Proctitis or other inflammatory changes.* These may be simple reddening (non-specific proctitis); ulcerative (ulcerative colitis, Crohn's disease); profusely productive (venereal diseases – gonorrhoea and chlamydia particularly); anteriorly situated ulcer in lower rectum (solitary ulcer syndrome). The last mentioned may raise suspicion of trauma or anal intercourse if accompanied by other suggestive pointers, e.g., patulous anus in a young male. Complete rectal prolapse can sometimes cause reddening of the anal and lower rectal mucosa, which has a sharp circumferential cutoff at its highest level; this may be the only sign discovered by a standard outpatient examination. *Neoplasms.* Usually proctoscopic examination will merely confirm what has already been expected as a result of the history, and digital and rectoscopic examinations, but occasionally a soft anal adenoma or other tumour (carcinoma, carcinoid, angioma, soft-tissue neoplasm) will be revealed by proctoscopy. Although in cases of overlooked tumours, the presence of haemorrhoids has been claimed to have hidden or disguised the neoplasm, in most instances the cause of misdiagnosis has either been lack of care or an inexperienced surgeon.

Haemorrhoids having been diagnosed by their characteristic appearance, as described earlier (p. 30) under visual inspection, in addition to confirming their presence, their size, position and number are noted, and a decision made as to their "best treatment". If they are suitable for immediate treatment, and the patient has been informed and agrees, the appropriate method is applied. For small haemorrhoids, this may be by injections or infrared thermocoagulation. For larger haemorrhoids, banding is usually the technique chosen for office treatment. For third-degree, or large second-degree piles, surgery is the best treatment.

Summary

As for all diseases, so for haemorrhoids the most important principle is that diagnosis precedes treatment. The diagnosis of haemorrhoids is made by taking a proper history, followed by examination. Examination falls into four categories – visual, digital, rectoscopic, anoscopic – and also by flexible endoscopy in selected situations, but is preceded by a general appraisal and abdominal examination. Diagnosis is made not only by positive identification of haemorrhoids, but also by ruling out any alternative or additional conditions which may be present, in particular carcinoma. This is achieved by a complete examination of the anal canal, rectum and lower sigmoid colon in all cases. Unless this is done, misdiagnosis is possible, sometimes with serious, and occasionally with tragic, consequences. At the conclusion of the diagnostic assessment, both the presence and the size of the haemorrhoids are known, and treatment can be decided. Office treatments for small haemorrhoids are possible at the time of anoscopy, which is the final examination carried out for diagnosis.

The status of a proctological surgeon can be estimated by the care and expertise which he exhibits for the diagnosis as well as the management of his haemorrhoid patients.

EDITORIAL COMMENT

Diagnosis precedes treatment. However, the diagnosis of haemorrhoids also establishes their size and distribution, and a precise knowledge of these physical characteristics is an essential guide to the best method for their treatment in the individual patient.

Equally important is the detection, or exclusion, of any other ano-rectal pathology (or of colonic disease as well in some cases).

Over many years, the Editor came to appreciate the importance of the case history for the diagnosis and evaluation of haemorrhoids.

The surgeon should take care to make his diagnostic techniques acceptable, and as user-friendly as possible, to both his patients and himself. He must also ensure that they are backed up by the appropriate instruments and facilities.

In busy clinics, there is pressure to increase patient turnover; this should be kept under control as a gentle, unhurried and thorough diagnostic evaluation is the key to successful treatment of haemorrhoids.

5 Indications for Intervention

Charles V. Mann

Introduction

It can be said that there are no absolute indications for surgical treatment of haemorrhoids, because haemorrhoids may cause inconvenient or unpleasant symptoms but are not responsible for serious health risks. Indeed, numerous patients make this assessment for themselves by never seeking out a doctor for any relief of their symptoms. Patients are well aware that haemorrhoids are a source of discomfort rather than risk, and are often afraid of medical treatments, which they apprehend to be at least embarrassing and at worst, extremely painful. Also, in certain families which are prone to develop haemorrhoidal disease, they know that recurrence of haemorrhoids after treatment is not uncommon.

In addition to creating a thriving market for "over-the-counter" remedies, many of them of dubious value, patients' fear of medical intervention has other consequences. Self-diagnosis can cause them to ascribe their symptoms (e.g., bleeding) to haemorrhoids rather than possible serious alternatives (which include ano-rectal carcinoma or major inflammatory bowel diseases). The prevalence of anal bleeding, even at a young age, can promote complacency not only by the patient but also by the family doctor. This, in turn, leads to incomplete examination and misdiagnosis. This has been stressed in Chapter 4 (p. 23).

If patients' fears can be reduced by better and less painful treatments, the problem of delayed diagnosis can be contained. Better standards of treatment, are materially promoted by increased specialisation of training in colo-proctological diseases. Only when the patient is confident that his surgeon will offer him accurate diagnosis, coupled to tolerable treatments, will haemorrhoidal disease become an accepted complaint. The challenge for the surgeon to convince patients to unhesitatingly attend for early diagnosis and treatment must involve removing any doubt in their minds that the cure may be worse than the disease.

Improved standards of treatment must be accompanied not only by impeccably accurate diagnosis but also by cures that rarely have complications, especially serious ones. Patients' expectations for their haemorrhoid treatment not only include that it should be almost pain-free, but also that they should suffer no injuries from it. With proper standards of investigation and treatment, the difficult balance between effective treatment and absence of risk can be achieved. The lurking figure of the lawyer lies in wait for any surgeon whose haemorrhoid treatments are attended by untoward consequences.

Proper attention has to be paid to selection of cases for any treatments that are available. This depends upon proper appreciation of the degree of discomfort that the patient is experiencing, as well as accurate assessment of haemorrhoid size, as will be discussed.

Any treatment offered should not be delegated to inexperienced juniors, and must be expert, compassionate and effective. But, to misquote Gilbert and Sullivan, "the object to be achieved in time is to make the treatment fit the 'crime'". In the treatment of haemorrhoids, this means cure of symptoms rather than cure of "disease".

Bleeding Haemorrhoids

Loss of bright red blood on defaecation is the symptom classically associated with haemorrhoids. However, such blood loss, although most frequently caused by haemorrhoids, cannot be assumed to be arising from them without proper investigation. In this regard, serious diseases occur in infants and young persons that can present with anal bleeding (e.g., familial adenomatosis coli (FAC)) and the author has experienced a young man of 23 years with advanced carcinoma of the rectum who had been treated for several years for "haemorrhoids". Therefore, blood loss per anum is always an indication for diagnosis in the first instance. "*Diagnosis precedes treatment*" was never more true. The diagnosis of haemorrhoidal disease should be established by exclusion of all other possible causes; by digital examination *in all cases*; by ano-rectoscopy *in most cases*; by colonoscopy and/or air contrast barium enema *in a few cases*. In the context of a hospital clinic, ano-rectoscopy should be done in all cases.

Some families have a strong association with haemorrhoidal disease. In these family members, bleeding can start during adolescence, and sometimes earlier than this. In young girls, early-onset haemorrhoid bleeding can be confused with menstrual losses, especially so because haemorrhoidal bleeding is frequently aggravated during this event; in their early stages, small haemorrhoids often bleed only during menstruation.

If a young man develops bleeding haemorrhoids, inherent susceptibility, or other contributory cause, can be assumed. But does such early onset of haemorrhoidal disease affect treatment? The answer to this question is in the affirmative. Young patients are not only less easy to cure; they also have a pronounced tendency for *early* recurrence after treatment. For this reason it has been the author's practice never to recommend a surgical operation to any patient below 35 years (and, preferably, 40 years) regardless of haemorrhoid size or the severity of their symptoms. In almost all cases, of course, effective non-operative management can and should be offered until the required age has been reached.

In female patients, menstruation, pregnancy and parturition aggravate haemorrhoids, and especially their associated bleeding (although prolapse and thrombosis can also be engendered). The greater tendency to bleed results from hormonal (oestrogen mainly) and mechanical factors, which result in 1) decreased coagulability, 2) diminished anal sphincter tone, 3) increased pelvic blood flow, 4) in pregnancy, pressure on the pelvic diaphragm by the gravid uterus, and 5) proneness to constipation, associated with increased straining. In the complex circumstances surrounding pregnancy and parturition, dietary factors and lack of exercise are particular constipating elements by which hard stools and/or straining cause increased bleeding which is not always linked to haemorrhoid enlargement. Because of the well-recognised tendency for pregnancy and labour to initiate or aggravate haemorrhoidal disease, it is the author's practice not to recommend a haemorrhoidectomy to female patients who are, or intend in the near future to become, pregnant. In addition to the fertility factor, there is the synchronous recommendation not to advise a surgical operation in patients who are below 35 years. It should not need stating (but unfortunately it does) that pregnancy must always be specifically ruled out if a potentially fertile woman, who is otherwise suitable for surgical management, is admitted for a haemorrhoidectomy: the possibility of this mistake, i.e., operating on a pregnant woman, is made more likely if there is a long preoperation waiting period for surgery.

Bleeding without prolapse is characteristic of small (first-degree) internal haemorrhoids. Such early haemorrhoids do not justify surgical treatment. If bleeding is slight (for example, spotty intermittent blood loss at defaecation), treatment should include correction of all factors which cause piles to bleed, such as hard stools, straining at defaecation, lack of exercise and faulty diet (see Ch. 6). The proctologist should not spurn the use of suppositories which are marketed as anti-haemorrhoid remedies (Anusol, Anugesic-HC, etc.). In some cases, these measures may be sufficient to stop the bleeding. However, in most cases, additional treatment by the measures outlined in Ch. 8 and Ch. 10 are required (e.g., sclerotherapy, infrared coagulation).

Before choosing any invasive non-operative treatment, the following should be acted upon: 1) no invasive treatment is entirely free from complications, so their recommendation should not be taken without the proper consideration, 2) the patient needs to be fully informed and give consent to any treatment, and 3) the patient should be reassured that the treatment should not cause great pain, or lead to social inconvenience or loss of earnings.

Injection sclerotherapy (Ch. 8) is the author's preferred method for treating first-degree bleeding haemorrhoids, but believes that infrared thermocoagulation is a suitable alternative. Dilatation (Ch. 11) is too severe, and can cause incontinence. Rubber band ligation (Ch. 9) is ineffectual as the small size of the haemorrhoids makes secure application of the bands very difficult. Since haemorrhoids are rarely cured by non-operative treatments, follow-up is always advisable. Provided the patients have not been hurt, and their bleeding has been stopped by treatment, they will return willingly for further injections as necessary.

Once haemorrhoids begin to prolapse, treatments directed solely against bleeding are increasingly ineffective and other treatments are better. However, there is one special case that needs to be discussed: some very large (third- and fourth-degree) haemorrhoids hardly bleed at all, probably because their surfaces become calloused. Such large haemorrhoids can only be treated by a haemorrhoidectomy but, in many cases, the patient is not unduly discommoded by the piles and is only worried about the bleeding. The surgeon should not impose a haemorrhoidectomy on a reluctant patient if all they require is reassurance that their bleeding is not due to cancer. Surgical operations are not recommended on the appearance and size of haemorrhoids but on the symptoms that are manifested: slight bleeding is an insecure basis for a haemorrhoidectomy for otherwise tolerated third- and fourth-degree haemorrhoids.

Despite the uncommon situation referred to in the previous paragraph, the degree of bleeding usually relates closely to the size of haemorrhoids. As their size increases, prolapse begins to occur, and treatments directed solely towards preventing bleeding become not only useless but also liable to complications. Treatments directed against haemorrhoids in which prolapse as well as bleeding are prominent features are discussed next.

Prolapsing Haemorrhoids

Just as with bleeding, prolapse, by itself, is not an indication for intervention unless it is symptomatic. However, as prolapse indicates increasing size, almost invariably associated with significant bleeding, there are very few cases of prolapsing haemorrhoids which should be left untreated.

If the extent of prolapse is slight, and seen by the examining surgeon rather than experienced by the patient (not by any means an unusual circumstance) non-operative interventions are very likely to produce excellent results and should be preferred, at least initially.

Early haemorrhoids with minimal prolapse (i.e., small second-degree piles) can respond to either sclerotherapy or infrared coagulation, although several treatments are usually required to produce worthwhile shrinking and binding down of the prolapsing tissues; bleeding will also respond.

Once a haemorrhoid has enlarged to the point that prolapse is a prominent symptom (i.e., a "mature" second-degree pile is present), sclerotherapy or infrared coagulation are so unlikely to have a good result that they are contraindicated. "Trials" of such methods should not be embarked upon as the results are not only negative but may be the cause of complications, e.g., prolapse/thrombosis, for which the surgeon will be blamed. Established second-degree haemorrhoids are treated best by banding. (See Ch. 9.)

If second-degree haemorrhoids do not respond to banding, haemorrhoidectomy is indicated. Some second-degree haemorrhoids are so large and fleshy, and their symptoms so troublesome, that the surgeon is justified in recommending surgical removal without delay, and this is always the case with third- and fourth-degree haemorrhoids in which the prolapse will never respond to lesser treatments.

There are other indications for haemorrhoidectomy as the treatment of choice which are not directly linked to the degree of prolapse. These are:

- large skin tags are present,
- lesser treatments (e.g., banding) have failed to produce worthwhile remission of symptoms (e.g., for up to a year),
- alternative management has resulted in complications,
- if additional pathology (e.g., a fissure) is present,
- if an attack of acute thrombosis has been experienced,
- if socio-economic factors prevent patient participation in multiple office treatments and follow-ups,
- there are no contraindications (e.g., age, see page 139).

If haemorrhoid prolapse is associated with reduced tone of the anal sphincters, great caution is indicated before haemorrhoidectomy is advised. Reduced sphincter tone may be due to age, general infirmity or complications around pregnancy (e.g., prolonged labour, episiotomy, application of forceps or multiple births) or previous anal operations. In some of these defective sphincters, the haemorrhoidectomy may be the final factor that precipitates incontinence to flatus and/or faeces.

Mucus Seepage. Pruritus

Haemorrhoid-linked mucus leakage problems may be caused by overproduction or inability to prevent mucus reaching the peri-anal skin.

Excessive mucus production is usually due to causes unrelated to any haemorrhoids that are found, e.g., inflammatory bowel diseases, non-specific proctitis, tumours (both adenomas and carcinoma), excessive nervous stimulation; their management does not include treatment of the haemorrhoids. Only if all such causes have been ruled out is therapy directed at the haemorrhoids justified.

More commonly, haemorrhoids cause mucus leakage either by preventing proper sealing of the anal orifice (by their bulk) or by producing mucus exterior to the anus (by their situation): in both cases the haemorrhoids will be large and other symptoms (bleeding, prolapse) are present which underpin the choice of haemorrhoidectomy as preferred treatment.

Mucus leakage is a prime cause of pruritus ani, and haemorrhoidectomy confers relief from the misery associated with a permanently irritating anus *when it is due to piles*. In cases where the cause lies with an incompetent sphincter rather than haemorrhoids, simple placement in the anal orifice of an absorbent tissue or pledget of cotton wool may provide excellent symptomatic relief. If there is 1) no evidence of another cause, 2) no evidence of reduced sphincter tone, and 3) large haemorrhoids are present, a haemorrhoidectomy can be advised, even if a mucus/pruritus link to piles is not unequivocally demonstrable. However, it is preferable if two elements are also present before surgery is resorted to: 1) other haemorrhoid symptoms are being experienced by the patient, and 2) the patient is aware that success cannot be guaranteed. The former will confer some benefits from the operation even if the pruritus is not abolished, and the latter will prevent the patient being resentful if a successful result is not achieved.

Long-standing mucus leakage is usually associated with severe dermatitis of the skin surrounding the anus, and skin tags are also present in many patients. Great efforts should be made to treat the dermatitis, as a soggy inflamed skin slows down postoperative healing. Skin tags should be removed at the time of haemorrhoidectomy. If the skin has responded preoperatively to appropriate measures (which can be greatly helped by the involvement of a dermatologist), it is wise to institute long-term postoperative treatment with protective barrier creams or ointments, which must never contain either hydrocortisone or antibiotics.

Faecal Soiling. Incontinence

Soiling and minor incontinence problems can be associated with haemorrhoids. It is important to establish their presence prior to any treatment so that they cannot subsequently be attributed to mismanagement, or even negligence; the author has defended a surgeon who was sued by one of his patients because minor soiling persisted following a haemorrhoidectomy; such is the current litigious environment in which surgery is carried out these days.

Mucus leakage is often accompanied by minor soiling problems, and can be the reason the patient seeks surgical help. The existence of soiling reinforces the case for surgical intervention if haemorrhoids are responsible for the mucus-soiling sequence.

Large prolapsing haemorrhoids, especially when they are accompanied by skin tags, can make post-defaecation cleaning a difficult and tedious process. This problem is cured by haemorrhoidectomy.

Faecal incontinence should never be attributed to haemorrhoids as the cause is invariably elsewhere, with sphincter weakness as the probable aetiological factor. If so, a haemorrhoidectomy is likely to make the incontinence worse. Other local causes of incontinence which may be confused with haemorrhoids, or co-existent, are anterior rectal wall prolapse, solitary ulcer syndrome and pedunculated adenomas.

Some deranged patients believe their faecal incontinence is due to haemorrhoids. True full-thickness rectal prolapse is often discovered in these cases. In other mentally unstable patients, undeclared laxative abuse may be responsible. Although their underlying abnormal mental state may be obvious, or betrayed on examination (e.g., by cathartic mucosal changes (melanosis) or by demonstrating the rectal prolapse), the surgeon should have a high index of suspicion for alternative causes if a patient presenting with haemorrhoids complains of faecal incontinence.

In specialist centres where facilities for anal manometry or a defaecating proctogram are available in addition to standard investigations such as radiography and colonoscopy, these can provide useful information for diagnosing the true cause of an incontinence problem in a patient with haemorrhoids. The worst possible outcome, as is stressed in other parts of this book (see Ch. 21) is to perform a haemorrhoidectomy on a patient with an undiagnosed colo-rectal malignancy.

Pain. Thrombosis

It must be recognised that *uncomplicated* haemorrhoids are not a cause of pain. This is underpinned by the longstanding histories that are provided by the great majority of patients, but also by frequent medico-legal actions when patients who have undergone an operation for "painful haemorrhoids" find that their symptoms persist after surgery because another condition was responsible for the pain. Ano-rectal causes of local pain in any patient presenting with haemorrhoids include anal fissure (common), anal sepsis (not uncommon), and anal carcinoma (rare). Only when it is recognised that anal pain is mostly due to other causes than haemorrhoids, and is never a symptom of uncomplicated haemorrhoids, will misdiagnosis, which can be serious, be avoided.

Once the above warning has been fully digested, it is safe to recognise that piles which prolapse on defaecation or after exercise can cause aching discomfort, which persists until they reduce or are manually replaced. This symptom accompanies large haemorrhoids which justify a haemorrhoidectomy on other grounds.

Anal pain which is due to another ano-rectal condition than haemorrhoids must be treated appropriately, but in the case of anal fissure it is often possible to treat the fissure (e.g., by sphincterotomy or dilatation) synchronously with the haemorrhoids. If an anal fissure is the prime reason for surgical intervention, especially by a sphincterotomy, any prolapsing haemorrhoids should be removed at the same operation.

If anal fistula surgery is being performed, it is permissible to remove any haemorrhoids that are present, except in the case of a high laying-open procedure which is likely to result in serious impairment of sphincter strength. In some of these patients, the haemorrhoids can assist post-operative sealing of the upper anal canal, and reduce problems of flatus and faecal incontinence. Furthermore, problems for healing a large fistula wound should not be increased by superimposition of haemorrhoidectomy wounds. If, after successful surgery for the fistula, residual haemorrhoids become symptomatic enough to justify treatment, banding or surgical removal both offer good prospects of effective treatment.

Internal haemorrhoids which are complicated by thrombosis (see also Ch. 22) cause anal pain, which may be severe in many cases. In the early stages of this complication, active intervention is indicated. For an acute attack of "strangulated piles" the author has employed anal dilation with good results; there is immediate relief of severe pain, early resolution of the thrombosis and long-term diminution of the piles. In other cases, and always for a recurrent attack or one that has been precipitated by large haemorrhoids, an immediate haemorrhoidectomy can also be carried out (see Ch. 22, pp. 150–151). The problem of a thrombosed *external haemorrhoid* is much simpler: if acute pain is present, sufficient to justify an immediate (office-based) thrombectomy, this should be done under local infiltration anaesthesia as described in Ch. 22, In those patients who have delayed presenting themselves for some days, conservative management is probably best, as spontaneous resolution is to be expected and further pain will be short lived.

Some patients with haemorrhoids suffer from "proctalgia". This is a poorly understood symptom complex that does not have a pathological basis. There is evidence that some cases are caused by spasm of the pelvic muscles, principally the levator ani muscle (with the pubo-rectalis portion particularly implicated) but objective data are lacking. Some patients can relate their attacks to stress. The condition causes pain, which can be so extreme that the patient may cry out or faint. The attacks come on without warning and may last just a brief period or for several hours. The pain is of "protopathic" rather than "epicritic" type. Relief is hard to obtain during an attack, but nitroglycerine has been helpful in some cases. Despite the severity of the pain, opiates are not suitable medicines to prescribe because of the danger of addiction. To perform a haemorrhoidectomy in a patient who suffers from proctalgia demands careful selection. The operation may not influence either the intensity or frequency of the attacks, and if the attacks should become worse, the patient may blame the operation. Providing the patients give informed consent, with complete acceptance that there is no proven link between their haemorrhoids and their proctalgia, treatment for their piles can be offered along the usual lines, including haemorrhoidectomy.

Anaemia

Very rarely, a patient with haemorrhoids is found to be anaemic. Although it is possible for blood loss from haemorrhoids to be severe enough to cause this, another explanation for the anaemia is usually found; for females, this is usually menstrual losses or a gynaecological disorder. In both sexes, a blood disorder may be identified, or another source of gastro-intestinal bleeding (e.g., peptic ulcer, inflammatory bowel disease, neoplasm). Within the author's personal experience, other diseases discovered in haemorrhoid patients which cause anaemia have included malnutrition, faulty diet, dental caries, drug and alcohol abuse and haemolytic anaemia. From these observations it follows that if a patient with haemorrhoids is found to be anaemic, in the first instance *investigation*, not surgery, is indicated.

Only when all other causes of the anaemia have been excluded by careful investigation should haemorrhoids be accepted as the prime cause and a haemorrhoidectomy performed.

Summation

The basis for any treatment of haemorrhoids is relief of symptoms rather than cure of the piles. Haemorrhoids do not cause ill health (with very rare exceptions) and do not demand "cure". With this in mind, treatment should not be worse than the disease. *Bleeding* usually responds to non-operative measures. *Prolapse*, which is usually associated with bleeding, may respond to banding, but often requires surgery (haemorrhoidectomy). Choice of the right procedure is decided principally by the size (degree) of the haemorrhoids. *Pain* is not caused by uncomplicated haemorrhoids, and is an indication for investigation rather than, and always prior to, intervention. *Thrombosis* can be treated by manual dilatation of the anus or an immediate haemorrhoidectomy, but in cases of delayed presentation, spontaneous resolution is usually the best treatment. *Mucus leakage* and *faecal soiling* can be associated with haemorrhoids, in which case they are relieved by haemorrhoidectomy. Care must be exercised not to overlook alternative causes of these symptoms, and sphincter weakness as a contributor to *incontinence* must not be overlooked. *Proctalgia* is a symptom complex not directly related to haemorrhoids, and does not respond to treatment directed towards any piles that are present in the sufferer. *Anaemia* is rarely caused by haemorrhoids.

Providing a surgeon takes proper care that the *indications* for any of his treatments are *proportional to the patients' symptoms*, he will not be guilty of inappropriately excessive interventions. Careful analysis of both patients' symptoms and expectations should be matched against the most effective techniques for their relief.

EDITORIAL COMMENT

This chapter emphasises the Editor's strongly held view that relief of symptoms rather than "cure" should be the aim of haemorrhoid treatment. In many cases, surgical intervention can combine the elements of symptomatic and structural elimination, and this constitutes ideal management. However, haemorrhoidectomy should never be performed for minor symptoms that can be relieved effectively by simpler office treatments. A proctological surgeon who is overenthusiastic for surgical treatment is either too attached to the exhibition of his surgical dexterity or (worse) additions to his bank balance.

6 Non-invasive Therapy

Charles V. Mann

Very little information is available (and usually nothing at all) in surgical textbooks or other literature concerning simple remedial therapies for the prevention and relief of haemorrhoids. Nor is instruction in their use given to medical students or surgeons in training; one has to assume that colo-proctologists attach little importance to this aspect of haemorrhoid treatment, despite the vast array of "over-the-counter" remedies and the frequency with which the public resorts to them. This attitude needs correction and unless colo-proctologists include these preparations in their practise, they will continue to lose an important part of management to mountebanks and practitioners of "alternative medicine".

Simple and straightforward treatments can assist in the office management of haemorrhoids in several particulars. Some can reverse many factors which promote the development of haemorrhoids (see Ch. 3). Others can be used alongside invasive treatments to increase the effectiveness of the treatment, and to reduce the chances of relapse. A few can be employed as "stand-alone" primary treatments for early haemorrhoids.

Some readily available preparations offered in pharmacies for haemorrhoid treatment can be harmful, especially so with regular long-term use. Colo-proctologists should always counsel their patients properly with regard to non-invasive remedies, and use them with due care in their own management strategies.

Diet

It is known that the *upright walk, sedentary life-style* and *constipated bowel habit* of urban man are major factors for the development of haemorrhoids. While we cannot advise patients to revert to walking on all four limbs, they can be educated on the value of *exercise* in the prevention and management of piles. Exercise is a stimulant of bowel activity, and should be encouraged as a natural way to avoid constipation. However, they should be counselled that too much exercise is as harmful as too little; physical (and mental) exhaustion reduces anal sphincter tone, and dehydration results in hard stools, and both can predispose to haemorrhoid prolapse and thrombosis. However, exercise is a minor contributor for the prevention of haemorrhoids, but diet is a major factor because of its all-important influence for the prevention of constipation.

Constipation causes and exacerbates haemorrhoids. It does this in two ways: (i) by producing hard stools (largely the result of sluggish colo-rectal motor activity), it encourages bleeding, (ii) by promoting prolonged and excessive straining at defaecation, prolapse and engorgement of haemorrhoids is increased.

It is important to emphasise that all patients with haemorrhoids need to avoid constipation, and that diet is the most significant factor in achieving this. However, a proper diet is also very important for the prevention of progression of anal cushions to symptomatic haemorrhoids (see Classification, p. 14).

Haemorrhoid patients should be advised to modify their diet in the following ways.

(i) *Increase fluid intake.* If sufficient water is drunk, constipation can be prevented (large volumes of water instilled by a intestinal tube ("antegrade colonic lavage") is used as a method of purging the colon of its faecal content preoperatively). The only difficulty is to persuade patients to take enough water (or other clear fluid) on a regular basis. Every patient should be advised to drink at least three pints (1,500 ml) of water daily, in addition to any other fluids. For men, beer is an acceptable alternative for some of this intake, although some women may also agree to this; however, any beer that is taken should be of low-calorie, low-salt type.

(ii) *Reduce tea/coffee intake.* Caffeine has constipating side effects, and intake of tea or coffee should be restricted to no more than two or three cups daily, unless decaffeinated brands are selected.

(iii) *Avoid starchy/sugary foods.* Such foods are constipating. Chocolate is a particularly powerful constipating confectionery.

(iv) *Avoid regular use of NSAIDs (e.g., aspirin, codeine) and/or tranquillisers (e.g., Valium).* These drugs are notorious for their constipating side effects. Their common indications, e.g., headache, stress, should indicate control of lifestyle rather than resort to these medications.

(v) *Increase fruit/fibre content of the diet* (Table 6.1). Fruits which are helpful include apples, dates, raisins, prunes and figs. Vegetables which are recommended include all pulses (peas, beans, lentils), cabbage, spinach, spring greens and rhubarb.

Fibre can be increased by taking bran supplements and by changing to wholemeal bread and flour. Muesli-based breakfast cereals should replace simple cornflakes.

In addition to the specific recommendations enumerated above it is useful to recall certain general principles which should underpin the regular daily intake. Foods with low fibre content (white bread, polished rice, potatoes, sweet or starchy foods) should be avoided or, at least, minimised (see Table 6.1). In some instances, large intake can compensate for low fibre content. Apart from the additional need to restrict calorie intake, foods with a high carbohydrate or fat content should not form the bulk of any meals. Meals should be regularly spaced every 3–4 hours and heavy meals eaten immediately prior to sleeping should be avoided. Alcoholic drinks increase peripheral blood flow, especially through arterio-venous connections and increase haemorrhoid bleeding; chronic excess alcohol abuse increases haemorrhoid size. Hot spicy foods irritate the ano-rectal mucosa and aggravate haemorrhoid symptoms.

Table 6.1. Fibre Content of Some Common Fruit and Vegetables

	Per Cent Weight per 100 g
Miller's Bran*	44
Wholemeal Flour*	9.6
Unpolished Rice	5.5
Polished Rice†	0.8
Wholemeal Bread*	8.5
Muesli*	7.4
All-Bran Cereal*	28.3
Nuts*	14.3–6.1
Spinach*	6.3
Cabbage*†	1.8
Lettuce†	1.5
Kidney Beans*	7.4
Potatoes†	2.0
Peas*	12.0
Beans*	7.4
Lentils	3.7
Dates*	8.7
Prunes*	7.4
Raisins*	6.8
Apples*†	2.0
Oranges†	2.0
Grapefruit†	0.6
Grapes†	0.9

1. * These foods are highly recommended. Prunes not only possess a high fibre content but laxative properties as well (shared with figs).
2. † Denotes *low* fibre content.
3. * The low fibre content of these foods (†) is partially compensated by being eaten in large quantities.

Bulking Agents, Laxatives, Purgatives, and Enemas

The ideal stool should be sausage-sized and shaped; it should have a soft putty-like consistency that is neither too dry nor too watery. The correct size and shape of the stool engages the physiological mechanisms which initiate and maintain an effortless and efficient expulsion of the stool(s), and a soft, pliant surface is non-traumatic to the ano-rectal mucosa. A stool with these optimum features is the product of many complex factors, including normal digestive processes, normal gastro-intestinal motility, and correct food and fluid intake, as described previously. It cannot surprise the reader that in consequence of the abnormal environmental, dietary and social conditions of modern urban-based life, the "ideal" stool is often the exception rather than the rule; however, it can be obtained if the patient is prepared to cooperate fully with expert advice (as described earlier).

Nevertheless, many patients require medications to assist in correction of constipation and/or an abnormal stool, especially for immediate or short-term purposes. Most medicines for achieving these fall into one of four categories: 1) bulking agents, 2) laxatives, 3) purgatives, and 4) enemas. Each of these will be discussed separately.

Bulking Agents

These act by increasing faecal mass. This is achieved by promoting faecal water content while the stool is forming but also in some instances by enhancing the amount of undigested material in the stools. The latter effect is hydrophilic, and mimics the properties of bran. Bulking agents are useful and very safe providing they are prescribed correctly. Two facts are important in this regard. First, they should not be over-prescribed, especially in older patients. If they are taken in excessive amounts, they can cause bolus obstruction. Second, increased quantities of fluid should be advised as these agents cannot obtain their full effects unless there is enough fluid available in the lumen of the colon.

Bulking agents have mild, gradual effects and may take time to produce a positive change. They have no direct action on intestinal smooth-muscle activity, but a stool of proper size is required to initiate peristaltic activity in the colon, as well as to set off normal defaecatory responses. They have no deleterious effects from long-term use, and are generally palatable. As discussed later, they can be combined with some laxatives to produce an enhanced symbiotic response that is an improvement on that achieved by either when used as a single agent.

Table 6.2 gives details of commonly prescribed bulking agents. A report by Senapati and Nicholls (1988) provided evidence of the value of bulk laxatives in the treatment of haemorrhoids.

Table 6.2. Bulking Agents

Products	*Notes*
Natural	
Bran	Excessive intake can cause bloating and flatulence
Manufactured	
Celevac. Fybogel. Fybranta. Ispaghula Husk. Metamucil. Methyl Cellulose. Normacol Sterculia [Karaya]	= Excessive intake can cause intestinal blockage due to bolus formation. = Should always be taken with extra fluid intake. = Should never be taken last thing at night. = Most have associated osmotic effects (c.f. Laxatives)

Laxatives

These act in two ways: 1) by stimulating increased intestinal activity, especially peristalsis and 2) by increasing intraluminal water in the colon, which is then absorbed by the faeces. By reducing the time spent by the faeces passing through the large bowel, there is less chance for water resorption from the stool, so that the net effect of increased exsorption and decreased resorption is to markedly increase the fluidity of the stools and also to encourage expulsion.

Whilst laxatives are safe for short-term (up to three months) use, they can cause serious side effects if used long term (years), as they often are by the uninstructed public. With prolonged habitual use, the neuromuscular mechanisms become dependent on their presence, and ever-increasing doses are required for a peristaltic response. In the end, even with huge doses, the large bowel remains inert ("cathartic colon") and partial or complete physiologic obstruction supervenes; this is a truly ironic conclusion for drug therapy originally taken to relieve constipation.

Senna and the anthra-quinone group of laxatives are especially prone to cause cathartic colon syndrome with excessive use.

Magnesium sulphate (and other similar salts) are very effective promoters of excess colon fluid content, through a combination of increased mucosal exsorption and osmosis. They can be used in small doses combined with a bulking agent to produce an enhanced effect, and, employed in this way, their long-term safety is increased (but not abolished).

Table 6.3 lists commonly prescribed laxatives, their indications and dangers.

Purgatives

While there is no precise distinction between a laxative and a purgative, their difference is characterised by their effects, which are mild and gradual for laxatives and violent and sudden for purgatives.

Table 6.3. Laxatives

Mode of Action	Names	Preferred Indications	Warnings
Osmotic attaction of fluid into gut lumen Makes stools softer and bulkier	Fibre Fybranta (bran fibre) Fybogel (ispaghula husk) Isogel (ispaghula husk) Methyl Cellulose Duphalac (lactulose) Lactulose	Persistent constipation associated with small hard stools Straining defaecation	Although these preparations are safe for long-term use they can produce bolus intestinal blockage if too much is taken, especially if fluid intake is not generous
Stimulation of neuromuscular activity, including peristalsis Lessened time for resorption of fluid from faeces Causes faster expulsion of more watery stools	Bisacodyl Dulcolax (bisacodyl) Cascara (hydroxyanthracene) Senna (sennosides) Agarol (phenolphthalein) Ex-Lax (sennosides)	A severe attack of constipation	These can be useful for relieving an episode of acute constipation but no more than a few doses should be used. Continual use leads to habituation, increasing dosage and, eventually, cathartic colon
Increase of exsorbed water available in colon lumen Softens and liquefies stools	Magnesium Sulphate "Salts" Epsom salts ($MgSO_4$) Glauber's salts (Na^2SO_4)	Rapid relief of faecal retention Can be combined with an osmotic laxative for enhanced effects of both drugs	Are not suitable for long-term use. Sodium salts should not be used because of fluid retention. Are a useful start-up for relieving severe constipation while long-term safer solutions (e.g., fibre) are established

Only a few examples of the many laxatives available on the market are given in the Table. Oil-based preparations (liquid paraffin, Petrolagar) should not be used as they 1) seep from the anus causing pruritus 2) interfere with absorption of fat-soluble vitamins and 3) can cause granulomas. They are also ineffective. Provided sufficient water and fibre are taken, laxatives should not be necessary. Coffee and tea promote constipation (see text) due to their caffeine content.

In some cases, the evacuation produced by a purge is so extreme as to cause incontinence.

In general, purgatives are best avoided in patients with haemorrhoids as they can cause bleeding (which may be profuse), as well as prolapse/thrombosis. Patients should be warned, when necessary, against these dangers, and purgatives should only be prescribed for serious indications under medical supervision. Some neurotic patients, and especially those inclined to illnesses such as bulimia, resort to regular use of purgatives, which aggravates haemorrhoidal tendencies; clinicians need to guard against this possibility in young patients presenting with symptomatic piles, especially if they are more than first degree.

In some circumstances faecal retention needs to be relieved by a purgative, mostly when it is caused by an acutely painful anal lesion. While this is commonly a fissure-in-ano or a peri-anal abscess, it can be necessitated by acute thrombosed haemorrhoids or post-haemorrhoidectomy (when it may not be possible to employ an enema).

Castor oil is still the most effective purge available, although it is unpleasant to take. Alternatives are available but they are not as reliable in their effect. The availability of enemas which can be administered through very fine tubes has reduced the need for purgatives (see next).

Enemas

If it is necessary to evacuate the distal bowel, enemas are generally more acceptable and safer than purgatives. For some disturbed individuals (e.g., bulimic or anorexic patients) or for others who are on abnormal diets in search of the "perfect" body (e.g., models), it may be necessary to resort to an enema to achieve this, usually in the form of a mechanical wash-out. (There have been well-publicised examples recently of high-society ladies who resort to colonic wash-outs on a regular basis.) Enemas, especially those which rely on stimulating the lower bowel, can aggravate haemorrhoids, and should be used with discretion.

Table 6.4 lists a selection of enemas that are used, together with some indications for their use (or avoidance) in patients with haemorrhoids.

Table 6.4. Enemas

1st Group. Rely principally on mechanical wash-out effects but also mild irritation of bowel mucosa
(i) *Soap and water enema.* The soap can inflame (redden) the rectal mucosa – a cause of misdiagnosis on endoscopy.
(ii) *Saline enema.*
(iii) *Tap water enema.* The large bowel can absorb water, with potential risk for cerebral oedema unless the water is (nearly) completely withdrawn.
2nd Group. Rely principally on osmotic effects but also on mucosal irritation
(i) *Sodium acid phosphate enema* (Syn. Fletcher's enema, fleet enema)
(ii) *Sodium citrate enema* (Syn. Micralax enema)
These enemas are made up in convenient plastic bags with a nozzle. The "micro"-enemas can be self-administered through their attached fine tubing.
3rd Group. Rely on stimulation of colonic neuromuscular activity.
(i) Oxyphenisation (Syn. Veripaque)
This enema works powerfully, and usually within 1 hour; it empties the colon and rectum of most of its faecal content.

Although enemas are safer to use than purgatives as they are less likely to cause prolapse and thrombosis of haemorrhoids, they have few indications in the treatment of piles. However, they can be used for emptying the distal bowel prior to investigation and for an episode of faecal impaction during treatment (which is usually engendered by pain from a concomitant fissure-in-ano or as an unintended sequel to an invasive treatment e.g., post-injection). They may also be required to initiate defaecation post-haemorrhoidectomy in an unusually nervous patient, for which the "micro" preparations are ideal as they have very fine tubing which can be inserted painlessly (almost) into the rectum.

Suppositories

These can be a valuable aid in the treatment of haemorrhoids.

1. *Small haemorrhoids which bleed.* Hard stools may be the major factor causing the bleeding, especially if it is of slight or occasional occurrence. The use of a lubricant suppository inserted prior to defaecation can cure the symptom. A suitable suppository (Anusol, glycerine) should be inserted a short time (up to one hour) prior to the usual time of defaecation. Use of the suppository should be combined with a stool softener (see under Bulking Agents, earlier). After a few days, when the stools are no longer hard, use of the suppositories may be discontinued.
2. *Haemorrhoids associated with pruritus.* Suppositories containing hydrocortisone can offer effective relief for the itching. The steroid is usually added to a lubricant base, for example in an Anugesic suppository. The anti-pruritic suppository is best inserted the previous night on retiring, so that the hydrocortisone is distributed on the anorectal mucosa, and is put in contact with the anal and peri-anal epithelium during defaecation the following morning. It is important to be certain that there are no infections (e.g., fungi) of the perianal skin before steroid-containing suppositories are used. Because of the risks of possible super-infection and thinning of the perianal skin, use of steroid suppositories should be discontinued after a maximum of 4–6 weeks, but can be resumed after a suitable interval (6 weeks).
3. *After sclerotherapy.* When haemorrhoids have been treated by injections (see p. 58) or infrared therapy (see p. 73), it may take a few days for the optimum effects to be achieved. In the case of submucosal injection therapy, it is also important that the injected material should not be disturbed by the passage of a constipated stool. The daily use of a lubricant suppository (Anusol, Anugesic) can assist in early relief of symptoms, and easier defaecation for the first few days after sclerotherapy treatment, while the haemorrhoids are responding to the injections.
4. *Haemorrhoids associated with a fissure.* In a few cases, a fissure is present in addition to haemorrhoids. If the haemorrhoids do not qualify for operative treatment, use of a local anaesthetic-containing suppository may be sufficient to allow the fissure to heal (by reversing the pain → spasm → pain cycle) and to permit office treatment for the haemorrhoids by the proctologist's preferred method (e.g., injection, banding) at a later date.
5. *Constipation.* Suppositories can be a useful substitute for oral preparations to relieve some types of constipation which may complicate haemorrhoid treatment. Many elderly patients experience difficulty in initiating defaecation, and resort to straining; straining habits of defaecation are also not uncommon in "urban man" (see under Diet, pp. 43–45). Pregnancy and post-parturition smooth-muscle inertia may also cause defaecatory problems for which oral preparation are unsuitable treatments and in which haemorrhoids are a frequent cause of symptoms. Here, suppositories are an excellent treatment; usually the haemorrhoids subside as the after-effects accompanying child-bearing and birth recede, and the need for continuing with suppositories also ceases.

Table 6.5 provides a list of some suppositories which are useful for haemorrhoid patients, together with suggestions for their use.

Table 6.5. Some Uses of Suppositories for Haemorrhoids

Suitable principal symptom	Suppository	Constituents	Actions
Difficult defaecation (straining)	Glycerine	Glycerine	Mildly stimulant to defaecation Lubricates anal canal & stools
Minimal intermittent anal bleeding	Anusol	Bismuth oxide Peru balsam Bismuth subgallate Zinc oxide	Lubricates stool surface Mild astringent effects
	Anosedyn	Ephedrine hydrochloride Lignocaine hydrochloride Allantoin	Mild vasoconstriction Local anaesthesia Astringent effects
Minor anal bleeding Itching Post-injection or infra-red treatment	Anugesic-HC	Benzyl benzoate Bismuth oxide Bismuth subgallate Hydrocortisone acetate Peru balsam Pramoxine hydrochloride Zinc oxide	Mild astringent effects Lubricates anal canal and stools Anti-inflammatory actions
	Proctosedyl	Cinchocaine hydrochloride Hydrocortisone	Local anaesthesia Anti-inflammatory actions
Anal pain e.g., from an associated fissure-in-ano	Xyloproct	Aluminium acetate Hydrocortisone acetate Lignocaine Zinc oxide	Lubricates and canal Anti-inflammatory actions Local anaesthesia Mild lubricant and astringent properties

Many varieties of suppository are produced. Most of their constituents are similar to those listed above. Lubrication and astringency are obvious desirable features of most suppositories but additional actions (e.g., vasoconstriction for bleeding, surface anaesthesia for pain) are provided for specific purposes, as seen in the Table. Suppositories containing hydrocortisone should only be used for short periods (7–21 days) and never if there is an anal infection or warts. Rarely, patients can have an allergy to some constituents e.g., Zinc oxide and the patient should re-attend promptly if untoward symptoms are noted.

Summary

It is recommended that colo-proctologists are not only aware of but also make greater use of the whole range of simple non-invasive remedies to improve their management of haemorrhoids. For small haemorrhoids with minor symptoms (bleeding especially), advice on fluid intake and a suitable diet may be all that is required. Most patients with haemorrhoids can benefit from correction of constipation, straining defaecation and pruritus, and restoration of normal effortless evacuation will reduce the chances of recurrence after treatment. Laxatives have a role for short-term correction of constipation, for which bulking agents are the best long-term treatment. Purgatives have very few indications, but may be required in specific situations; they should be carefully supervised when they are prescribed. Suppositories have an important role in treatment that is often ignored (but not by haemorrhoid sufferers or their pharmacists!). For some cases of small bleeding haemorrhoids, they are the only treatment required; in other patients they make treatments more effective, or permit their application.

Surgeons should play a more active part in the teaching and application of non-invasive remedies described above. This would allow them to repossess treatments that are often the province of non-medical practitioners and help their patients both to understand and participate in their haemorrhoid management.

EDITORIAL COMMENT

Simple remedies (e.g., dietary modifications, laxatives, suppositories, etc.) can *sometimes replace* invasive treatments for haemorrhoids, but they can *always supplement* every treatment. Therefore, it is necessary to incorporate the benefits of simple remedies into surgical management: why should cranks, quacks and pharmacists receive credit for the results of such medications, especially as resort to them exposes patients to the risk of misdiagnosis? Dentists include hygiene as an integral part of their treatment; surgeons should learn from their example with regard to non-invasive treatments.

References and Further Reading

Broader JH, Gunn IF, Alexander-Williams J (1974) Evaluation of a bulk-forming evacuant in the management of haemorrhoids. Br J Surg 61:142

Keighley MRB, Buchmann P, Minervum S, Arabi Y, Alexander-Williams J (1979) Prospective trials of minor surgical procedures and high-fibre diet for haemorrhoids. BMJ 2:967–9

Senapati A, Nicholls RJ (1988) A randomised trial to compare the results of injection sclerotherapy with a bulk laxative alone in the treatment of bleeding haemorrhoids. Int J Colorectal Dis 3:124–6

7 Anal Dilation Treatment

P.H. Lord

Introduction

The theoretical background to the employment of dilatation for the treatment of haemorrhoids depends principally on the following precepts:

1) Haemorrhoids consist of loose connective tissue which contains thin-walled sinusoids fed with oxygenated blood via small arterioles. The sinusoids drain via vessels which run upwards in the submucosa of the lower rectum for at least three centimetres before they penetrate the muscular lamina propria to eventually link with the portal system (Fig. 7.1). While the draining vessels are in the submucosa they are easily obstructed by any raising of intrarectal or intra-abdominal pressure, causing backflow and rapid engorgement of the haemorrhoid plexus (Fig. 7.2). Much of our current understanding of the nature of haemorrhoids, and their relation to anal cushions – normal structures present from birth – stems from the work of W.H. Thomson.
2) That, in cases of haemorrhoids, a band (or bands) of fibrosis can be felt in the circular muscle of the anal sphincter and lower rectum. Attention to the existence of this band was originally drawn by Ernest Miles (1919) who named it the "pecten band", although he thought wrongly that the band lay in the subcutaneous tissue. As a consequence of the fibrous ring(s), even when the anal sphincter relaxes to allow stool to pass, the lumen remains restricted, thus generating higher intrarectal pressures.
3) Chronic persistent rise in pressure in the lower rectum and anal canal during defaecation causes permanent stretching and enlargement of the haemorrhoid veins and other supporting tissues, converting normal cushions to abnormal haemorrhoids. Straining habits of defaecation contribute an important element for backpressure on the pelvic and haemorrhoidal veins, increasing the degree of engorgement.
4) Once the presence of a haemorrhoid is established, mechanical pressure, as when a hard constipated stool is squeezed through the constricted anal outlet, dislocates the pile in a downward direction, causing progressive problems of prolapse as well as aggravating venous engorgement of the anal veins.

One way to reverse the interlocking causes of increased ano-rectal pressure responsible for greater venous engorgement would be to permanently lower the element of outlet obstruction by stretching the fibrotic bands in the anal sphincter muscle. This is achieved by digital dilatation according to the method described below.

Indications

It is most important to stress that *elective dilatation is a treatment that is reserved for symptomatic haemorrhoids that would justify a haemorrhoidectomy* (i.e., third- and fourth-degree piles).

The procedure can be used for the management of acute prolapsed thrombosed haemorrhoids ("strangulated piles") as described in Ch. 7.

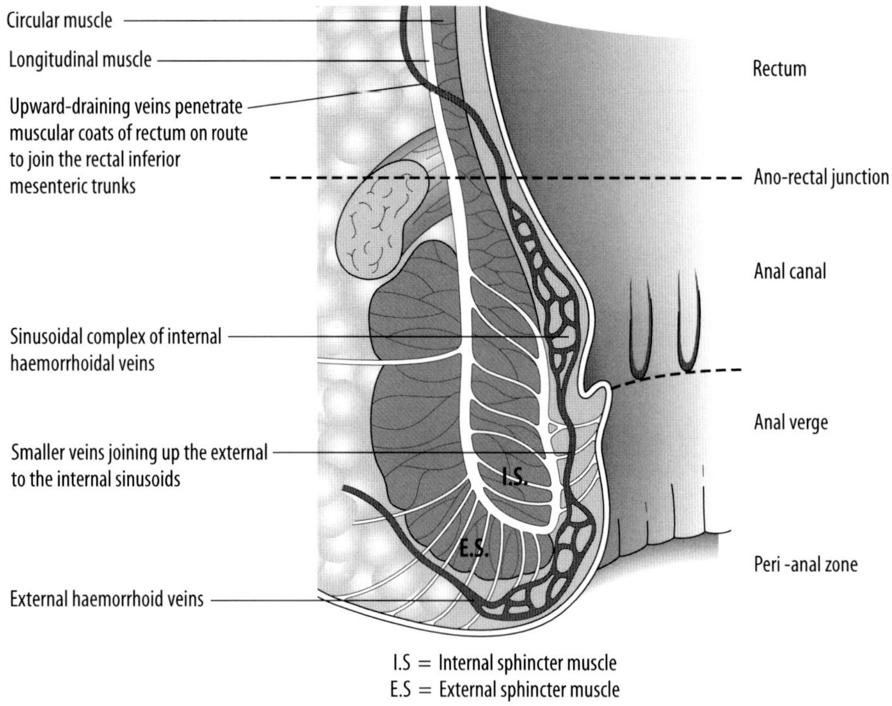

Figure 7.1. Note that the normal route of the blood draining from the haemorrhoidal venous sinusoids is upwards, and that the blood exits by penetrating the circular muscle coat of the rectum above the ano-rectal junction. The squeezing effect of **increased muscle tone** or a **constricting band** in the upper anal canal will cause back flow and engorgement of the veins of the anal cushions and haemorrhoids. Prevention of high anal sphincter tone or dilatation of any constricting ("pecten") bands will abolish the causes of abnormal venous engorgement. There are veins which connect the external and internal veins which can allow involvement of the external veins by engorgement factors which start in the internal (haemorrhoidal) veins.

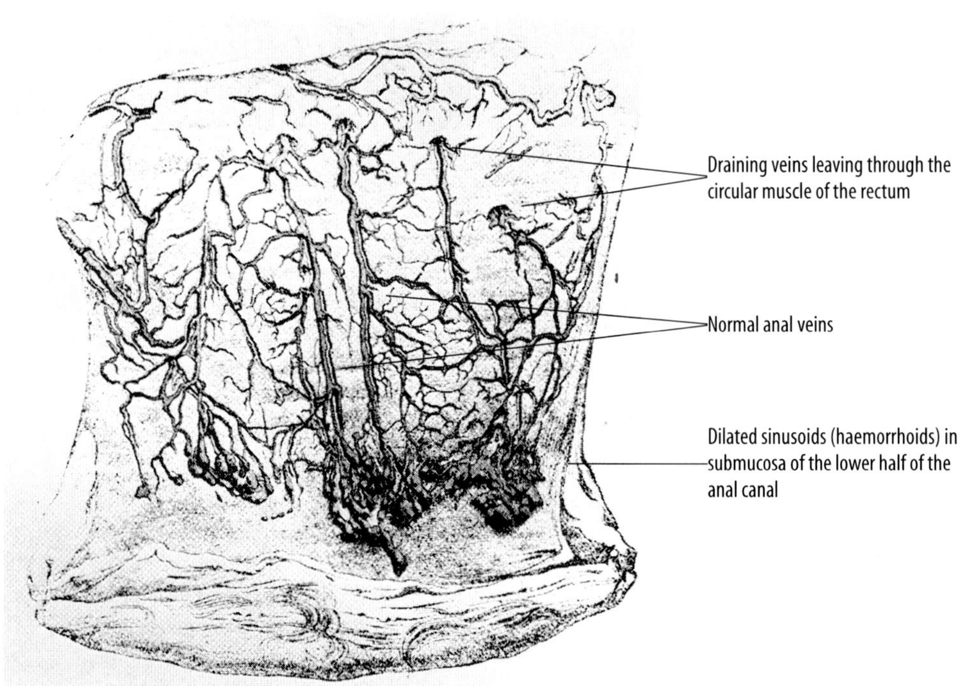

Figure 7.2. After injection of the anal veins with a resin solution, the anal canal has been opened out and the overlying mucosa removed to display the veins. Note the dilated sinusoids in the lower half of the anal canal – the haemorrhoidal plexus.

Contraindications

Haemorrhoids which would not qualify for treatment by a haemorrhoidectomy are not suitable for treatment by dilatation.

First- and second-degree haemorrhoids should be treated by other methods (e.g., sclerotherapy, banding, or cryotherapy).

Asymptomatic haemorrhoids should not be treated by dilatation.

If the patient has large piles but the symptoms are not due to haemorrhoids but arise from another source (e.g., mucous leakage causing pruritus; mucosal prolapse), dilatation is contraindicated, not only because the symptoms will persist, but also because they may be worsened, after dilatation.

Patients with a weak sphincter should not undergo dilatation, not least because their prolapsing tissue will consist of ano-rectal mucosa rather than haemorrhoids (although associated haemorrhoids may well be present). Whenever mucosal prolapse is responsible for the symptoms rather than haemorrhoids, and most especially if a weak sphincter is the cause of the problem, a surgical answer is indicated (e.g., haemorrhoidectomy) although stapling may be used as an alternative (see Ch. 14).

No patient should undergo dilatation who has not passed through strict diagnostic procedures, which should include a careful history, expert examination, and procto-sigmoidoscopy plus colonoscopy and/or barium enema when necessary. The surgeon should have a low threshold for arranging a colonoscopy or barium enema (see Ch. 4: Diagnosis).

Technique

1. Preparation.
Provided due attention has been paid to correct diagnosis by examination of the patient, which must include a satisfactory (i.e., complete) sigmoidoscopy, no special preparation is required.

Informed consent should be obtained and signed for by the patient. Possible complications should be discussed, even if they are unlikely.

2. Anaesthesia.
A general anaesthetic is often used, and the anaesthetist should be experienced. The anaesthetist must take all necessary precautions to ensure that the patient is fit for anaesthesia. It helps if the surgeon and anaesthetist are accustomed to working as a team and have a pre-arranged system in place for carrying out the procedure.

A caudal block can be used as a very effective alternative to general anaesthesia, but takes more time, both pre- and post-operation. A caudal block can be a good choice for patients who are unsuitable for, or unwilling to undergo, a general anaesthetic.

Pre-medication is not required.

3. Position.
As the patient is fully conscious, positioning is easy. The patient is settled comfortably on the left side (left lateral position), with the knees drawn up and the buttocks projecting well over the edge of the table. Once the patient is in the correct position, the anaesthetic is commenced. Dilatation should not start until the anaesthetist is sure that the patient will not react to the dilatation in a dangerous way (e.g., by laryngeal spasm), as tracheal intubation is not employed.

4. Dilation technique.
Standing at the patient's back, the surgeon ensures that the anus and his gloves are well lubricated. Two fingers of the left hand are inserted, and, with the digits partially hooked, they are lifted to open out the anal canal. The right index finger is now slipped in and pressed downwards, thus identifying all constricting bands. It must be remembered that some bands may be present as high as the fingers can reach.

Having ascertained the positions of all bands that are present (usually only one – the "Pecten Band"), the dilation can begin. This is usually done with the surgeon standing near to the bottom of the table. Only the two index fingers are used for initial dilation, and it is done with a gentle ironing out motion – like "ironing out the perineum when delivering a baby's head". *Care is taken not to damage the sphincter muscles.* Gradually the constricting bands are felt to give way. As the dilation proceeds, extra fingers are *fully* inserted as required to achieve the required end result, which should be abolition of all constrictions, leaving *an unobstructed passage from mid rectum to the exterior* such that even a well-formed stool could be extruded without any build-up of rectal pressures by straining (Fig. 7.3).

During the dilatation, the surgeon should remember that the anal sphincter is thinner and weaker at front and back and should concentrate stretching at the sides (i.e., 3 o'clock and 9 o'clock positions). *It*

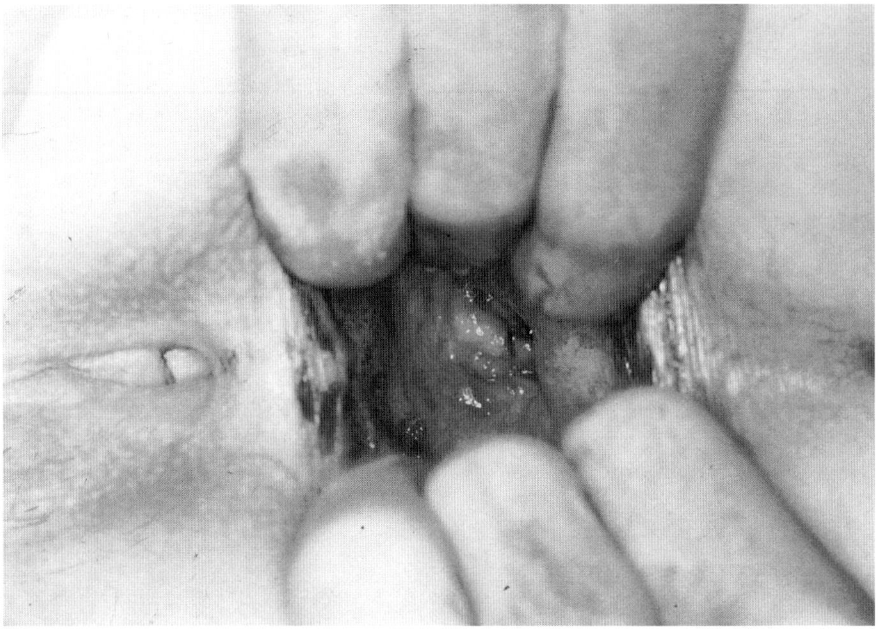

Figure 7.3. Note the following features. 1) That there is an unimpeded passage between the anal orifice and the rectum; the lumen of the latter is clearly seen. 2) That in this case, three fingers of each hand have been deemed sufficient for the dilatation. 3) That the fingers are only slightly curved, i.e., not hook-shaped. 4) That the anal mucosa and perianal skin are undamaged, i.e., that the dilatation has been gradual and gentle.

is always better to do too little rather than too much. If the dilatation is done gradually and gently, rather than abruptly and forcefully, sphincter muscle should be preserved from damage, and the anoderm should not be torn.

When the procedure is concluded, a decision is made as to whether insertion of a sponge is needed. A soft sponge can help to minimise post-stretch haematoma formation, but its removal (after the patient has woken up from the anaesthetic) can be the most unpleasant part of the procedure for the patient. Nor is there any evidence that its insertion makes any difference to the end results. The surgeon should make his own decision on use of a sponge as judged at the end of each dilatation.

Post-dilatation Care

Once the patient has recovered from the anaesthetic, and any sponges have been removed, they are allowed home. They are warned that defaecation may be a different experience, especially for the first few weeks. Straining should be abolished, and stool passage may be so effortless that it will occur quickly, almost without warning. In the early days after dilatation, incontinence may occur, especially on exertion, sneezing or straining; recovery from these initial effects can be speeded up by simple medications (e.g., codeine phosphate tablets) and sphincter exercises. Provided patients have been properly briefed on what to expect, and what action to take, they are able to manage any early problems without difficulty, and are happy to accept any temporary complications until normal control is re-established; a pad may be needed for the first few weeks until full control returns.

Once the patient has established normal post-dilatation defaecation, they are advised to add bran to their diet, along with plentiful fluids (see Ch. 6), to prevent recurrence of straining habits of defaecation and/or the hard stools that promoted their haemorrhoidal complaints in the first place.

If a patient continues to be troubled by prolapsing tissue (usually with mucosa as its principal component) this should be treated appropriately. In many cases, prolapsing mucosa can be treated effectively by banding (Ch. 9) or cryotherapy (Ch. 19). Skin tags which are symptomatic (pruritus ani, difficulties with anal cleaning post-defaecation) can be excised under local anaesthesia, although in some cases this can also accompany the dilatation.

The author devised a special dilator to be used post-operatively on a long-term basis, as a means to ensure that no return of the pecten band (or other narrowings) was possible. The dilator was large, and there is suspicion that only a minority of patients persisted in its use. There is no information on this point, and the present position would be that use of this dilator is not essential to a successful outcome.

Every patient should be reviewed at two weeks postoperatively, when any persisting symptoms can be treated. In the majority of cases, the patient is discharged, but others may require additional measures, as described earlier. Inadvertent passing of flatus may persist for several months, but should respond within two or three months to sphincter-tightening exercises that can be practised within the home; these cases are reviewed at two months post-operation, when most are discharged.

Complications

In contrast to haemorrhoidectomy, the following complications do not occur: **1)** postoperative bleeding, **2)** urinary retention, **3)** faecal impaction, and **4)** anal stenosis (see Ch. 20: Complications).

Faecal incontinence has been reported. *The author has knowledge of two cases of incontinence but in both cases there was evidence that the dilatation procedure had been wrongly applied*; in one case, too much force was used, leading to sphincter disruption with a keyhole anal deformity; in the other case, the wrong indication was used. Providing anal dilatation is treated with serious respect; carried out for the right indications; and performed with due regard to gentleness and avoidance of sphincter disruption (see Technique), faecal incontinence should not occur.

Finger perforation of the lower rectum has been reported. This is always iatrogenic, being due to forceful pulling with the fully hooked index finger against the rectal wall.

Minor complications (haematomata, small anodermal tears) occur in many cases but require no special treatment other than hot baths and applications of a bland cream (e.g., Nivea); any bruising disperses and the tears heal within a few days.

Despite the simplicity and safety of the dilatation method, it is strongly recommended that informed consent, with full knowledge of all possible complications, should be obtained before carrying out anal dilatation.

Results

For the elective management of *symptomatic* haemorrhoids that cannot be treated by alternative (office) methods, the results are excellent. Symptoms disappear immediately, and the patient is expected to (and does) return to normal activities the next day. A surgical colleague who was treated by dilatation on a Friday morning under general anaesthesia was able to perform a full operating list on the next day (Saturday). Such dramatic results are not uncommon, but rather the expected outcome. The worse the symptoms, the more gratifying the result.

After an initial report of the immediate results in 100 patients (1969), the method was used widely, and became the standard treatment (in the local catchment area) for haemorrhoids that would otherwise have needed a haemorrhoidectomy. Between 1961 and 1970 (Table 1) the number of haemorrhoidectomies performed in the Wycombe Hospital Group dropped to almost vanishing point, despite increasing attendance for treatment.

Because the method proved so successful, the author did not feel justified in carrying out a con-

Table 7.1. Haemorrhoidectomies Performed in the High Wycombe Hospital Group 1961–1970

Years	Total Number of New Patients	Total Number of haemorrhoidectomies	Number to be expected on basis of 1961–1964 figures
1961–1964 (average per year)	2,850	54	
1965	3,364	52	63
1966	3,411	38	64
1967	3,955	9	75
1968	3,725	6	71
1969	4,290	6	81
1970	4,381	3	83

Note the abrupt decline of the need for surgical haemorrhoidectomy after 1966, when the method had been accepted by the patients and their family doctors. This was achieved despite rising numbers of patients attending the surgical clinics.

trolled clinical trial of the technique, and no long-term results have been collected so patients did not return for further treatment.

For the emergency treatment of *strangulated haemorrhoids* (see Ch. 22 for details) the results are excellent; pain vanishes at once, and there is rapid resolution of oedema and thrombosis, both of which almost disappear after the first week.

It must be emphasised that dilatation treatment is directed towards the relief of symptoms rather than complete disappearance of all anal masses. Although the haemorrhoid component may shrink post-dilatation, prolapsing anal mucosa (as well as other tissues) and skin tags will remain, both of which may require subsequent treatment.

While complications have been reported, particularly faecal incontinence, these are extremely uncommon, and can be attributed in almost all instances to either faulty selection or poor technique. The author has continued to use the method.

EDITORIAL COMMENT

In the great majority of specialist centres, anal dilatation is no longer used as a mainstream treatment for haemorrhoids. Fear of complications, especially faecal incontinence, played a major role in its unpopularity. Nevertheless the Editor believes that anal dilatation can still play a useful, if limited, role in the management of haemorrhoids, especially in younger patients with hypertonic sphincters who must otherwise undergo haemorrhoidectomy.

Anal dilatation can dramatically relieve the pain of acutely thrombosed prolapsed haemorrhoids and accelerate their resolution. It was used regularly by the Editor in such cases, with no ill effects.

Complications can be avoided by careful patient selection and correct technique. Patients who are elderly, or have weak sphincters at any age, should not be offered this treatment. Known or potential obstetric trauma (e.g., difficult labour, forceps delivery, episiotomy) is a contraindication to anal dilatation.

Summation

Anal dilatation is a safe, quick and efficient method for treating patients whose haemorrhoids would otherwise require a haemorrhoidectomy. The method can be applied as a day-case procedure under general or caudal anaesthesia. Patients are expected to return to normal activities the following day. Complications are rare; the most important potential risk is of faecal incontinence, but this can be avoided by careful selection of patients and meticulous gentle technique. Skin tags and mucosal prolapse may require their own treatments post-dilatation.

References and Further Reading

Buchmann P, Babotai I (1984) Why do patients with haemorrhoids benefit from Lord's procedure? pages 166–168 in Coloproctology, 1984. [Editors. J. Cl. Givel and F. Saegesser] Springer-Verlag. Berlin Heidelberg. New York

Hancock BD, Smith K (1975) The internal sphincter and Lord's procedure for haemorrhoids. Brit J Surg 62:833–36

Hardy KJ, Wheatley IC, Heffernan EB (1975) Anal dilatation and haemorrhoidectomy. A prospective study. Med J Austral 2:88–91

Lord PH (1969) A day case procedure for the cure of third-degree haemorrhoids. Brit J Surg 56:747

Lord PH (1977) Approach to the treatment of ano-rectal disease, with special reference to haemorrhoids. Surg. Ann. 9:195–211

Miles WE (1919) Observations upon internal piles. Surg Gynec Obst 29:496–7

Sun WM, Read NW, Shorthouse AJ (1990) Hypertensive anal cushions as a cause of the high anal pressures in patients with haemorrhoids. Brit J Surg 77:458–62

8 Sclerotherapy

Charles V. Mann

Introduction

Bleeding associated with the presence of internal haemorrhoids may come from two sources: 1) small vessels in the overlying rectal mucosa, and 2) the venous radicles of the haemorrhoidal plexus. Although evidence from directly observed bleeding is surprisingly sparse, it is reasonable to surmise that slight bleeding (seen mainly on the toilet paper or faecal surfaces) is derived from torn mucosal vessels. This is supported by the usual cause, which is surface trauma from passage of a hard stool. If the bleeding is more than slight, and especially if it is profuse, as exemplified by blood dripping into the pan after defaecation, it is assumed to arise from torn haemorrhoidal veins. The colour of the blood does not distinguish between the two sources as it is bright red in both cases (the blood in the haemorrhoidal veins having a high oxygen content, see Ch. 2, p. 7).

The principal purpose of sclerotherapy is to stop bleeding. Since it is also possible to achieve this in a substantial proportion of cases who present with bleeding arising from small internal haemorrhoids by a correct diet supplemented by a bulk laxative or other simple medicines (e.g., suppositories), it is sensible to add these precautions to any patient who undergoes sclerotherapy, as the combination of injections with such adjuvant measures will be more effective than either management by itself.

Sclerotherapy stops bleeding by virtue of causing a low-grade, long-standing, inflammatory reaction which, in turn, binds down the mucosa and scleroses the submucosal tissues, thus shrinking the haemorrhoids. The solutions used for sclerotherapy should not necrose the tissues, and should be free from the risk of septic complications. The technique should be painless and free from side effects.

Because sclerotherapy is designed for office treatment of large numbers of patients, the method used should be easy to learn, simple to execute, rapid and safe. Nevertheless, any method needs to be learnt from an experienced practitioner, as only good techniques will give good results and avoid complications.

Some sclerosant solutions are more injurious than others, and only small quantities are injected into the tissue at the base of each haemorrhoid. Other solutions are less powerful but longer lasting in their effects; larger quantities are injected, which distribute around the submucosa in circumferential fashion, and achieve a wider submucosal sclerosis. There is no evidence as to which choice is preferable, but less powerful solutions have a lesser risk of mucosal necrosis, and the wider submucosal area affected is probably an advantage. In this chapter, the solution used falls into the latter category (five per cent phenol in almond oil).

Despite the fact that injection treatment is simple, safe, and rapid, it should produce a response that is worthwhile. In general, it should stop the bleeding for a period of at least twelve months, after which the treatment can be repeated if necessary. If symptoms do not remit for a reasonable period, a dissatisfied "customer" is likely to result. However, all sclerotherapy treatment is subject to failure, and patients should be warned that no guarantee can be given of a successful outcome. The success of treatment is also dependent on a correct method and proper selection of cases for treatment (see next). As with all techniques, the skill and experience of the operator is a vital ingredient for achieving the best possible results.

Selection of Cases

Sclerotherapy should be restricted to smaller haemorrhoids (first-degree and early second-degree piles). Treatment by sclerotherapy of prolapsing haemorrhoids is always associated with a high incidence of failure, and better treatments (e.g., banding) are available for these cases.

If bleeding from first-degree haemorrhoids is pronounced, it is necessary to exclude contributory causes for the bleeding (e.g., NSAIDS such as aspirin or the contraceptive pill). Provided no other cause is found, however, even profuse bleeding from first-degree haemorrhoids usually responds to sclerotherapy, although several treatments may be required.

For early second-degree piles, in which prolapse is slight or unnoticed by the patient, sclerotherapy is an appropriate treatment, as cessation of bleeding is all that is required. However, as haemorrhoids get larger, the chance of a successful response becomes smaller, and the necessity for multiple treatments increases. If the surgeon has reason to believe that the size of the piles raises suspicion of failure, two responses are appropriate: 1) initial treatment should consist of multiple injections (three separate treatment sessions at three-week intervals is usual), and 2) the patient should be asked to return for review after twelve months for follow-up treatment even if symptoms have not recurred.

Larger second-degree haemorrhoids should not be treated by sclerotherapy for the following reasons: 1) there is too high an incidence of treatment failure, 2) better office treatments are available for these cases (e.g., banding), as stated previously, and 3) there is a small risk of acute prolapse-thrombosis complications.

Third-degree haemorrhoids should never be treated by sclerotherapy, not only because treatment is never successful in such patients, but also because the risk of acute prolapse-thrombosis following treatment is high.

If ano-rectal inflammatory bowel disease (ulcerative colitis, Crohn's disease) is present, and most especially if active disease is identified, sclerotherapy should not be carried out since it may be followed by mucosal ulceration and/or severe bleeding. The risk of septic consequences is also increased, and an anal abscess or a fistula may be caused. The presence of other ano-rectal pathology, such as a fistula, crypt abscess or recently healed fissure-in-ano, is also a contraindication to sclerotherapy, although this should not need saying to a competent proctologist. AIDS does not contraindicate sclerotherapy.

Providing proper selection of cases is carried out, and sclerotherapy restricted to the treatment of small haemorrhoids in which bleeding is the only (or, at least, predominant) symptom, a high degree of patient satisfaction can be guaranteed. Attention to the details of the technique is also essential.

Technique

Preparation

No bowel preparation is required; however, defaecation soon after sclerotherapy may disperse the solution and reduce its effectiveness; therefore, the patient should be advised to defaecate shortly before treatment (at least, on the same day as treatment will be carried out) and to avoid passing stool for 24 hours afterwards.

The anal canal should be properly lubricated, and the use of a local anaesthetic gel for this is recommended (Lidothesin-Gel). Local anaesthetic lubricants probably do little to prevent pain but informing the patient that an anaesthetic cream is being used is of great help for reducing patient anxiety, and a relaxed patient is a considerable aid to an untroubled treatment session.

Position

Excellent illumination must be provided, and the proctoscope should have an efficient lighting system that does not impinge on the lumen. The proctoscope should have a wide bore, and an oblique or slotted tip. The patient is conveniently placed in the left lateral position with the buttocks pulled out, but the prone or lithotomy positions can also be used if this is the preferred position by the operator. Whatever position is used, there must be easy and complete access to all quadrants of the anal canal, and total visual and physical control of the injection.

Injection

Each haemorrhoid is injected in turn, with a maximum of three sites. With the haemorrhoid

1. The needle

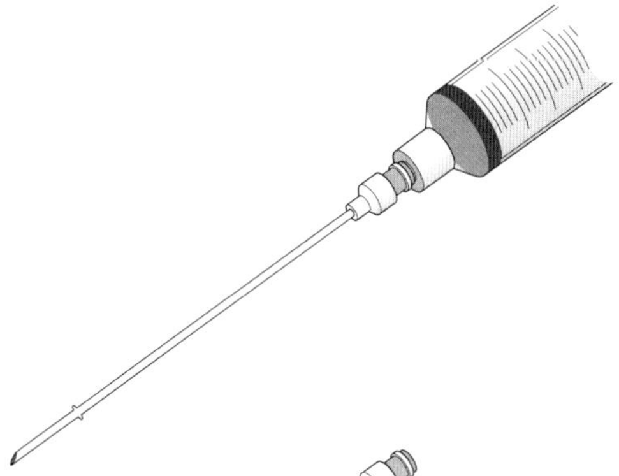

The needle should be:-

1. Long.
2. Large bore.
3. Securely fixed to the syringe (e.g., by a Luer-Lok device).
4. Robust ("unbreakable").
5. Have a shoulder near the end to prevent overpenetration.

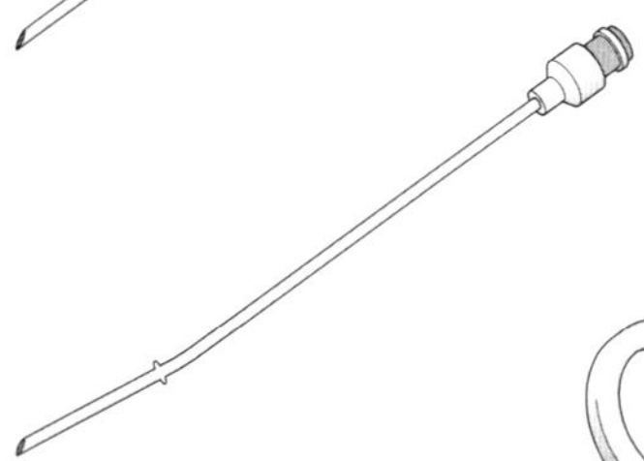

Angle-tip needles are also available.

2. The syringe

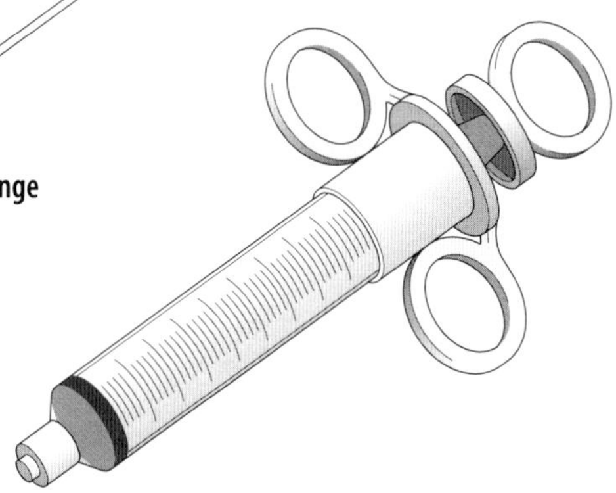

The syringe should have:-

1. Plunger with finger and thumb sockets to aid forcible injection.
2. Pressure resistant barrel (i.e. not glass) to prevent bursting.
3. Luer-Lok needle fitting to prevent needle separation.

3. The sclerosant (example 5% phenol in almond oil)

The solution should be:-

1. Provided in ampoules.
2. Safe to use { no tissue necrosis. / no septic complications. / non-toxic. }
3. Self-sterilising.

Figure 8.1. Some equipment features for Sclerotherapy. An angled needle tip is no longer considered necessary, and some surgeours believe it increases the likelihood of deep penetration into, and beyond, the rectal wall. Disposable injection sets are now available, and are preferred over re-use syringes and needles which could spread AIDS.

isolated in the end of the proctoscope, *the base of the haemorrhoid is identified just above the dentate line* (which delineates the wavy junction between sensitive squamous epithelium (below) and insensitive columnar epithelium (above). Columnar epithelium is characteristically pink.

The loaded syringe is taken up and the injection is given through the basal columnar epithelium into the tissues around the base of the haemorrhoid. Suitable instruments and solution are shown in Fig. 8.1. If a viscous oil-based solution is employed, a wide-bore needle, Luer-lock connection and special finger–thumbs syringe sockets are advisable, as the material requires considerable force to eject from the needle and it is necessary to guard against needle separation and bursting of the barrel of the syringe. These warnings apply to the use of the author's favoured solution, viz., five per cent phenol in almond oil. The original Gabriel's syringe incorporated all the necessary features, and disposable versions of this are now available. All injection solutions must be sterile and available in sealed ampoules. The solution should also be self-sterilising, as the injection is being put in through an infected mucosa, with consequent risks for abscess formation.

When the point of the needle penetrates the mucosa, it is a neat trick for the operator to tell the patient that "he is testing that the local anaesthetic gel is working". If the patient does not feel the prick, both operator and patient are reassured, the former knowing that he has correctly identified the site for the injection. On those uncommon occasions when the patient has clearly felt pain, the needle should be withdrawn and another site chosen, usually at a slightly higher level.

If all is well, the needle is gently advanced in the submucosal plane, parallel to the long axis of the anal canal, to a distance of 1–2 cm (Figs. 8.2 and 8.3). Between three and five ml of solution is now injected into the tissues at the base of the haemorrhoid, the patient being asked to report any pain. If the patient feels pain, the injection should be stopped immediately.

When the solution has been injected, the needle should not be withdrawn immediately, as this may lead to release of solution (and blood) back through the needle track; instead, if the needle is allowed to stay in place for a minute or two, this release is substantially reduced, or averted altogether.

If the injection is performed slowly enough, a raised bleb of solution is not formed, and the overlying mucosa does not blanch. If the mucosa blanches, or develops an intense white discolouration, the solution is being put into the intraepithelial layers and should be stopped, otherwise mucosal necrosis and ulceration will be caused. If the solution appears to be injected too easily, or the patient notices an unpleasant taste or pain in the area of the liver, these symptoms indicate that the needle has inadvertently entered an anal vein and the injection has entered the portal and/or systemic circulation. The injection should, of course, be stopped at once, but (surprisingly) no harmful effects have been reported from this rare, but well-known, complication.

In most patients, three separate injections to the bases of haemorrhoids in the classical positions (left lateral (three o'clock); right posterior (seven o'clock) and right anterior (eleven o'clock)) are given, to a total quantity of not more than 9–15 ml if the phenol and oil solution has been used. Although this is a large quantity, provided the injections are given slowly, the tissues (which are loose) accommodate this quantity without difficulty, and the patient should not experience more than mild discomfort, usually described as an ache. After all sites have been injected, a minute or two should be spent checking them through the proctoscope to confirm that all is well, and that bleeding is not persisting (see Complications). When he is satisfied, the operator should withdraw the proctoscope, once again slowly and with maximum gentleness.

Throughout the entire course of the injection treatment session the operator should be in verbal contact with his patient, offering advice and reassurance. If there is evidence that the patient is

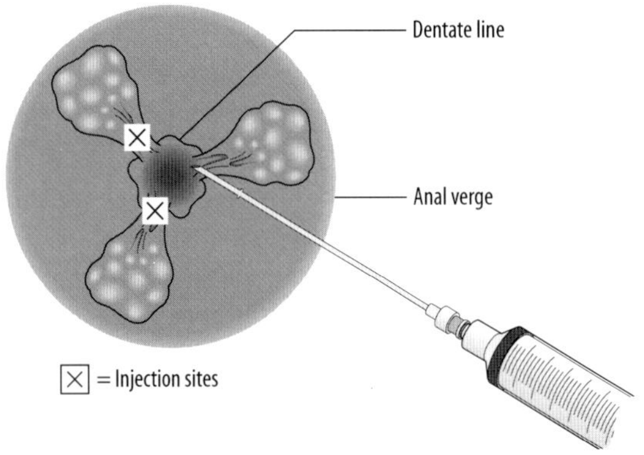

Important elements

1. Each haemorrhoid is visualised and isolated in the end of the proctoscope.
2. The needle is introduced close to the origin of the haemorrhoid *above* the dentate line (x in the diagram).
3. The needle is advanced for 1–2 cms in the submucosal plane parallel to the wall of the anal canal.
4. The solution (5% phenol in almond oil) is injected *slowly*, allowing time for dispersion in the submucosal tissues.
5. The injection is stopped immediately if the patient complains of pain or mucosal blanching is noted.
6. 3–5 mls is put into each haemorrhoid origin.
7. The needle is withdrawn *slowly* to facilitate sealing of the track.
8. If there is profuse bleeding from the needle puncture, pressure or banding may be needed.

Figure 8.2. Injection technique. 1. [as viewed through a proctoscope].

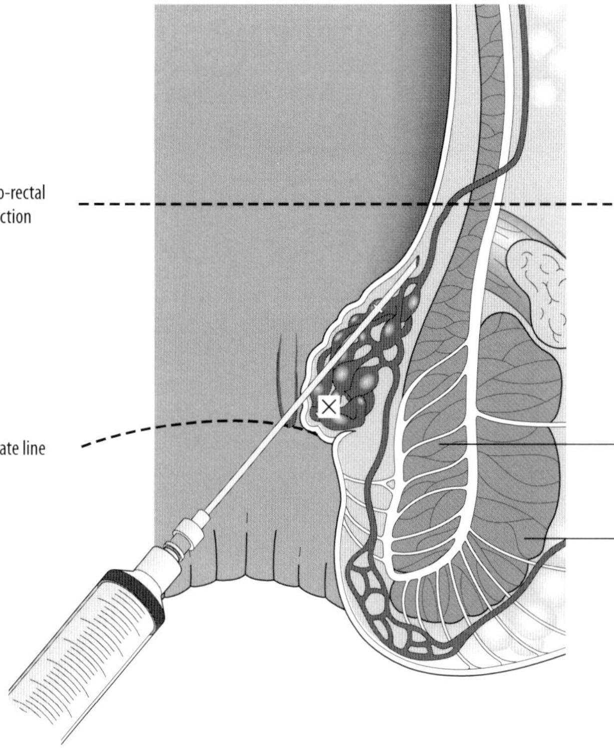

1. Note how the needle is introduced above the dentate line at the base of the haemorrhoid.
2. If the needle is kept parallel to the long axis of the anal canal, too deep injection is avoided.
3. If pain is experienced the injection is misplaced and is stopped immediately.
4. The injection must never be made into the prominence of the haemorrhoid. (X)

Figure 8.3. Injection technique. 2. [diagram of cross section of *sagittal view*].

experiencing unusual levels of discomfort, or even pain, treatment should be discontinued at once. Occasional serious complications which can arise from an injection can be mitigated or avoided by this simple rule. Observance of rules, simple ones or not, are essential if grave consequences, invariably followed by medico-legal actions, are to be avoided (see next section).

Complications

Some complications are relatively common and minor. Serious complications are extremely rare – possibly as few as one per 5,000 injections – and do not constitute an argument against the use of injection treatment, especially as most of them are preventable by good technique.

Bleeding at the Injection Site

Immediate. Withdrawal of the needle can be followed by brisk bleeding, sometimes pulsatile (i.e., arterial in origin). Almost always, such haemorrhage can be stopped by immediate pressure with a small pledget of gauze soaked in adrenaline solution (1 : 1,000). Pressure should be maintained for five minutes for greatest effect. If pressure does not stop the haemorrhage, the bleeding site should be seized with tissue forceps and banded (as described in Ch. 9).

Delayed. If too much solution has been injected, or it has been put *into* the mucosa rather than beneath it, mucosal sloughing can ensue, and an ulcer be caused. This can lead to secondary haemorrhage between 7 and 14 days after the injection, which can be profuse. Although the patient should be admitted to hospital, and may need a blood transfusion, the bleeding usually responds to conservative management, which should include broad-spectrum antibiotics combined with Metronidazole. This complication is extremely rare.

Pain

Providing the injection is correctly sited at a point beneath insensitive mucosa, real pain, as opposed to discomfort, should not be experienced by the patient. Occasionally, despite the injection being given above the dentate line, severe pain is experienced because tongues of squamous epithelium are present in the upper half of the anal canal, although sometimes it is due to spread of the solution below the dentate line. Provided injection is stopped once pain is experienced, it is usually short-lived and responds to simple analgesics. In exceptional instances, opiates may be needed.

In most patients, questioning may reveal that they have experienced some aching discomfort for the first 24 hours post-injection, which has responded to self-administration of analgesics, usually aspirin, codeine or paracetamol. In the author's practise, no patient has refused further injection treatment on grounds of severe pain.

Intravenous Injection

This has been referred to earlier and despite symptoms that are unpleasant and/or painful ("liver pain"), does not result in ill-effects. However, it is not to be expected that the injection will improve haemorrhoid symptoms if the solution has been dissipated into the circulation, and an early appointment should be made for repeat injection. Reassurance of the harmless nature of the symptoms should be given to the patient in terms that do not increase anxiety.

Prostatic Injection

The occasional misplaced injection is to be anticipated when the length of the needle used is set against the thickness of the ano-rectal lamina propria. It is made more likely if an enlarged prostate is pressing upon the rectal wall. One authority (Sir Clifford Naughton-Morgan) has also ascribed penetration of solution into the prostate to venous communications between the prostatic and haemorrhoidal venous plexuses.

Depending upon the quantity of solution that enters the prostate, and the depth of its penetration into the substance of the gland, the consequences vary from a minor inconvenience to an extremely serious problem, as follows:

(i) Retention of urine. This is the commonest response to intraprostatic injection, and usually relieves itself spontaneously. In a few patients, temporary catheterisation is required. It is wise to give the patient antibiotics to prevent septic complications, and to keep him under close observation for a few days until the situation is resolved.

(ii) Epididymo-orchitis. Occasionally the seminal vesicles are involved and retrograde spread of the solution may occur to the testicle or epididymis, which (fortunately) is usually unilateral. The condition usually responds to conservative management, which again includes antibiotics as well as bed rest and pain relief. In subsequent years, testicular atrophy may be noticed, and infertility may be confirmed.

(iii) Prostatitis. Sometimes long-lasting prostatitis may be caused, with symptoms of urinary frequency, dysuria and urgency: partial incontinence may be experienced, together with aching perineal pain. The symptoms may be aggravated by sexual intercourse. No treatment is possible other than symptomatic relief, although in the first few weeks antibiotic cover to prevent secondary infection should be considered. The symptoms usually last weeks, sometimes last months, and may last years. While intraprostatic injection is always rare, it is commoner when an inexperienced operator has used poor technique; however, it is the author's observation than even experienced operators employing good technique can experience this complication, and he has had one case in his own practise, fortunately a minor example which resolved rapidly without serious consequences.

(iv) Intraprostatic abscess. A deep-seated intralobar injection can cause a prostatic abscess – usually sterile. This requires treatment by a urological specialist, and often involves drainage by closed or open techniques.

(v) Acute thrombosis. If a large second-degree, or, worse still, a third-degree pile has been wrongly treated by sclerotherapy, an acute attack of thrombosis may be precipitated ("strangulated haemorrhoids"). This can either be left to settle spontaneously, but may require more active intervention (anal dilation p. 53; surgical removal p. 147). Although the patient may be resentful of this painful consequence (and the proctologist should be ashamed of causing it), the end result may be substantial resolution of the haemorrhoids for a long period. Nevertheless, proper selection will prevent this complication.

Aftercare

After a short period to recover, and to check that there are no untoward after-effects (e.g., bleeding), the patient can leave the clinic, having made a follow-up appointment a few weeks ahead.

The patient may notice some mild aching pain which may persist for up to 24 hours. Mild painkillers will control this, but they should be of a non-constipating brand (e.g., codeine-containing compounds should be avoided). A stool softener should be prescribed, and any tendency to constipation should be prevented by appropriate advice, extra fluids, dietary precautions and any indicated medication (see Ch. 16).

Since it is important that the injection solution should not be dispersed by straining to pass a stool in the early post-injection days, it can be helpful to prescribe a lubricant suppository for a few nights after treatment (the author prescribes an Anugesic-HC suppository).

The patient is asked to return to the clinic three weeks after injection treatment. It is not advisable to repeat the treatment earlier than this, even if further injections have been planned (larger haemorrhoids may need three treatment sessions to stop the bleeding). If there has been complete relief of symptoms, no further treatment is required, unless this has been preplanned. Although re-attendance at three weeks is the minimum recommendation, it is permissible for the patient to return at any time within six weeks of the injection.

Because sclerotherapy is designed to provide symptomatic relief rather than cure, it is best to warn patients that further treatments may be required in the future, and that early re-attendance is advisable, as the piles may enlarge beyond the size suitable for injection treatment if they are ignored. Provided their experience of sclerotherapy has been dignified, pain-free and effective, they will be willing to re-attend promptly should bleeding recur.

Results

A study showed that injection treatment for early haemorrhoids stopped bleeding in three-quarters of the patients, and this could probably be raised to nearly 100 per cent of cases with stricter selection, as some prolapsing haemorrhoids were included in the cases reported. (Mann et al., 1988.) Although in some patients short-lasting pain is experienced post-injection, this has not been sufficient to deter patients from re-attendance for further treatment. Overall, the patients respond very favourably to the treatment, provided their bleeding is stopped. With sufficient care to put the injection below insensitive mucosa, and to make the injection slowly, pain can be reduced to minimal levels.

Although rare serious complications of the technique are recorded, these are usually the result of poor selection or faulty technique. The incidence of serious complications is so low that, even if some can never be eliminated, they do not contraindicate use of injection sclerotherapy for early haemorrhoids.

Summation

Sclerotherapy is a simple, safe and cost-effective treatment for small internal haemorrhoids. Good results depend upon strict case selection and careful technique. Repeat treatments are possible for recurrent symptoms. Rare serious complications are known to occur, but most are preventable. The technique is not suitable for haemorrhoids in which prolapse is more than slight, and the ideal case for sclerotherapy is a patient with small (first-degree) haemorrhoids presenting with bleeding as the only, or predominant, symptom.

EDITORIAL COMMENT

Injection treatment is a cheap, safe and effective method for stopping bleeding from small (first-degree) haemorrhoids. It is less helpful for larger (second-degree) haemorrhoids, and is both useless and potentially risky for treatment of third-degree piles. Once haemorrhoids possess any bulk, especially if prolapse is a prominent symptom, treatment by other methods (e.g., banding, infrared) should be preferred.

Injections do not cure piles, and repeat treatments are to be expected. Unless the injections offer a substantial period of symptom relief (e.g., one year), they should not be persisted with.

Good technique is needed to achieve the best effects and avoid complications. The Editor has used phenol injections as his principal treatment for first-degree piles for forty years without a major incident, and the patients were satisfied with the results.

References and Further Reading

Blanchard CE, (1928) A Textbook of Ambulant Proctology. Medical Success Press, Youngstown, Ohio, USA, p. 134

Broader JH, Gunn IF, Alexander-Williams J (1974) Evaluation of a bulk-forming evacuant in the management of haemorrhoids. Br J Surg 61:142

Goh Hak-Su (1993) Management of uncomplicated haemorrhoids in operative surgery. 5th. edn. In: Fielding LP, Goldberg SM (eds) Surgery of the Colon, Rectum and Anus. Butterworth-Heinemann, Oxford London Boston, pp 784–8

Keighley MRB, Buchmann P, Minervium S, Arabi Y, Alexander-Williams J (1979) Prospective trials of minor surgical procedures and high-fibre diet for haemorrhoids. BMJ 2:967–9

Mann CV, Motson R, Clifton M (1988) The immediate response to injection therapy for first-degree haemorrhoids. J R Soc Med 81:146–8

Santos G, Novell JR, Khoury G, Winslet MC, Lewis AAM (1993) Long-term results of large dose, single-session phenol injection sclerotherapy for haemorrhoids. Dis Colon Rectum 36:958–61

Senapati A, Nicholls RJ (1988) A randomised trial to compare the results of injection sclerotherapy with a bulk laxative alone in the treatment of bleeding haemorrhoids. Int J Colorectal Dis 3:124–6

9 Rubber Band Ligation

Sridhar Chalasani and L. Peter Fielding

Introduction

This book is devoted to a description and analysis of the many treatments for symptomatic hemorrhoids. One of these methods, which has been the preferred technique for non-prolapsing symptomatic hemorrhoidal disease, is that of rubber band ligation (RBL). Initially performed in the nineteenth century, the original technique involved a ligation of the hemorrhoidal mass with surrounding mucosa and skin, which was obviously a very painful method not frequently used until its reintroduction in modern times by Blaisdell in 1958. Blaisdell suggested that simple ligation of hemorrhoidal tissue resulted in hemorrhoidal sloughing. This technique was modified by Barron in 1963 who introduced his own instrument modification. Several studies have shown that RBL is superior to other non-operative modalities in the treatment of Grades 2–3 symptomatic hemorrhoids, although enthusiasm for the technique has been tempered by occasional reports of death secondary to pelvic sepsis (Salvati, 1967; O'Hara, 1980; Russell and Donohue, 1985; Scarpa et al., 1988; Bat et al., 1993).

Principle of the Method

Hemorrhoidal banding works by local obliteration of submucosal hemorrhoidal vessels leading to ulceration. The subsequent healing is associated with fixation of the mucosa by scarring following this ischemic necrosis process. Typically, the ulcer forms about 7–10 days after banding and the area is healed by 3–4 weeks.

Equipment

Barron designed the original instrument, which is still frequently used, and consists of two closely fitting concentric barrels connected by a long shaft to a handle that operates the movement of the barrels over each other. Squeezing the handle moves the outer over the inner barrel, and thereby pushes the rubber band forward so that it deploys over the base of the hemorrhoidal complex. The rubber O-rings are about one mm in their inner diameter. The O-rings are supplied in the form of a long tube, cut into segments approximately 2.5 mm wide. They are loaded onto the applicator by using a cone, which gradually dilates the O-ring as it is moved into position around the inner metal barrel. Each O-ring can be separated from the others quite easily.

The McGiveny ligator incorporates a modification of the original Barron apparatus and consists of a short cylinder at the end of a shaft (Fig. 9.1). The rubber band is stretched around the shaft and the hemorrhoid is pulled into the cylinder. The rubber band is applied using a rod that passes down the hollow shaft of the instrument to maneuver the band into position. Similar devices have been introduced that employ a vacuum to suction the hemorrhoidal plexus into the barrel of the apparatus so that a rubber band may then be applied. These devices are attractive because they need only one

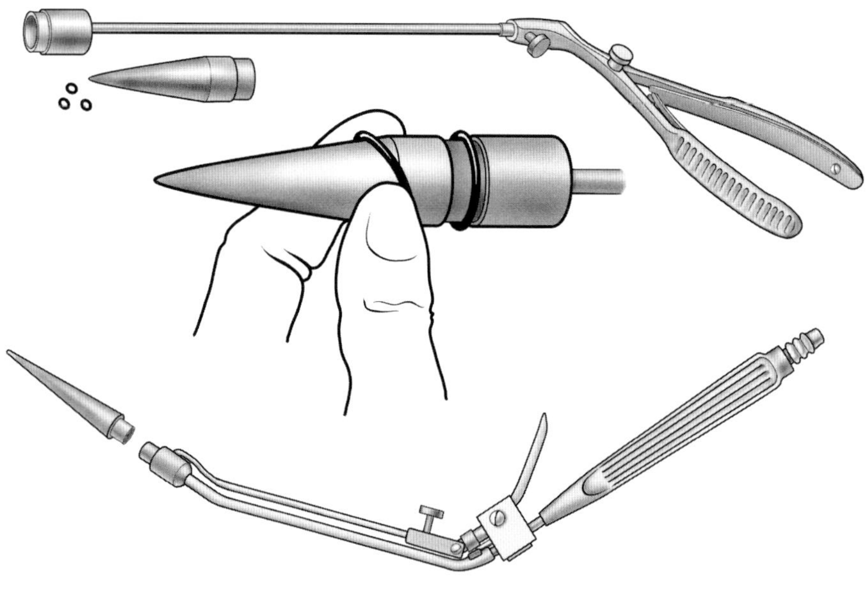

Figure 9.1. McGiveny modification of original Barron apparatus. The suction apparatus (below).

hand to operate, thereby obviating the need for an assistant during the procedure (Fig. 9.1).

Positioning and Preparing the Patient

The patient does not need a full bowel preparation, but ideally there should not be any stool in the rectum. Patients can be given either a Dulcolax® suppository or a Fleet® enema before arrival at the physician's office. In addition, patients are advised not to take any medications such as aspirin or Coumadin, which may cause bleeding. In our opinion, preoperative antibiotics are unnecessary for the majority unless the patient has an immune deficiency disorder; a patient on steroids or one who has a congenital or acquired immunodeficiency syndrome. In addition, preoperative antibiotics should be given to patients who are at risk of developing septic embolization onto previously implanted prosthetic devices such as artificial joints or heart valves. Most patients, therefore, can be treated at the time of initial visit and diagnosis. The great majority of patients do not require preoperative sedation or analgesics, but these can be used for the occasional patient who is experiencing unusual levels of anxiety.

Operative Technique

The patient is usually placed in the left lateral position with the operator seated, although the jack-knife position can be used according to surgeon preference. A grooved proctoscope is warmed and smeared with a small amount of lubricant and then passed into the rectum where the whole internal hemorrhoidal plexus is allowed to prolapse into the lumen of the proctoscope. It is easier to recognize the base of the hemorrhoidal complex by allowing this prolapse to take place. It is very important to identify the dentate line so that the rubber band may be applied entirely above this sensate part of the anoderm. Thus, the band should be applied at least one cm above the dentate line to avoid pain. The most common error in the technique is to place the band too low in the anal canal, causing immediate and postoperative pain. Once the dentate line and the base of the hemorrhoid have been identified, the hemorrhoidal mass is grasped with an Allis forceps, which has been placed through the barrel of the applicator; the tissue is then firmly pulled down into the instrument. If the patient complains of pain at this time, then the hemorrhoidal mass should be released and grasped a second time at a higher level further away from the dentate line. The cylinder is then gently advanced over the tissue held in the Allis clamp until the distal

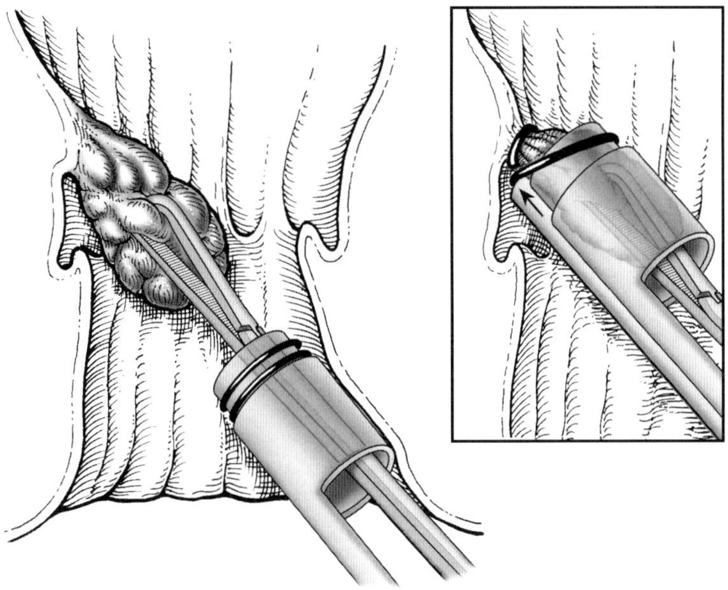

Figure 9.2. Pulling hemorrhoidal tissue into apparatus and placement of bands.

end of the cylinder is at the base of the elevated mucosa. The handle of the applicator is then squeezed and the rubber band thus deployed (Fig. 9.2). (When the suction-aided apparatus is used [Fig. 9.1], the negative pressure is activated by the thumb which obliterates the venting hole on the handle of the band applicator and draws the tissue into the instrument.) If the patient complains after the banding procedure, it must then be assumed that the band has been placed too low involving the sensate part of the anoderm. The band should be cut, taking care not to incise the mucosa, and reapplied at a higher level.

In our practice, we apply two rubber bands at each location so that there is protection against mechanical failure sometimes associated with the failure of one of the bands. Furthermore, it is felt by some surgeons that there is better strangulation of the tissue when two bands are used. Khubchandani in 1983 stated that the diameter of the banded hemorrhoid should ideally be about one cm. Some authors prefer to inject a local anesthetic (bupivacaine or lidocaine) into the site of banding in order to reduce immediate post-banding pain. Local anesthetic should not, however, be used to treat any sharp pain that occurs due to an improperly placed band involving sensate anoderm. Under these circumstances, the band should be removed promptly and reapplied.

Results

Several studies have shown that RBL is an effective mode of treatment of hemorrhoids when compared to other forms for Grades 1–3 symptomatic lesions: sclerotherapy (Cheng et al., 1981; Gartell et al., 1985); photocoagulation (Weinstein et al., 1987); anal dilatation (Cheng et al., 1981; Keighley et al., 1977; Lewis et al., 1983); and cryotherapy (Keighley et al., 1977). Other studies have not demonstrated any significant advantage of RBL over other therapies such as photocoagulation (Ambrose et al., 1983; Templeton et al., 1983; Leicester et al., 1981) and sclerotherapy (Greca et al., 1981), although the statistical power in these studies has been compromised by the small numbers of patients investigated.

Several meta-analyses have shown RBL to be superior to or as effective as other modalities (Johanson and Rimm, 1992; MacRae and McLeod, 1995; 1997). The current consensus seems to be that RBL is a safe and effective method of managing Grades 1–3 symptomatic hemorrhoids. Up to 60–80 per cent of patients who have undergone banding are satisfied with the clinical outcome (Cheng et al., 1981; Gartell et al., 1985; Weinstein et al., 1987; Leicester et al., 1981; Greca et al., 1981; Murie et al., 1980; Wrobleski et al., 1980; Mattana et al., 1989; Savioz et al., 1998).

Complications

Pain

The most common complication of RBL is severe pain immediately after band application. As has been explained, this eventuality needs to be treated by the removal of the band and its placement higher in the anal canal. If the band is not removed immediately, edema of the surrounding tissues can make it difficult to visualize. Consequently, the operator must decide immediately after band placement whether it should be removed or not. With experience, this action is rarely needed. Some operators believe that the mild pain/pressure feelings after a well-placed band can be mitigated by the injection of local anesthetic into the base of the hemorrhoidal complex on the patient side of the obliterating band. Even when well placed, there is a short period of pressure or discomfort experienced by the majority of patients, and this persists for 1–2 hours after band application. This pain is usually quite mild and controlled by the use of simple analgesics.

Bleeding

Secondary hemorrhage may occur 7–10 days after a successful banding and results from tissue necrosis and local infection. The bleeding is usually self-limiting, but if it persists, local pressure, local application of adrenaline, or a single stitch (a chromic or Vicryl suture) may be necessary. Patients should be warned that some bleeding quite often occurs at the time of first bowel movement and is usually self-limiting.

Severe bleeding is rare and less than one per cent of patients may need to be admitted for blood transfusion and control of bleeding (Bat et al., 1993).

Pelvic Sepsis and Infection

This is a very rare event but the most serious and feared complication that can occur following RBL. O'Hara (1980) reported the first case of death secondary to pelvic sepsis following rubber band ligation of hemorrhoids. Russell and Donohue (1985) reported another series of four patients who developed pelvic sepsis. Murphy (1978) reported a single case of tetanus infection following RBL.

Some authors report that patients typically present with symptoms of pain, urinary retention and fever. Awareness of this potential complication and this constellation of symptoms should allow early recognition so that the patient may be treated by broad-spectrum antibiotic regimen, and when necessary, local tissue debridement. The most important aspect to prevent serious pelvic infection is for the patient, and those caring for the patient, to be told of this rare eventuality and its symptoms, which should cause the patient to seek immediate assistance.

Thrombosis of External Hemorrhoids

This occurs in about five per cent of patients secondary to internal hemorrhoidal plexus banding. The patient should be treated on merits and may require the thrombosed hemorrhoid to be excised if there is significant pain.

Band Slippage

This complication can easily be avoided by placing two bands on each hemorrhoidal plexus at the time of first application. If slippage occurs, rebanding of the hemorrhoidal plexus and patient reassurance are all that are usually required.

Anal Fissure

This occurs in about one per cent of patients and is a result of sloughing of the hemorrhoid. This can usually be managed initially by non-operative means, but if persistent, an internal sphincterotomy may be indicated.

Controversies

Single Band Application vs. Multiple Band Application

Barron (1963a; 1963b) advocated ligation of a single hemorrhoid at a time, and suggested that if other hemorrhoidal masses are present, they should be banded at future sessions at three-weekly intervals. By contrast, other authors have advocated that up to three hemorrhoidal plexuses may be banded at a single session without any increased complication or failure rate (Khubchandani, 1983; Poon et al., 1986; Lau et al., 1982; Lee et al., 1994). Initial concerns about the risk of developing anal stenosis have not been borne out. It is our practice to band up to three hemorrhoidal plexuses at a single session for both patient convenience and economic reasons. Khubchandani (1983) has shown that there is no significant increase in the level of discomfort with multiple banding for up to three hemorrhoidal plexuses.

Injection of a Local Anesthetic

Attempts made to decrease the amount of discomfort following RBL by injecting a local anesthetic at the time of banding (Hooker et al., 1999) have shown that injection of 0.5 cc of bupivacaine with 1:20,000 of epinephrine into the mucosa on the rectal side of the band effectively decreased the amount of pain at the site of banding in the immediate postoperative period. Injection of lignocaine into the banded hemorrhoidal mass has little effect on post-procedural pain (Law and Chu, 1999). We do not use local anesthetic at the site of banding on a routine basis. However, we would caution that if injection of an anesthetic agent is thought warranted, the needle must not be placed in a vascular structure because it is well established that bupivacaine may induce complete heart block if more than 3.0 cc is injected directly into the circulation.

Summary

Rubber band ligation is an effective method to manage symptomatic Grades 1–3 hemorrhoids. It is a simple procedure that can be performed in the office or in an outpatient surgical center. Results are very favorable compared to other non-operative forms of hemorrhoidal plexus obliteration. Patient education is very important in order to avoid the rare but significant adverse outcomes of complications such as pelvic sepsis.

EDITORIAL COMMENT

Rubber band ligation was instantly accepted for the treatment of hemorrhoids when it was introduced twenty-five years ago. Worldwide, it is still the most widely used office treatment for second-degree hemorrhoids, despite the development of other methods (e.g., infrared, cryotherapy). Banding has not replaced surgery for treatment of bulky second- and third-degree hemorrhoids, although some surgeons have extended its use on a selected basis.

The Editor used a phenol injection to distend each banded hemorrhoid as this both protected against early slipping of the bands, and sterilized the necrotizing process (septic complications, including fatalities, had been reported in the literature). The Editor had some failures and complications arising from faulty selection or technical error. These included *severe pain* (bands applied to sensitive anal mucosa), *band separation* (not enough pile tissue beyond the bands), *failure* (piles too large for the technique), and *prolapse-thrombosis* (mistaken use of the technique for third-degree hemorrhoids).

After some clumsy attempts to use a one-man ligator, the Editor abandoned its use, having concluded that in his hands, the instrument did not give the best chance for accurate band placement; this may not be so for more dexterous practitioners.

Banding can be difficult, and sometimes impossible, if the mucosa has been tethered by previous sclerotherapy.

References

Ambrose NS, Hares MM, Alexander-Williams J, Keighley MR (1983) Prospective randomised comparison of photocoagulation and rubber band ligation in treatment of haemorrhoids. BMJ (Clin Res Ed) 286(6375):1389–91

Barron J (1963a) Office ligation treatment of hemorrhoids. Am J Surg 105:563–70

Barron J (1963b) Office ligation of hemorrhoids. Dis Colon Rectum 6:109–13

Bat L, Melzer E, Koler M, Dreznick Z, Shemesh E (1993 Complications of rubber band ligation of symptomatic internal hemorrhoids. Dis Colon Rectum 36(3):287–90

Blaisdell PC (1958) Prevention of massive hemorrhage secondary to hemorrhoidectomy. Surg Gynecol Obstet 106:485–8

Cheng FC, Shum DW, Ong GB (1981) The treatment of second-degree haemorrhoids by injection, rubber band ligation, maximal anal dilatation, and haemorrhoidectomy: A prospective clinical trial. Aust N Z J Surg 51(5):458–62

Gartell PC, Sheridan RJ, McGinn FP (1985) Out-patient treatment of haemorrhoids: a randomized clinical trial to compare rubber band ligation with phenol injection. Br J Surg 72(6): 478–9

Greca F, Hares MM, Nevah E, Alexander-Williams J, Keighley MR (1981) A randomized trial to compare rubber band ligation with phenol injection for treatment of haemorrhoids. Br J Surg 68(4):250–2

Hooker GD, Plewes EA, Rajgopal C, Taylor BM (1999) Local injection of bupivacaine after rubber band ligation of hemorrhoids: prospective, randomized study. Dis Colon Rectum 42(2):174–9

Johanson JF, Rimm A (1992) Optimal non-surgical treatment of hemorrhoids: A comparative analysis of infrared coagulation, rubber band ligation and injection sclerotherapy. Am. J. Gastroenterol 87(11):1601–6

Keighley MR, Buchmann P, Minervini S, Arabi Y, Alexander-Williams J (1977) Prospective trials of minor surgical procedures and high-fibre diet for hemorrhoids. Br J Surg 2:967–9

Khubchandani IT (1983) A randomized comparison of single and multiple rubber band ligations. Dis Colon Rectum 26(11): 705–8

Lau WY, Chow HP, Poon GP, Wong SH (1982) Rubber band ligation of three primary hemorrhoids in a single session. A safe and effective procedure. Dis Colon Rectum 25(4):336–9

Law WL, Chu KW (1999) Triple rubber band ligation for hemorrhoids: prospective, randomized trial of use of local anesthetic injection. Dis Colon Rectum 42(3):363–6

Lee HH, Spencer RJ, Beart RW Jr (1994) Multiple hemorrhoidal bandings in a single session. Dis Colon Rectum 37(1):37–41

Leicester RJ, Nicholls RJ, Mann CV (1981) Infrared coagulation: a new treatment for hemorrhoids. Dis Colon Rectum 24(8): 602–5

Lewis AA, Rogers HS, Leighton M (1983) Trial of maximal anal dilatation, cryotherapy and elastic band ligation as alternatives to haemorrhoidectomy in the treatment of large prolapsing hemorrhoids. Br J Surg 70:54–6

MacRae HM, McLeod RS (1995) Comparison of hemorrhoidal treatment modalities. A meta-analysis. Dis Colon Rectum 38(7):687–94

MacRae HM, McLeod RS (1997) Comparison of hemorrhoidal treatments: a meta-analysis. Can J Surg 40(1):14–17

Mattana C, Maria G, Pescatori M (1989) Rubber band ligation of hemorrhoids and rectal mucosal prolapse in constipated patients. Dis Colon Rectum 32(5):372–5

Murie JA, Mackenzie I, Sim AJ (1980) Comparison of rubber band ligation and haemorrhoidectomy for second- and third-degree haemorrhoids: A prospective clinical trial. Br J Surg 67(11):786–8

Murphy KJ (1978) Tetanus after rubber-band ligation of haemorrhoids. BMJ 1(6127):1590–91

O'Hara VS (1980) Fatal clostridial infection following hemorrhoidal banding. Dis Colon Rectum 23(8):570–1

Poon GP, Chu KW, Lau WY, et al. (1986) Conventional vs. triple rubber band ligation for hemorrhoids. A prospective, randomized trial. Dis Colon Rectum 29(12):836–8

Russell TR, Donohue JH (1985) Hemorrhoidal banding. A warning. Dis Colon Rectum 28(5):291–3

Salvati EP (1967) Evaluation of ligation of hemorrhoids as an office procedure. Dis Colon Rectum 10(1):53–6

Savioz D, Roche B, Glauser T, Dobrinov A, Ludwig C, Marti MC (1998) Rubber band ligation of hemorrhoids: relapse as a function of time. Int J Colorectal Dis 13(4):154–6

Scarpa FJ, Hillis W, Sabetta JR (1988) Pelvic cellulitis: a life-threatening complication of hemorrhoidal banding. Surgery 103(3):383–5

Templeton JL, Spence RA, Kennedy TL, Parks TG, Mackenzie G, Hanna WA (1983) Comparison of infrared coagulation and rubber band ligation for first- and second-degree haemorrhoids: a randomised prospective clinical trial. BMJ (Clin Res Ed) 286(6375):1387–9

Weinstein SJ, Rypins EB, Houck J, Thrower S (1987) Single-session treatment for bleeding hemorrhoids. Surg Gynecol Obstet 165(6):479–82

Wrobleski DE, Corman ML, Veidenheimer MC, Coller JA (1980) Long-term evaluation of rubber ring ligation in hemorrhoidal disease. Dis Colon Rectum 23(7):478–82

10 Treatment of Haemorrhoids by Infrared Thermocoagulation

Roger J. Leicester

Thermal methods for the treatment of haemorrhoids have been used for many hundreds of years, ranging from heating, using various forms of cautery or heater probe, to freezing, as in cryotherapy. Most coagulation procedures, including the infrared technique, cause tissue coagulation by the action of heat increasing the temperature of the tissue. Historically speaking, infrared coagulation developed as a spin-off of medical laser technology. Both infrared and laser photocoagulation have decided advantages over procedures that use high-frequency electric current. Diathermy electrocoagulation uses the human body as the electrical conductor and a dissipater or neutral electrode is therefore necessary in most cases. Due to the variation in water content causing irregular distribution of electrolyte conductors in the tissue, it is not possible to predict the depth of necrosis when using electrocoagulation. In rare cases, burning may occur at areas of the body away from the point of application, where several current paths converge. In addition, metallic coagulation probes tend to adhere to the tissue.

In contrast, coagulation, using laser or infrared radiation, can be controlled and reproduced. The effect of an infrared or laser beam on tissue can be determined simply and accurately by regulating the duration of exposure, producing exact depths of necrosis whilst avoiding damage to the adjacent tissue. Infrared radiation penetrates the tissue to a predetermined depth virtually at the speed of light and is instantly converted into heat in this layer. This allows very brief coagulation times (approximately one second) when high-power laser or infrared radiation is employed. By selecting the optical wavelength, it is possible to vary the depth of penetration into the tissue. Depths from one to three millimetres are usually adequate for coagulation and haemostasis. The optimum depth is obtained when the wavelength of the radiation employed is in the near infrared spectrum. Unlike the laser, the infrared coagulator employs a non-coherent, multispectral light source whose spectral maximum, however, is 10,000 Å (similar to that of the neodymium-YAG laser), which has proved effective for coagulation. Another distinctive feature of the infrared coagulator compared to the laser is its high beam output divergence; this allows high power density to be generated only at the focal point of the focussing mirror assembly. This focal point can undergo translational movement through light-guiding systems so that endoscopic procedures can be conducted even with divergent, incoherent radiation. Unlike the laser, the infrared coagulator does not effect non-contact coagulation; the end of the light conductor must be pressed against the tissue. To prevent adhesion, the tip of the light conductor is coated with a fluorocarbon copolymer that is transparent to infrared light. By pressing the tip of the light conductor against the tissue, blood flow is reduced, allowing easier access to the vessel to be coagulated and with no cooling effect of the circulating blood during coagulation. Haemostasis is therefore possible with a minimum energy dose and at coagulation intervals which are frequently substantially shorter than those for non-contact laser coagulation.

Infrared coagulation differs from all other known coagulation procedures because of its reliability and simplicity of operation. It is especially reliable

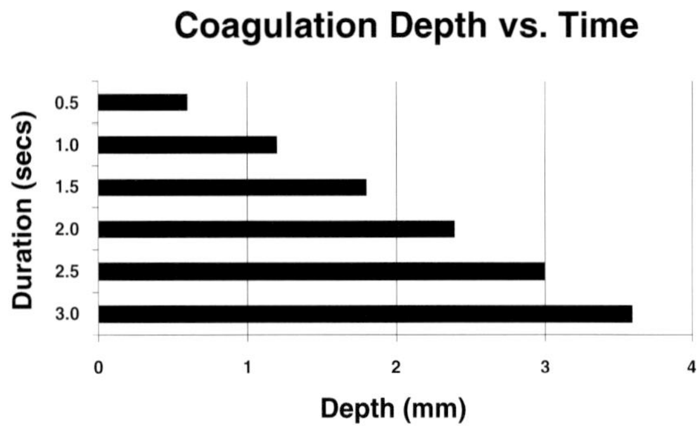

Figure 10.1. Tissue effects of infrared coagulation.

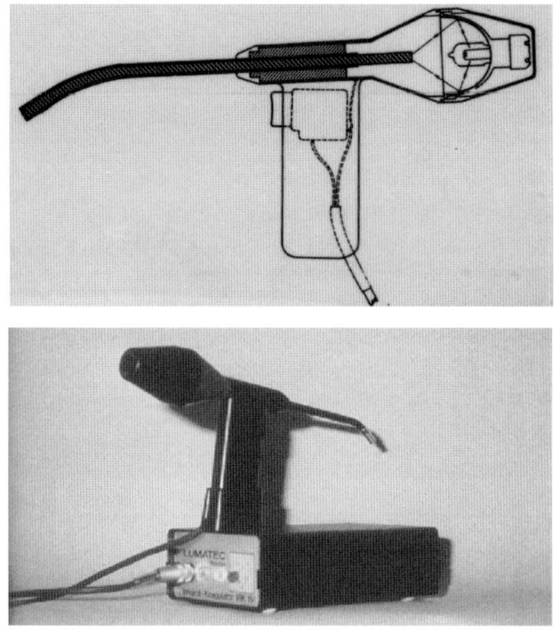

a

b

Figure 10.2. **a** Infrared generator. **b** Infrared coagulator for haemorrhoid treatment.

because the exact depth of necrosis can be pre-set using a timer adjustment (Fig. 10.1).

The infrared coagulator also has the added advantage of not causing high-frequency electromagnetic interference that could affect other devices such as pacemakers. Infrared coagulation operates at temperatures only slightly above 100°C. Tissue coagulation with infrared radiation is based on the denaturation of proteins by elevated temperature. After approximately one second exposure to the infrared coagulator, a hissing noise will be heard which indicates that the intracellular fluid has reached boiling point. The superficial cellular fluid has now reached a temperature in excess of 100°C. The maximum temperature is generated at the tissue surface owing to the exponential decline in radiation power in the tissue. Longer exposure times lead to desiccation and subsequent carbonisation, which may be useful when using to arrest acute bleeding. The most common form of infrared coagulator is a pistol with interchangeable light conductors and a trigger release. A standard projector bulb, focussed to a quartz light guide by a gold-plated reflector, generates infrared energy (Fig. 10.2a). Quartz light conductors with diameters varying between two and ten millimetres are available, the latter usually being used for haemorrhoids (Fig. 10.2b).

Before conducting any therapy for haemorrhoids, a complete evaluation of the patient should be made, including a full history and careful physical examination. In particular, any patient taking anticoagulants should have their clotting parameters checked and, if necessary, anticoagulants adjusted or stopped prior to treatment, in order to avoid secondary haemorrhage. Ano-rectal examination should be performed in the Sims' position (lateral decubitus with knees flexed). Assessment should begin with a careful inspection of the perianal area to look for rashes, lesions, discharge, or evidence of fistula or fissure. Digital rectal examination of the anal canal and distal rectum is then performed to palpate for lesions. Sigmoidoscopy should be performed to detect any more proximal cause for the patient's symptoms. Proctoscopy should then be performed to visualise any palpable abnormality and to evaluate and grade the haemorrhoids.

Haemorrhoids are classified by their relationship to the dentate line, which marks the transition between the rectal mucosa and the anal canal. Internal haemorrhoids are located above the dentate line. They occur most commonly in the right posterior, right anterior, and left lateral positions, and typically present with painless bleeding or pruritis ani. As they enlarge, prolapse occurs. Whilst traditionally graded in four levels (Table 10.1), this is a symptomatic grading and the presence of prolapse is best assessed by asking the patient to strain whilst the proctoscope is placed at the anal margin and grading made on the basis of non-prolapsing or prolapsing. Infrared coagulation is suitable for both types, although prolapsing haemorrhoids may require repeated treatment sessions. If the haemorrhoids are irreducible then formal haemorrhoidectomy is likely to be the only successful form of treatment.

All methods of outpatient treatment should also include patient education regarding diet and defaecatory behaviour. Recommended dietary changes include an increased intake of nonabsorbable fibre and increased fluid intake. Fibre can be in the form of raw fruits and vegetables, cereal, or fibre products. Most patients consume well below the recommended 25–30 g of insoluble fibre per day. Fluid intake of caffeine-free beverages should be increased to six to eight glasses per day. Prolonged periods in the toilet, straining during defaecation and excessive use of toilet paper should be discouraged.

Table 10.1. Classification and Treatment of Haemorrhoids

Grade	Symptoms	Treatment
1	Painless bleeding	Infrared Coagulation
2	Prolapse with spontaneous reduction	Infrared Coagulation
3	Prolapse requiring manual reduction	Infrared Coagulation or Rubber band ligation
4	Irreducible haemorrhoids	Haemorrhoidectomy

Technique of Infrared Coagulation

The infrared coagulator is set to a duration of coagulation of between 1.0 and 1.5 seconds. The base of the haemorrrhoid, at the site also used for injection

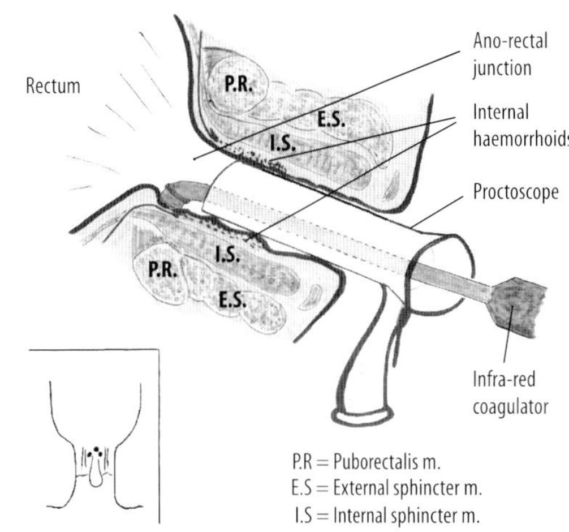

Figure 10.3. Note how the tip of the coagulator is applied at the superior apex of the haemorrhoid, close to the ano-rectal junction. It is recommended that each haemorrhoid should have at least three applications ("triangulation") as shown in the inset. The treatments can be repeated if necessary.

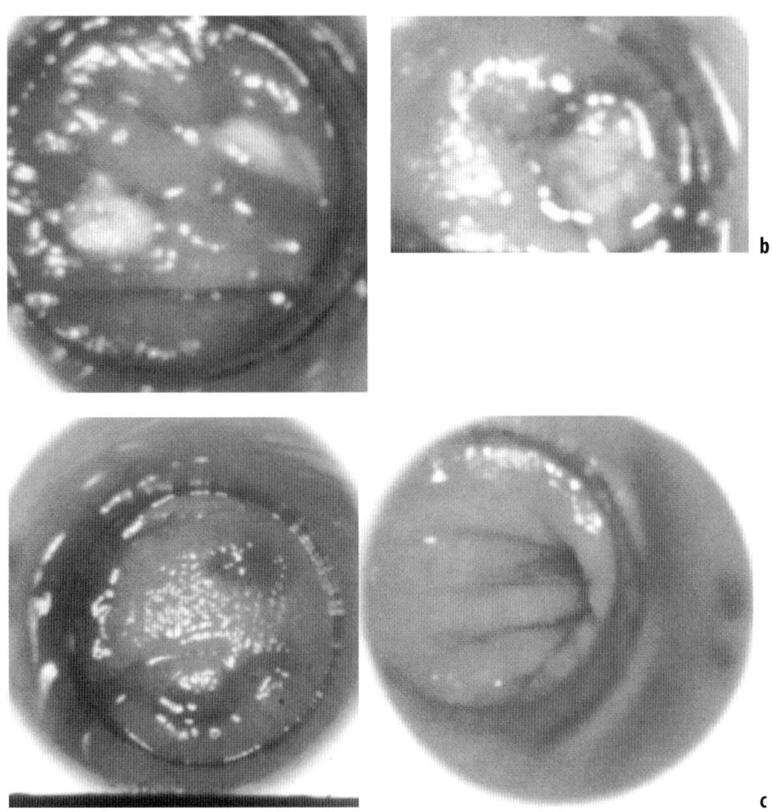

Figure 10.4. **a** Appearance immediately post coagulation. **b** Appearance at one week. **c** Healed areas four and six weeks later.

or rubber band ligation, should be brought into the proctoscopic view; four areas of coagulation are then made in a diamond shape, around the base of the hemorrhoid (Fig. 10.3). If the hemorrhoid is particularly large, this diamond-shaped configuration can be repeated along the haemorrhoidal column. Before applying the infrared energy, the patient should be warned that they might feel a sharp pricking or burning sensation, which lasts only momentarily. The process is then repeated for the remaining haemorrhoids. Rotating the probe facilitates direction of coagulation. There is no limit to the number of haemorrhoids that may be treated in one session.

The points of coagulation can be seen as a small white spot (Fig. 10.4a), underneath which coagulation of blood vessels in the hemorrhoid occurs, resulting in decreased blood flow and often an immediate reduction in bleeding from the hemorrhoid. Over the course of the next week, a small ulcer appears at each coagulation point (Fig. 10.4b), which heals by cicatrisation, resulting in tethering of the mucosa to the underlying muscle and thus reducing prolapse (Fig. 10.4c). Patients should be warned that they may experience some bleeding seven to ten days after treatment, when the area coagulated undergoes ulceration. This is usually of a minor nature and rarely requires any intervention. Following use, the distal end of the probe should be wiped clean with an alcohol-soaked swab and then disinfected in a solution such as glutaraldehyde, taking care not to immerse the proximal end.

In the case of small haemorrhoids, one treatment session is usually sufficient but, if symptoms persist, treatment can be repeated at intervals of four to six weeks.

Infrared coagulation has been found to be as effective as both injection sclerotherapy and rubber band ligation in two English studies, and is significantly less painful for the patient, incurring less time off work. Whilst usually completed in one session, repeated treatments have been found to be required for large prolapsing haemorrhoids, where the long-term results are not as good as rubber band ligation.

EDITORIAL COMMENT

Infrared thermocoagulation is one of the alternatives for small haemorrhoids (first and early second degree). It is safer than phenol injection as it does not have dangers of deep rare misplaced injection, but the apparatus is expensive. The triangulation technique requires skill and know-how to apply, and multiple treatments may be needed for complete remission of symptoms. Follow-up treatments after one year are commonly needed.

Poor technique can cause burnout of the detachable tips of the instrument, which is both inconvenient and expensive.

Minor bleeding between the seventh and fourteenth post-treatment days was often experienced by the Editor's patients, but was not harmful, as Professor Leicester confirms.

The treatment is not painful, and surgeons who adopt the technique may wish to start on a selective basis, with an initial emphasis on nervous patients or those whose experience of other treatments (e.g., sclerotherapy) has been less than ideal.

Further Reading

Leicester RJ, Nicholls RJ, Mann CV (1981), Infrared coagulation: a new treatment for haemorrhoids. Dis Colon Rectum 24(8): 602–5

Templeton JL, Spence RA, Kennedy TL, Parks TG, Mackenzie G, Hanna WA (1983) Comparison of infrared coagulation and rubber band ligation for first- and second-degree haemorrhoids: a randomised prospective clinical trial. British Medical Journal Clinical Research Ed. 286(6375):1387–9

11 Open Haemorrhoidectomy (St Marks Milligan–Morgan Technique)

Charles V. Mann

Introduction

Treatment for haemorrhoids, including surgical methods, has a history extending back for centuries (see Ch. 1). Their physical removal by tying-off their bases or by cautery is described in texts in the Middle Ages, but the search for a surgical treatment that combined cure of the haemorrhoids with acceptable levels of pain and complications has continued into the twentieth century and is still being pursued at the present time.

In 1935, two surgeons at St Marks Hospital (E.T.C. Milligan and C. Naughton Morgan) described a surgical treatment that satisfied the three criteria of acceptable pain levels, low risk and few recurrences, and is still used extensively throughout the world. Their method, with some modifications, is described in this Chapter; it is still considered the procedure that initiated modern surgical treatment for haemorrhoidal disease.

Selection of Cases

There is no degree of internal haemorrhoid that cannot be treated by the Milligan–Morgan method. However, small haemorrhoids (first or second degree) can be handled effectively by simpler techniques, and since such treatments (e.g., sclerotheraphy, banding) can often be carried out as office procedures with minimal pain, inconvenience and expense for the patient, it is usual to restrict surgery by the Milligan–Morgan method to large second-degree or third-degree haemorrhoids. In essence, this restricts case selection to haemorrhoids in which prolapse is a pronounced feature, with haemorrhoids that are permanently prolapsed being ideal subjects. Haemorrhoids which are too bulky for banding or for which other treatments have failed can also qualify for "open" haemorrhoidectomy.

The age of the patient has an influence on selection. While it can be stated with confidence that recurrence of haemorrhoids following open haemorrhoidectomy is extremely rare, there are cases of young patients (less than 35 years of age) who present with haemorrhoids which are large enough to justify haemorrhoidectomy if they were older. However, it is a matter of experience that if young patients of 35 years or less are operated upon, recurrence is much more likely to occur. It is possible that familial predisposition, or other factors (e.g., social, environmental) may be responsible for this increased likelihood of recurrence. For this reason, whenever possible those patients who present with large haemorrhoids at an earlier age than usual should have haemorrhoidectomy postponed until they are 40 years of age of more, and be managed as best as can be until the requisite age is attained.

There are occasions when open operation is contraindicated despite the piles being of appropriate size. The operation should not be carried out if active inflammatory bowel disease (ulcerative colitis, Crohn's disease) is present in the ano-rectum. For both diseases, if the inflammation is quiescent, it is possible to consider surgery, but the decision is one that requires extremely delicate judgement, for which no guidance can be offered other than the advice that great caution should be exercised before proceeding.

The presence of *autoimmune deficiency*, most notably due to AIDS, is a contraindication to open haemorrhoidectomy (see Ch. 23).

Pregnant women, or those who are likely to become so, should be advised against open haemorrhoidectomy, as recurrence of haemorrhoids is likely if labour is difficult, or further pregnancies occur. Most such cases also fall within the general caveat that open haemorrhoidectomy is inadvisable in younger subjects.

The presence of a *fissure* does not contraindicate an open haemorrhoidectomy (see p. 151). The existence of a *fistula in-ano* likewise does not necessarily contraindicate surgical removal of the haemorrhoids (see p. 41), and it is important not to leave large haemorrhoids after a fistulectomy, as the fistula surgery inevitably aggravates the degree of prolapse.

Some cases of acute prolapsed thrombosed haemorrhoids presenting as an emergency are suitable for immediate treatment by open haemorrhoidectomy. Although the condition will settle spontaneously after ten to fourteen days, and may be followed by substantial shrinking of the haemorrhoids (usually only temporary), conservative management involves as much pain (often more) and expense as surgical removal, and it is sensible to offer the chance of immediate, *permanent* relief, if this can be done safely. For the first 48 hours after thrombosis, the anatomy is usually not obscured by oedema and inflammation to an extreme extent, and the degree of sepsis is not prohibitively high; during this period, and in some cases even longer, operation can be undertaken. The surgeon should cover the operation by antibiotics active against both aerobic and anaerobic bacteria, and should take special care that adequate skin bridges are preserved during the operation.

Extreme care must be exercised not to perform an open haemorrhoidectomy in the presence of a neoplasm situated proximally in the large bowel or rectum. Live cancer cells can implant in any open wound exposed to them, and if this occurs in an anal wound, there ensues the disastrous conjunction of two tumours requiring treatment, the lowest of which (in the anal canal) will require treatment by excision of the rectum and anus.

Preparation

Prior to hospital admission, the patient should receive advice for establishing correct bowel habits. Ideally, all patients should come to surgery with daily effortless passage of soft stools of adequate size (see Ch. 6). The usual precautions to stop all potentially harmful medications (e.g., contraceptive pill) and to diagnose (and treat, when indicated) any chest or heart disease that could cause perioperative dangers, should be carried out. Chronic diseases and disorders (e.g., diabetes) should be under proper supervision, and the anaesthetist should be informed of any potential hazards to a safe anaesthetic. Heavy smokers should be advised to eliminate, or at least reduce, their nicotine use over the operative period, which should include a 14-day preoperation abstention.

During the pre-admission period, efforts should be made to achieve a clean, healthy anal and perianal skin. Some patients with large haemorrhoids have copious mucus and faecal contamination of the anal verge, producing a soggy, excoriated and inflamed perianal skin. Suitable treatment with cleansing and drying applications should be instigated, but too-frequent bathing should be avoided. In some patients, the self-application of noxious chemical or sensitising ointments may be a cause of perianal skin damage; these should be stopped, and suitable treatment with protective or desensitising agents given, with advice from a skin specialist when necessary. The presence of any atopic or other skin disease (e.g., psoriasis) should be noted, together with any ongoing treatments which might complicate healing (e.g., hydrocortisone).

The presence of anal skin tags and/or co-existing anal pathology should have been established at the initial diagnostic workup, but it is important that such adjuvant conditions should be considered at every stage of preoperative management.

When the patient is admitted to hospital, it is very important not to assume that no changes in the patient's state of health have taken place since their last appearance in the clinic. A session is required to ensure that the patient is fit for surgery, with special attention being paid to any recent illnesses, and medication being taken. No patient should be operated upon who is suffering from an active respiratory tract infection, or who has diarrhoea from any cause (some anxious patients overdose on laxatives prior to admission).

The patient should arrive in the operating theatre with a “clean” (i.e., empty) lower rectum and anal canal. This can be achieved by preoperative administration of a stimulant suppository (Bisacodyl) or a mini-enema (Fleet phosphate enema).

Position

The operation can be done in either the lithotomy or the prone position. In both positions, the access is improved by strapping back the buttocks with adhesive tape, and in obese patients, this is essential.

For the *lithotomy position*, the buttocks should be raised by a firm pad under the sacrum which elevates the perineum free from the table surface and, incidentally, allows the drapes to slide easily underneath the buttocks. The buttocks should be pulled well forward so that they project beyond the edge of the table. This not only increases exposure and access to the perineum and anal region, but also facilitates the use of a small instrument table pushed against the buttocks below the operation area, which reduces the need for constant turning around for instruments. Finally, the table should be adjusted in height, with a moderate head-down position, so that the anal area is at eye-level with the surgeon seated.

The head-down position materially reduces vascular congestion of the pelvic and perineal regions (so reducing bleeding during the haemorrhoidectomy) and also allows easy run-off of any blood during the dissection of the piles (which increases the accuracy of the excision). It is worth remembering in this context that the buttocks in obese subjects should not be pulled out to an extreme degree because this squeezes the thighs onto the abdomen, with consequent raising of intra-abdominal pressure; in turn, this impedes venous return from the perineum and increases congestion in the pelvic and anal veins, causing increased bleeding during haemorrhoidectomy. It also aggravates problems with maintaining proper inflation of the lungs by the anaesthetist.

The *prone position* materially assists venous return from the ano-rectum, and is associated with the lowest propensity to bleeding from anal wounds; however, this advantage is not sufficient in degree to make a compelling reason for preferring the prone position. The prone position requires cushions beneath the upper chest and the pelvis to prevent restriction of respiratory movements, and the extra difficulties of access to the face and mouth make intubation desirable, or even essential. If the surgeon or anaesthetist favour the use of caudal or epidural anaesthesia, the prone position provides excellent access to the spine, but the risks of the anaesthetic solution reaching higher than intended levels must be guarded against.

Once the patient is correctly positioned it is the author’s practise to shave the operation area. While this is not essential, it makes the procedure tidier to perform, and helps to keep the area clean during postoperative healing.

Nothing is more important for the optimum performance of anal surgery than swift, efficient and careful positioning of the patient, which sets the whole tone for the subsequent operation.

Technique

Before the skin is prepared and the drapes applied, the anal canal and lower rectum should be digitally cleansed of faecal residues using soft moist tissues or cotton wool pledgets. The swabbing should be done gently to avoid starting bleeding. If significant residues are encountered they may need to be sucked out through a proctoscope, or a rectal washout may even be performed. While digital cleansing proceeds, there is a final opportunity for observing the size and location of the haemorrhoids and the presence of an (unexpected) adjuvant condition.

Once the ano-rectum and surrounding skin have been thoroughly cleaned, antiseptic preparation of the entire area (buttocks, perineum and perianal skin) is performed; the solution used should be water-based and inert (the author uses Betadine). This point may seem trivial but is important because the solution has a tendency to pool around the periphery of the operative field, and a spirit-based solution many ignite with, for example, subsequent use of the diathermy. Allergenic or chemical preparations must also be avoided as pooled concentrations of these may cause severe dermal blistering or sensitivity reactions.

Next, the drapes are put on in such a way as to allow generous unimpeded exposure of the operative field. Towels made to provide a preformed “window”, often with leg drapes attached, are

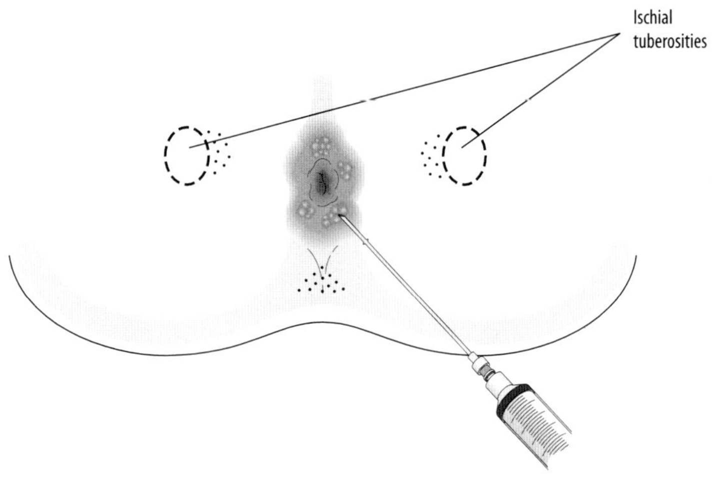

The solution is injected subcutaneously and submucosally at three or four different sites around the anal verge, concentrating on the known sites of the piles (**a**).

Note:-

1. The solution is injected slowly and should not raise a bump that distorts the anatomy of the haemorrhoids.
2. Not more than 15 mls should be used.
3. The anaesthetist may need to be reassured that the solution will not produce anaesthetic-related complications.
4. Time must be allowed (3–5 minutes) for vasoconstriction to take place.
5. Any excess solution can be usefully injected near the inner surfaces of both ischial tubercles to induce a local block of the pudendal nerves (**b**).

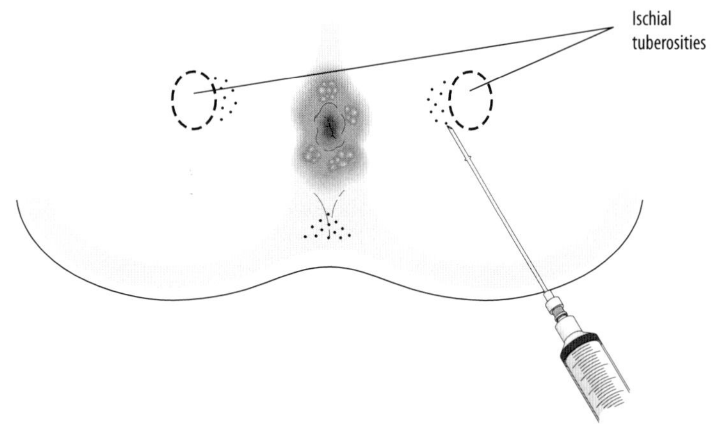

Figure 11.1. Injection of weak adrenaline (1/200,000) and bupivacaine solution.

attractive in theory, but in the author's experience they are clumsy to apply, and the "window" is subject to movements which obscure the dissection at critical moments. For these reasons, the author continues to use separate drapes fastened with clips to the leg poles and the patient's skin.

Once the drapes are secure, the surgeon comfortably seated, and good illumination achieved, the tissues of the anal verge and the exposed surfaces of the haemorrhoids are infiltrated in the subcutaneous/submucosal plane with a weak solution (1: 200,000) of adrenaline in bupivacaine or lignocaine (1%). This solution is strong enough to achieve vasoconstriction but sufficiently weak to allay fears that cardiac irregularities might be caused; it has been in regular use at St Marks Hospital for many decades without such complications.

During the three-to-five minutes that must elapse to allow the adrenaline solution to work, the surgeon should begin to plan the operation. In particular, he should decide on the location and number of the skin bridges that he must preserve. This is a most important step because the guiding principle of a satisfactorily complete haemorrhoidectomy should *not* be to remove the haemorrhoids and hope that skin bridges may be conserved, but rather *to preserve skin bridges and remove all haemorrhoid-related tissue between them.* Application of this rule prevents any risk that the haemorrhoids may not be totally removed, or that insufficient skin bridges remain at the end of the excision of the piles. In most cases, including very large haemorrhoids, three skin bridges 2.0 cm in width can be preserved between the locations of the main haemorrhoidal masses, which is ideal. In exceptional cases when most or all of the anal circumference is affected by haemorrhoids, special techniques are required to preserve skin bridges (see pp. 82–83 and Figs. 11.6 and 11.7).

After deciding on the skin bridges to be preserved (which can be marked out to good effect in difficult cases), the haemorrhoids are teased out gently to their full extent with the index finger. Any skin tags to be included in the dissection are noted. In most cases, an anal dilation is unnecessary as sphincter tone is not initially high, and has often been reduced even further by the anaesthetic, especially if spinal, epidural or caudal techniques have been utilised. In a few cases, anal sphincter tone remains high and a gentle two-finger anal stretch is indicated. A four-finger dilatation is not only unnecessary but may contribute to loss of continence postoperatively, although this is usually temporary.

Small artery forceps are now applied to the base of each haemorrhoid, and they are pulled down to expose their apices (identifiable by their pinkish rectal-type mucosa) (Fig. 11.2, 1). A second clip is now applied to each base (Fig. 11.2, 2). Consistent with the usual distribution of haemorrhoids, three separate pile masses have now been demarcated; gentle traction on each set of forceps produces a triangular shape to the pulled down piles, with the apex of each in the upper anal canal. This is the so-called "triangle of exposure", which marks out the shape of the haemorrhoid tissue to be removed (Fig. 11.2, 3). It is important not to extend upward dissection of the haemorrhoids above the apex of the triangle, as this is known to result in narrowing (and even stricturing) of the upper anal canal postoperatively, and haemorrhoidal disease is developed in the lower half (i.e., below the dentate line).

Commencing at the skin just outside the anal verge, each triangular mass of haemorrhoidal tissue is dissected free of the underlying sphincter muscles of the lower anal canal (Fig. 11.3). This is done slowly in the submucosal plane, and small blood vessels are dealt with as they present. In fact, the dissection should not be particularly bloody if the recommended infiltration with weak adrenaline has been carried out. If large skin tags are being removed along with the internal haemorrhoids, the exterior line of dissection commences slightly farther out on the perianal skin; skin tags on the bridges are not dealt with at this point, but are removed last of all, as discussed on p. 83.

At conclusion of the dissection of each of the (three) haemorrhoidal masses, three triangular-shaped wounds are created with a wide base 1.0 cm or so outside the anal verge, which narrows down to a smaller apex, with the haemorrhoids still attached, just above the dentate line. Keeping the haemorrhoids elevated, time is now spent achieving a completely dry wound. If the dissection has been carried out just superficial to the internal anal sphincter, identifiable by its whitish circular muscle fibres, minimal use of diathermy or plain catgut ligatures will provide a dry field without difficulty.

Finally, dissection excision of the haemorrhoid masses is completed by transfixion/ligation and division of their apices. This is done with needle-mounted fine (00) chromic catgut, which is supplemented by an additional tie if the base is bulky (Fig. 11.4).

Although in many instances ligation of the apices of the haemorrhoids may not be required (c.f. Diathermy Haemorrhoidectomy p. 120), the author prefers to retain this step. Providing it is done correctly, ligation of the pedicles does no harm, and in some cases they contain vessels of sufficient size that ligation is absolutely necessary. The author has personal experience of some haemorrhoidectomies which justify the old name "arterialised piles", in which large pulsatile arteries can be not only seen, but also felt, in the pile base; nor has the experience of re-operating on cases of slipped ligatures causing severe bleeding postoperatively been anything other than a strong reinforcement of the conviction that pedicle ligation is essential.

However, apex ligation should observe the following rules: (i) it should be done with absorbable material; (ii) the size of the material should be medium strength, i.e., 00 grade; (iii) the material should be delayed-absorption type, i.e., chromic catgut/polyethylene, etc.; (iv) the ligature should not contain any fibres of the internal anal sphincter, and (v) sufficient tissue should be left distal to the

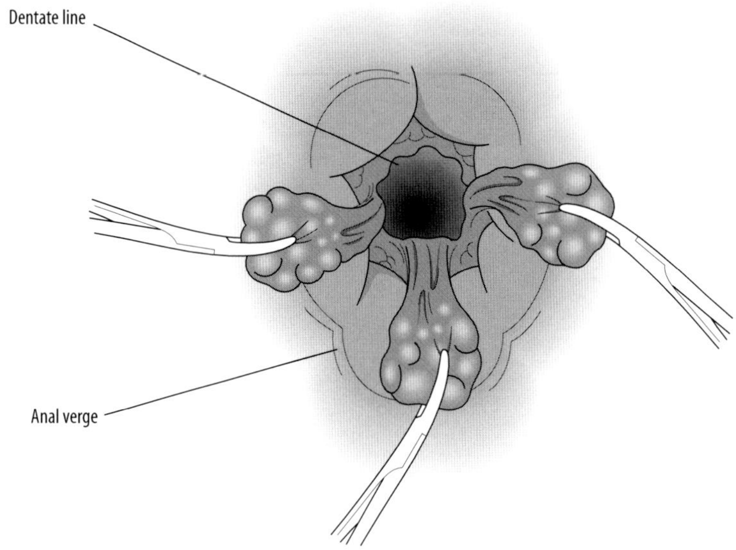

Step 1

The haemorrhoids are gently teased out (no anal dilatation involved) and clips applied to their lowest prominence (bases).

Step 2

The haemorrhoids are pulled down, and a second clip is put on at a higher level (not shown).

Step 3

Traction on both sets of forceps exposes the full length of the haemorrhoids as a triangle ("triangle of exposure") with their apices at the mid-point of the anal canal.

Note that the apex of the haemorrhoids is near to the dentate line and further upward dissection is unnecessary and has risks.

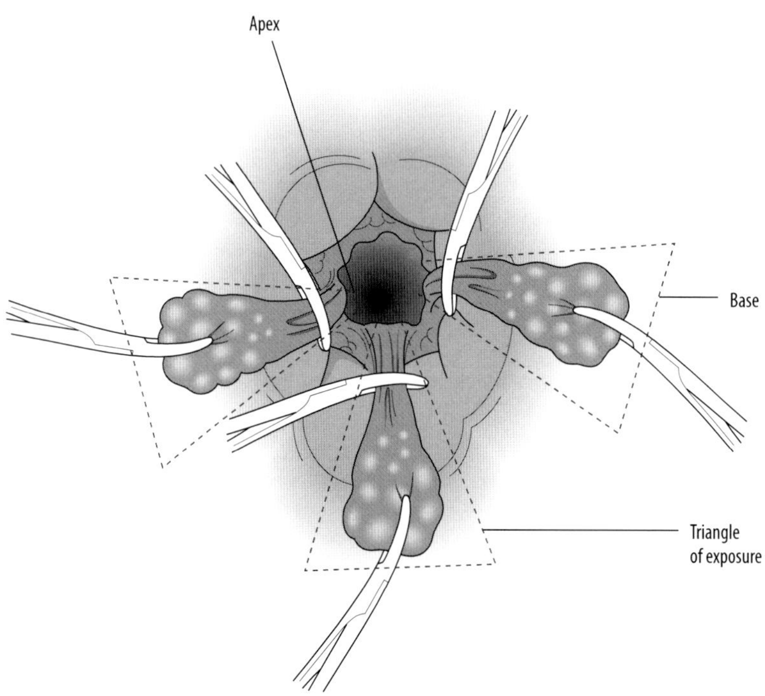

Figure 11.2. Exposing the haemorrhoids.

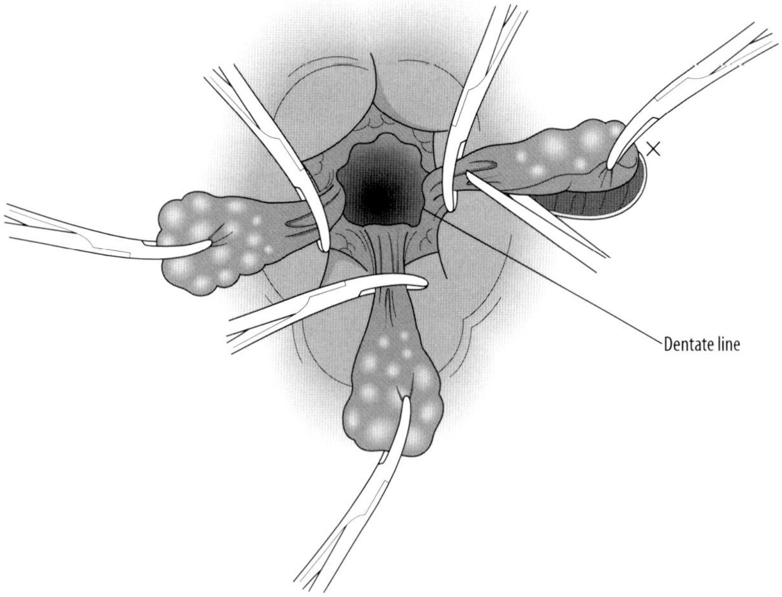

1. Starting at the wider external base of the haemorrhoid close to the anal verge, each haemorrhoid is freed from the underlying anal sphincter muscle (×).
2. Traction on the other undissected haemorrhoids keeps them out of the way and exposes the field to view.
3. A dry field is achievable, using diathermy spot coagulation or the occasional ligature, as dissection proceeds.
4. Dissection is not continued beyond the narrow apex of the haemorrhoid adjacent to the dentate line.
5. The apex of the haemorrhoid is transfixion ligated (see text) before it is cut through.
6. Any bleeding is stopped before proceeding.

Figure 11.3. Dissection of each individual haemorrhoid.

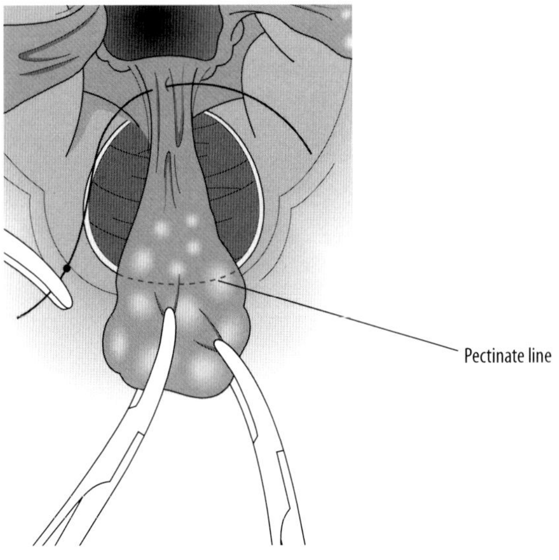

Note the following:-

1. the transfixion is carried out not flush with the anal wall: this prevents incorporation of internal sphincter muscle.
2. the transfixion stitch is supplemented by an additional (non-transfixion) ligature – "double ligation".
3. the ligation is performed with fine (00) delayed absorption material (e.g. chromic catgut, Ethicon). Fine material reduces foreign body reaction, pedicle abscess formation, secondary haemorrhage, and fistulation.
4. the ends of the ligatures are left 2.0 cms or so long to guard against slipping of knots.

Figure 11.4. Transfixion – ligation of the pedicle.

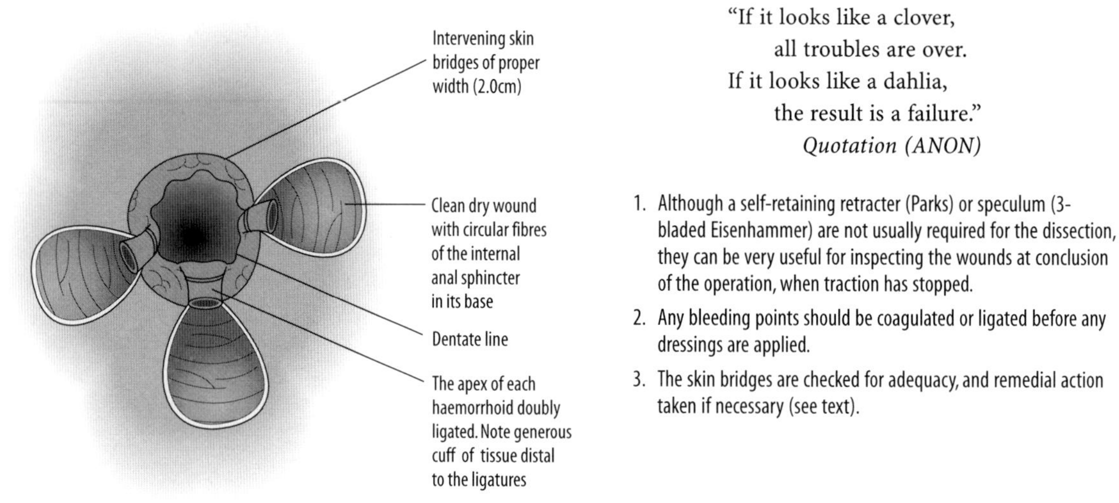

Figure 11.5. Final appearance.

ligatures to safeguard against early dislodgement by defaecation.

Providing these rules are followed, pedicle ligation will not be responsible for complications such as *secondary haemorrhage* (sepsis around a large unabsorbable ligature); *fistula* (inclusion of muscle in the ligature); *foreign-body reaction* (use of unabsorbable suture material) and there would seem to be nothing to gain, and much to lose in some cases, by omission of this precautionary step.

At conclusion of the dissection, ligation, excision process, three clean, dry triangular wounds are left, separated by three healthy skin bridges of the required width (2.0 cm or more) (Fig. 11.5). The operation is not finished, however, until complete haemostasis has been confirmed by careful, unhurried observation.

The problems created by (i) circumferential extension of haemorrhoids beneath the skin bridges, (ii) pleating and prolapse of skin bridges, (iii) residual skin tags, and (iv) profuse bleeding will now be considered in turn.

(i) Residual Circumferential Haemorrhoids

These can be handled by one of two alternative methods, as follows.

(a) "Filleting" (Fig. 11.6 I). If there are only a limited number of residual haemorrhoids, they can be teased out from beneath the edges of the skin bridges. This should not result in the skin bridges being separated from their attachment to the wall of the anal canal (in which case it would be better to use the technique (b) below).

(b) Skin bridge division and resuture (Fig. 11.6 II). If there are numerous residual haemorrhoids beneath the skin bridges, the skin bridges should be divided in their upper half, and all haemorrhoidal tissue removed from beneath each end. The skin bridge is then reconstituted by suturing the ends together with fine interrupted unabsorbable sutures (e.g., 00 silk or Vicryl). Sometimes, the skin bridge that remains after the haemorrhoids have been removed is excessively long, and prone to prolapse, in which case an appropriate length can be removed before resuture. *Any division and/or partial removal of a skin bridge should always be done in the upper portion of the divided bridge*, so that when it is replaced, squamous epithelium is taken up into the anal canal rather than mucus-secreting mucosa brought down to the anal verge (which can cause problems with mucus contamination of the perianal skin). It is wise never to divide and reconstitute all the skin bridges in case the sutures cut through or the bridges necrose, posing dangers for postoperative anal stenosis.

1. By "filleting" out the haemorrhoids from beneath the edges of the skin bridges.

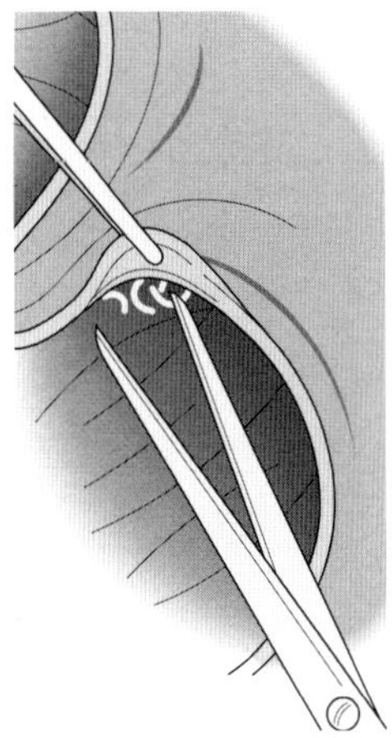

2. By division and reconstitution of skin bridges. (This technique should not be applied to all 3 skin bridges).

(a) Raising and division of skin bridge.

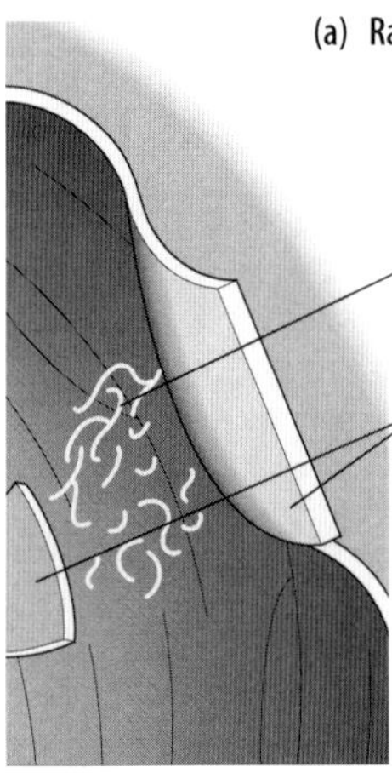

(b) Reconstitution of skin bridge.

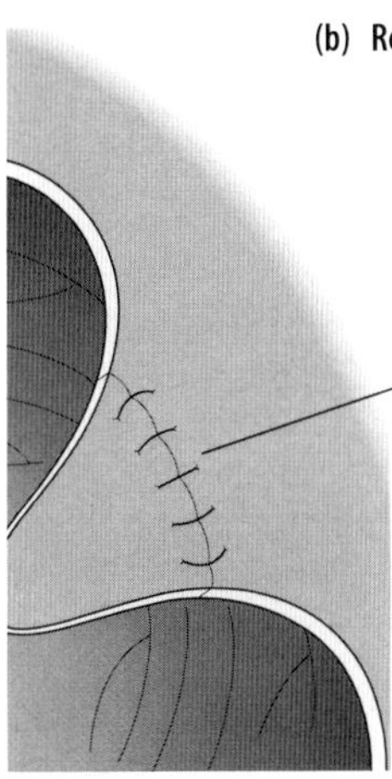

Figure 11.6. Removal of residual haemorrhoids.

(ii) Prolapsing Skin Bridges (Fig. 11.7)

Long, narrow skin bridges are prone to prolapse, and this problem can also be caused by too-enthusiastic filleting (cf. above). This can be corrected in two ways: (i) the skin bridge can be shortened by removing a segment and reconstituted, as in method (Fig. 11.6, 2) above, or (ii) if the prolapse is not severe, the skin bridge can be held back by two (or more) restraining hitch-stitches between the anal mucosa at each side of its upper end and the sides of the skin bridge at its midpoint.

(iii) Residual Skin Tags (Fig. 11.7)

After removal of any haemorrhoids, residual skin tags cause an untidy appearance and may be respon-

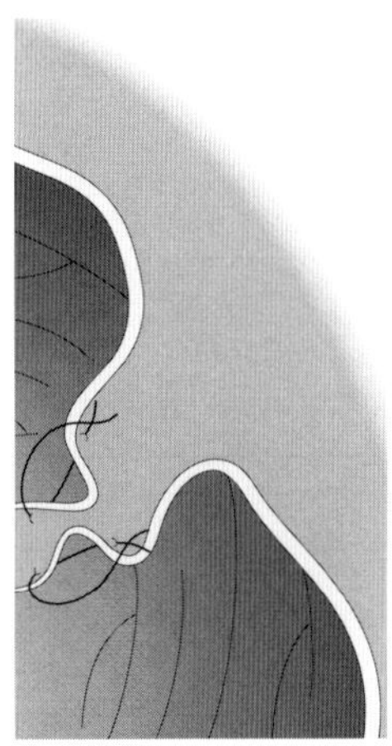

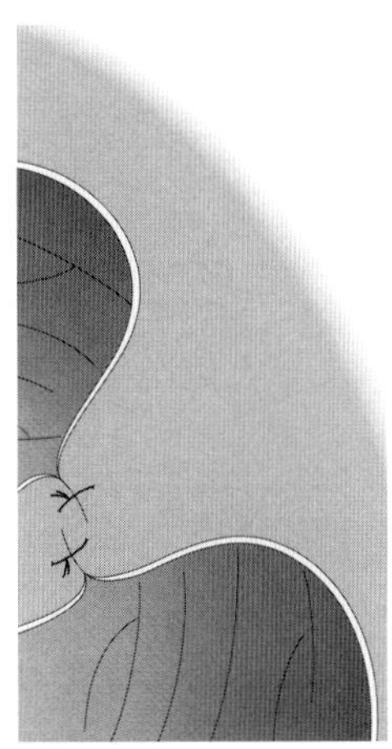

Figure 11.7. Correction of prolapsing redundant skin bridge by insertion of hitch stitches.

sible for postoperative symptoms (post-defaecation cleansing problems, pruritus ani). They may also lead the patient to believe that not all his haemorrhoids were removed! Whenever possible, they should be removed. The best method is to pluck them off individually by slicing through their bases; any small wound created can be left to heal. This method is similar to that employed in scissor dissection to remove anal warts, except that full-thickness skin need not be excised. If the skin tag is on, or adjacent to, a skin bridge it is important that the base is shaved off mostly through the epidermis so that there is no interference with the blood supply to the bridge itself.

(iv) Difficult Haemostasis

In some patients, dissection is accompanied by unexpectedly severe bleeding. This is always in patients who have florid intero-external haemorrhoids, usually with a pronounced congested appearance.* In some of these patients, excessive alcohol intake is clearly a contributory cause of their increased peripheral vascularity, although hepatic disease is not usually apparent. Multiple repeat applications of the diathermy or multiple ligations are time-consuming, or ineffective, or both. Furthermore, the risk of continuing bleeding postoperatively is high. Although the bleeding can be stopped by an anal pack, this has to be removed within 24 hours, and bleeding may restart. The anal pack is also a cause of intense discomfort, and removal may involve giving an anaesthetic.

The author's individual answer to this problem has been to settle for as much haemostasis as can be reasonably achieved under the circumstances, and to close the wounds with a continuous running suture using 00 chromic catgut. Having thus converted the open wounds to closed ones, a *small* cigar-shaped cylinder of moist antiseptic-soaked tissue is left in the anal canal. This not only applies sufficient pressure to stop any bleeding, but is also easy to remove after 12 to 24 hours without risk of bleeding restarting and with an acceptable degree of pain.

There is one other circumstance which justifies resort to the use of a postoperative intra-anal dressing to prevent postoperative haemorrhage, namely, the patient who comes to haemorrhoidectomy with subnormal anal tone, amounting to a patulous anus. In these patients, the recovery of anal sphincter tone (which is a significant contribution to haemostasis by its squeeze/closure of the anal canal) does not take place, and there is an increased risk of early re-bleeding. This risk can be averted by use of a light postoperative anal plug (also moistened by antiseptic), which can be removed while the patient is still within the period of postoperative analgesia, i.e., as soon as initial haemocoagulation has taken place.

* It is assumed that any general cause contributing to a bleeding tendancy has been excluded by the pre-operative work up.

Aftercare

To the Anal Wounds

At the end of the operation, when haemostasis has been achieved, a single layer of *non-adhesive* gauze or tissue should be laid flat on the surface of each wound, the end being tucked upwards into the anal canal to avoid early displacement of the dressing; Jelonet, Tulle-gras or Sofra-tulle are all suitable materials, and each surgeon will have his own preference. On top of these dressings, a large absorbent pad should be put over the anus and perineum to collect any discharges that may be released; the author has found large-size female sanitary pads to be excellent for this purpose. Finally, a large square of Gamgee tissue is applied to the buttocks to prevent blood and other fluid losses soiling the bedclothes; this is held in place with a "T" bandage or jockey shorts.

Once the patient has been taken down from the lithotomy position and placed on the trolley, the buttocks should be squeezed together: this is a valuable trick to assist haemostasis, and prevents separation of the dressings.

An indwelling catheter is not used as a routine, but in male patients with enlarged prostates it is often wise to empty the bladder with a fine catheter before the patient leaves the theatre suite as a precaution against postoperative retention.

The dressings are not changed for 24 hours, but they should be inspected from time to time in case postoperative haemorrhage has become significant. It is to be noted that blood loss always appears greater than it really is and that minor persistent oozing from the exposed wounds can be stopped by topical application of 1 : 100,000 adrenaline solution. If the haemorrhage is profuse, no delay should be allowed to prevent prompt return to the theatre for thorough re-appraisal of the wounds under anaesthesia and appropriate haemostasis.

On the day following surgery, the dressings are taken down in the ward dressing room. If the non-adhesive dressings do not separate easily, there is no need to tug them free at this stage, as they will usually separate spontaneously after baths are instituted or defaecation occurs. An intravenous, small dose of opiate immediately prior to taking down the dressings can materially reduce pain, and should always be considered in an anxious patient.

After the first wound dressing, the anal wounds are kept clean by daily bathing (or by warm saline irrigations if the patient has still not fully recovered mobility). Each bath is followed by a generous application of a water-soluble cream, which prevents pads or clothing sticking to the wounds; a flat Gamgee pad completes the wound toilet, held in place by elasticated shorts. Patients should be encouraged to apply the cream themselves, especially when they are fully ambulant, and can take baths as often as they wish. Once defaecation has started, a bath should follow each action.

Keeping the wounds clean by bathing is all that is required until healing is complete. No direct dressings applied to the wounds are necessary or desirable, although a perineal pad is required to protect clothing and household linen and furniture. Once the patient has learnt how to keep his wounds clean, and to use the cream and pads, it is not necessary to keep him (or her) in hospital for an unnecessary meddlesome regimen of postoperative wound care.

Restoration of Defaecation

Every patient dreads the pain that is associated with postoperative defaecation, and regard most attempts at reassurance with scepticism. They should be reassured that their pain will be regarded compassionately and treated promptly.

There is no need for the first postoperative stools to be firm (and certainly they should never be hard). The author has usually prescribed frequent doses of magnesium salts to encourage early ("irresistible") passage of liquid or semi-solid stools. Extra oral fluids should be encouraged (beer is excellent). If defaecation has not occurred after 72 hours, a mini-enema should be administered through a fine well-lubricated tube.

Once defaecation has been initiated, attention is turned to obtaining daily passage of formed stools of regular size. This is vital to reduce the chance of postoperative anal stenosis, for which the only alternative management would be daily passage of a finger or an anal dilator. The required stool type is achieved by giving a bulking agent (Isogel), but naturally occurring osmotic compounds (bran, muesli) are useful additions to the diet, as are certain fruits (e.g., prunes, figs). The patient must not be allowed to continue taking laxatives.

If the patient has not started defaecation by the end of the third postoperative day, digital examination is advisable. If the patient is retaining faeces, an immediate mini (Fleet) enema should be given, and, if this is ineffective, a rectal washout is required – under anaesthesia if necessary. Providing proper bowel care has been given, this should be a very uncommon occurrence.

On extremely rare occasions, the surgeon may encounter a patient who is resistant to restoration of normal postoperative bowel habits. For such exceptional circumstances, the patient should be trained on regular daily self-passage of a dilator (St Marks no. 2 size (medium) is suitable for this purpose); this "old-fashioned" remedy will prevent any risk for postoperative anal stenosis, and should not be taken as a reproach of the surgeon's technique.

Once the patient has resumed normal activities, supervision should ensure that normal bowel actions continue indefinitely. Diet, frequent exercise, enhanced fluid intake (see Ch. 6) and bran are the mainstays of therapy, which can be supported with isphagula husk on occasion. Straining habits of defaecation must be eliminated, and sedentary life styles and large intake of caffeine-containing drinks should be cut down to an acceptable level.

Providing a technically proficient operation has been performed and normal bowel actions are established postoperatively, the results of open haemorrhoidectomy are excellent.

Complications

If complications occur, they should be very much the exception rather than the rule. If this is not the case, either the surgeon's technique is substandard or aftercare is of poor quality. Nevertheless, even in the best hands, complications occur, and these must be handled efficiently to reduce both suffering and costs, as follows.

Postoperative Haemorrhage

Provided a good technique has been used and unhurried, meticulous haemostasis has been carried out, postoperative haemorrhage should be rare. Significant bleeding is usually obvious when the wounds are inspected after the patient has returned to the ward, but occasionally hidden bleeding occurs into the rectum and the only signs of bleeding are those of diminished blood volume (pallor, rising pulse rate, falling blood pressure) and shock.

The usual source of the bleeding is persistent oozing from smaller vessels, often in the external surfaces of the wounds. Such bleeding can be controlled by gauze soaked in 1:1,000 adrenaline pressed onto the wounds, but sometimes an individual "spurter" may need to be clipped and ligated. If a larger vessel, as from the ligated apex of one of the haemorrhoids, is responsible for the haemorrhage this will require accurate ligation under anaesthesia, and the sooner this is done, the better. It is to be noted that bleeding from the tied-off base is a preventable error. Restoration of circulating blood volume should be carried out, by a blood transfusion if necessary. Packing the anus and rectum should not be used to control early postoperative haemorrhage, but may be required for secondary haemorrhage, as discussed later.

Acute Retention of Urine

This is not uncommon in male patients, especially if they have had spinal anaesthesia. It is treated in the usual way initially, by catheterisation. A fine-bore, indwelling catheter should be used, and left in place until the patient is fully ambulant and free from pain. If the patient has an enlarged prostate, and retention does not respond to catheterisation, a prostatectomy may be required.

Faecal Retention

This can be prevented in the great majority of patients by adequate management of anxiety and pain, together with giving stimulatory laxatives in the early postoperative period (see postoperative care, "irresistible" defaecation, p. 85). The acutely nervous disposition of some patients causes them to suppress all defaecatory urges, and in these, faecal overloading of the rectum may occur. Once the condition is confirmed by digital examination, prompt cure by a thorough distal washout of the rectum and sigmoid colon under anaesthesia should be performed. Delay is both useless and harmful. In selected patients with anal spasm contributing to faecal retention, an anal dilation can be added, but this must be done very gently and slowly, so that the anal wounds are not unduly disrupted.

Secondary Haemorrhage

Rarely, septic manifestations in the anal wounds, usually around the basal ligatures, produces conditions which cause secondary haemorrhage, often profuse. This can occur any time between the seventh and sixteenth postoperative days, and usually after the patient has left hospital. In the past, deaths have resulted, but this should not happen nowadays. Prompt readmission and immediate transfusion provide control of the situation, and, once the patient's condition is stable, exploration of the wounds under anaesthesia is performed. Any obvious bleeding vessel is transfixion ligated, but in many instances, a single source of the bleeding is not identified. In this circumstance, packing the rectum with gauze may have to be resorted to, but this should be removed after 24 hours. Antibiotic cover should be given.

Fissure-in-ano

Sometimes, the anal wounds narrow down to a fissure, especially if bowel supervision has been inadequate to keep the anus properly dilated by defaecation. On other occasions, an almost-healed wound is split by a hard stool. Treatment is by anal dilation under anaesthesia, but an internal anal sphincterotomy is also good treatment.

Fistula-in-ano

This is another rare complication that has been recorded. If a transfixion ligation of the apical vessels has mistakenly included some muscle of the lamina propria, and this error is compounded by the use of unabsorbable bulky ties, an entry point for faecal organisms is created, and a fistula may result. The author has dealt with two such cases referred to him. Presentation is usually long after the haemorrhoidectomy (4 and 32 months, respectively in the author's cases). Treatment is by the appropriate surgical method – usually a standard laying-open procedure.

Incontinence

This is not a risk unless haemorrhoidectomy has been performed in a patient with a patulous anus. It should be noted that routinely combining internal anal sphincterotomy with a haemorrhoidectomy increases the risks of postoperative incontinence, and is not recommended as it neither diminishes pain nor assists healing. Likewise, anal dilation as a first step in haemorrhoidectomy is unnecessary and harmful, except in those exceptional cases that have a hypertonic sphincter.

Anal Stenosis

Provided regular passage of a formed stool is established within the first week after haemorrhoidectomy, this should not occur unless inadequate skin bridges have been preserved at surgery. If the condition is discovered early, treatment by anal dilatation, followed up by passage of a St Marks dilator twice daily for three months is usually successful. For patients who have a dense stenosis in the upper anal canal, special surgical measures may be required, including surgical division of the stricture and flap advancement to cover the resulting wound (see also Ch. 20; Complications).

Recurrent Haemorrhoids

Although recurrence of haemorrhoids is known to occur, it is almost unknown for a patient to require a further haemorrhoidectomy, although some patients may need treatment by sclerotherapy or banding. The author cannot recall a single example of a repeat open haemorrhoidectomy (see next).

Results

Although open haemorrhoidectomy by the Milligan–Morgan technique has occupied a central position in the surgical treatment of haemorrhoids for fifty or more years, there is little published material on the results. By proper scientific standards, this could be considered a criticism, but it can also be taken as an endorsement of its value.

The following statements can be made without causing controversy:

1. The operation is very safe; patients do not die from the operation.
2. The operation has few complications, most of which are preventable by good technique.
3. With few exceptions, the complications that occur respond to simple remedies which are well understood.
4. The technique is easily taught and requires no delicate or expensive equipment.
5. Studies have confirmed that pain and rate of healing are comparable to other techniques (such as closed haemorrhoidectomy, Ch. 12).
6. Pre- and postoperative care is straightforward and does not require unusual medical or nursing expertise.
7. Recurrence of haemorrhoids is acceptably uncommon, and does not usually require a repeat haemorrhoidectomy.

Control of pain is necessary postoperatively but the degree of pain is not unacceptably high, and is kept within bounds by normal postoperative medications.

Length of hospital stay is greater than for closed haemorrhoidectomy, but this is not a concern for countries where healthcare costs do not overwhelm all other considerations. Overall, open haemorrhoidectomy remains a cost-effective procedure. The proper aim is to give the patient the best operation, and procedures that claim to offer less pain and quicker healing are often associated with more complications, more recurrences, and more litigation.

Summary

Open haemorrhoidectomy is a straightforward, effective and safe treatment for large prolapsing haemorrhoids. It deserves to retain its position as a well-regarded operation until other techniques have been demonstrated to be superior by long-term experience and randomly allocated controlled clinical trials.

EDITORIAL COMMENT

Open haemorrhoidectomy is used widely in the UK and parts of Europe. In North America and other important geographical areas (South America, Asia) open has been replaced by closed haemorrhoidectomy. Why should this be so? Nobody can be entirely certain of the answer as comparisons of the results of treatment do not show an overwhelming advantage for either technique; nor is case selection for haemorrhoidectomy identical in all surgical cultures. Perhaps more attempts should be made to identify which patients requiring an operation should be allocated to one or the other technique. Closed haemorrhoidectomy should be preferred for day-case surgery.

Open haemorrhoidectomy gives excellent results, and recurrence rates are low – around five per cent. The technique is straightforward and complications are few, and preventable by good technique allied to proper after-care. Postoperative pain remains a problem but can be kept to a reasonable level by sensible management. The claim of surgeons who advocate closed haemorrhoidectomy because it is significantly less painful than the open technique has not been confirmed by a randomised clinical trial.

Despite repeated exposure to the closed technique, the Editor continued to use the open technique for most cases, but turned to the closed technique for some (e.g., piles with no skin tags or other external manifestations, extremely florid piles, unusually bloodsome surgery).

Further Reading

Allen-Mersh TG, Mann CV (1993) Open haemorrhoidectomy (St Marks ligation excision method) in operative surgery. In: Fielding LP, Goldberg SM (eds.) Surgery of the Colon, Rectum and Anus, Fifth Edition. Butterworth-Heinemann, Oxford London Boston

Bennett RC, Friedman MHW, Goligher JC (1963) The late results of haemorrhoidectomy by ligature and excision. BMJ 2:216

Cormie J, McNair RJ (1959) The results of haemorrhoidectomy. Scot Med J 4:571

Mazier WP (1973) Emergency haemorrhoidectomy: a worthwhile procedure. Dis Colon Rectum 16:200

Milligan ETC, Morgan CN, Jones LE, Officer R (1937) Surgical anatomy of anal canal and operative treatment of haemorrhoids. Lancet 2:1119

Soderlund S (1962) Results of haemorrhoidectomy according to Milligan: a follow-up study of 100 patients. Acta Chir Scand 124:444

12 Closed Hemorrhoidectomy

Indru T. Khubchandani

Indications

With the newly available techniques for nonsurgical hemorrhoidectomy, surgical hemorrhoidectomy is being practiced much less frequently. However, for fourth-degree hemorrhoids and some third-degree hemorrhoids, a well-performed hemorrhoidectomy, with removal of the pathology and correction of the associated conditions, still remains the procedure of choice. A technique of closed hemorrhoidectomy with primary closure of the incisions and local anesthesia is described.

Preoperative Preparation

Unless the history indicates otherwise, no preoperative testing is needed, especially if the patient has had some other procedures performed in the past. An ECG is performed in the elderly only when there is a history of cardiac problems. A chest radiograph is not necessary. Unless the patient has previously been on anticoagulants, the preoperative coagulation workup is not necessary. The patient should be approved for anesthesia preoperatively during the preadmission testing. The patient should fast after midnight the day before surgery and report to the Ambulatory Surgical unit on the morning of surgery, after having self-administered a disposable phosphosoda enema. An intravenous line is established with a 250 ml solution of 0.5% normal saline in 5% dextrose. The patient is delivered to the operating room either in a wheelchair or by foot.

Position and Anesthesia

A prone jack-knife position is used in which the buttocks are retracted with adhesive tape on both sides (Fig. 12.1). The hips are flexed, and both arms are extended. The patient is sedated with Propofol® (Zeneca) and Midazolan® (Roche). The local anesthesia is prepared by mixing two ampoules of 150 USP units of hyaluronidase in a 50 ml solution of 0.5% lidocaine with 1:200,000 epinephrine. About 15 ml of this solution is used per procedure. A subcutaneous, circumferential infiltration is performed with a no. 30 needle using approximately 5 ml of this solution. Another 8 ml are then deposited in the submucous plane, 2 ml in each of the four quadrants with a finger or a pediatric Hill-Ferguson retractor in the anal canal (Fig. 12.2). If the solution is inadvertently deposited in the plane outside of the sphincter muscle, no ill effects are encountered. The anesthetic effect is instantaneous and complete with adequate relaxation of the sphincter.

Procedure

The surgical technique (Khubchandani et al., 1972) is considerably modified from the original description of Ferguson and Heaton (1959). A medium-sized Hill–Ferguson retractor is inserted, and the anal canal is inspected. A plan is outlined for the extent of required dissection. As a rule, three classic primary hemorrhoidal complexes (i.e., left lateral, right posterior, and right anterior quadrants) are

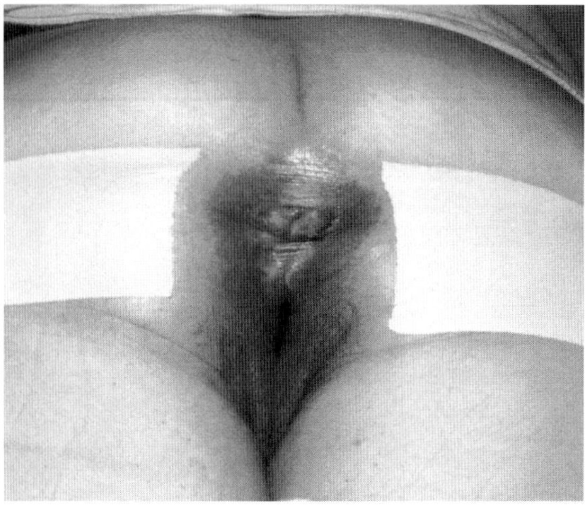

Figure 12.1. Patient in prone (jack-knife) position with buttocks retracted with adhesive tape.

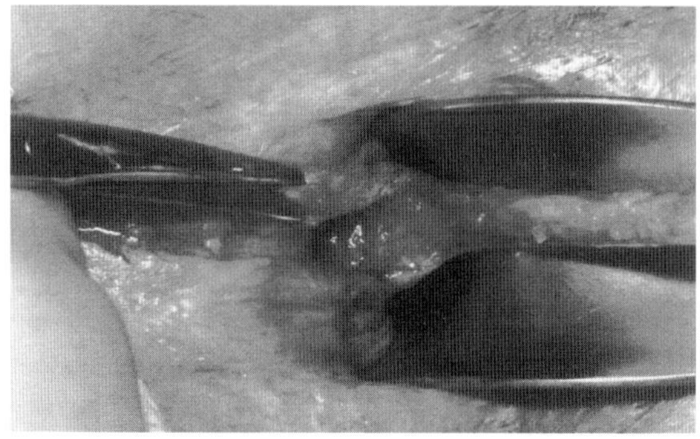

Figure 12.3. Dissection of hemorrhoidal mass, well proximal to the dentate line.

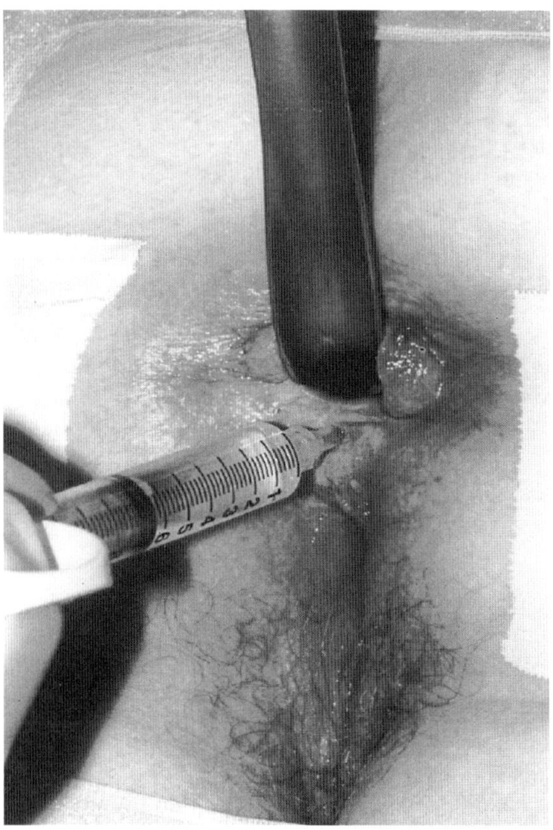

Figure 12.2. Infiltration of local anesthetic solution in the submucosal plane.

excised. Care is taken to avoid making excisions in the anterior and posterior midline, where an unhealed wound may result. A knife is used to make a radial elliptical incision, encompassing the primary hemorrhoidal complex, starting at the point proximal to the dentate line and extending well beyond the anal verge. Using scissors, the skin is lifted from the underlying external sphincter, and the mucosa is freed from the internal sphincter cephalad, proximal to the dentate line. With local anesthesia, the tissue planes are remarkably easily demarcated, and the anatomic definitions are perfect. Due to vascular constriction, the blood loss is minimal, often requiring only a few 4×4 sponges for the entire procedure. A suction device is not necessary. The proximal point is reached when the attachment of the muscle of Treitz is seen to anchor the internal sphincter to the mucosa. Using scissors, this mucosal suspensory ligament is divided, the salmon-colored proximal part of the internal sphincter is dissected free, and the hemorrhoidal complex is excised (Fig. 12.3). This is the so-called "pedicle" described in the literature, and it does not bleed. Except in the very elderly, a superficial, partial internal sphincterotomy may be performed in the base of one or both lateral wounds. This procedure would accomplish three results: relief of pain; facilitation of closure without tension; and, most importantly, division of the fibrotic, thickened band which may be an etiologic factor in the proximal high-pressure zone genesis of hemorrhoidal disease. The wound is closed primarily with one continuous, simple over-and-over suture of 5–0 polyglycolic acid, beginning at the apex, the most proximal point of the excised tissue, and ending at the external verge, where no attempt is made to leave any open area for drainage (Fig. 12.4). Reinforcing sutures are not used.

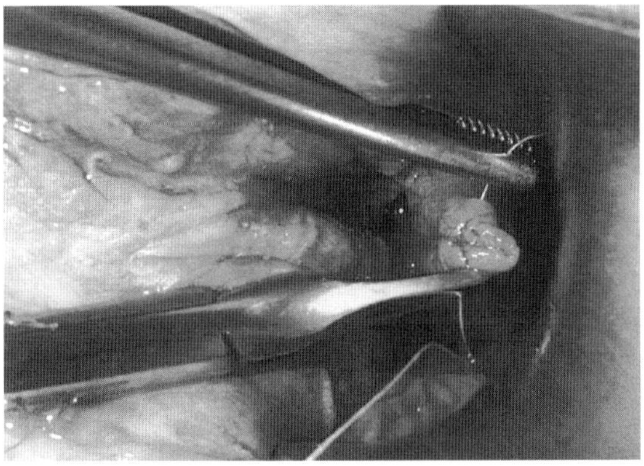

Figure 12.4. Closure of the wound, commencing at the proximal cut edge of the "pedicle".

The suture should not be pulled tight. It is intended to approximate the tissue, rather than act as a hemostatic constriction. Contrary to the traditional surgical axiom, no attempt is made to eliminate the potentially contaminated deep space. The underlying sphincter muscle, therefore, is not incorporated into the suture. No drainage tubes or hemostatic packs are inserted, and no compression dressing is considered necessary. Only an external Telfa® dressing may be applied. A completed three-column hemorrhoidectomy is shown in Fig. 12.5.

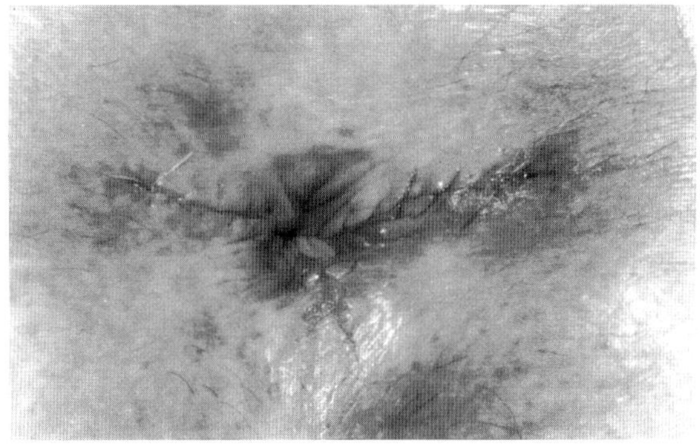

Figure 12.5. Complete closure of the wounds.

Table 12.1. Complications of closed hemorrhoidectomy in 3,274 cases

Complications	Number (%)
Bleeding:	
Requiring packing	16 (0.49)
Requiring reoperation	0 (0)
Abscess formation:	
Opened in office	4 (0.12)
Requiring reoperation	2 (0.06)
Suture line dehiscence:	
One-quarter only	163 (4.97)
Circumferential	2 (0.06)
Urinary retention	121 (3.70)
Excessive edema requiring reoperation	199 (6.08)

Postoperative Management

The patients are returned directly to the Ambulatory Suite, either via a wheelchair or on a stretcher. They are given a snack and a drink soon afterwards, and if necessary, an oral analgesic. Patients are discharged one-half to one hour after surgery with appropriate instructions.

The follow-up regimen consists of sitz baths (patients are given a disposable sitz bath to be placed over the commode with connections for plumbing), and patients are advised to take an oral analgesic as necessary. They are given two tablets of Ducolax® on the evening of surgery to promote a bowel movement. In addition, patients are advised to take a bulk supplement, such as psyllium seed, to facilitate bowel activity. An appointment is scheduled 10 days postoperatively, when the sutures will have been absorbed. The next visit is scheduled for three weeks later, when the wounds are completely healed.

Results

Table 1 lists the complications in a series of 3,274 cases. The low incidence of urinary retention (3.7%) is explained by the limited use of intravenous hydration during the procedure (Ferguson and Heaton, 1959). There is a low incidence of infection and abscess formation (0.16%). Postoperative pain is always difficult to evaluate. However, most patients do not finish a 30-tablet prescription for analgesic medication (oxycodin). Postoperative follow-up (one to seven years) of 441 patients who underwent closed hemorrhoidectomy showed that 7.5% needed further treatment for hemorrhoids (McConnell and Khubchandani, 1983). Patient satisfaction was 92.6%.

Discussion

Closed hemorrhoidectomy with local anesthesia is the preferred choice for surgical management of hemorrhoidal disease in the United States. A questionnaire sent by Wolfe et al. to members of the American Society of Colon and Rectal Surgeons revealed that 65.6% of surgeons who performed a closed hemorrhoidectomy used local anesthesia (Wolfe et al., 1979). This author prefers the closed hemorrhoidectomy technique because it affords faster healing (per primum), less pain, and fewer complications. The procedure can be performed in an ambulatory setting, requiring about a two-hour stay at the hospital. Resumption of full activity, particularly in the motivated patient, occurs in about one to two weeks.

EDITORIAL COMMENT

As stated in the comments on Ch. 11, the Editor retained the open technique as his routine method of hemorrhoidectomy, but used the closed technique for special cases. As time passed, closed hemorrhoidectomy was used more frequently but never predominantly.

In the hands of an expert, such as Professor Khubchandani, closed hemorrhoidectomy gives excellent results.

References

Ferguson DJ, Heaton JR (1959) Closed hemorrhoidectomy. Dis Colon Rectum 2:176–9

Khubchandani IT, Trimpi HD, Sheets JA (1972) Closed hemorrhoidectomy with local anesthesia. Surg Gynecol Obstet 135:955–7

McConnell JC, Khubchandani IT (1983) Long-term follow-up of closed hemorrhoidectomy. Dis Colon Rectum 26:797–9

Wolfe JS, Munoz JJ, Rosin JD (1979) Survey of hemorrhoidectomy practices: Open versus closed techniques. Dis Colon Rectum 22:536–8

13 The Treatment of Haemorrhoids by Submucosal Haemorrhoidectomy (Parks Method)

Giovanni Milito and Francesco Cortese

Introduction

Alan Parks conceived and described this operation in 1952 in order to avoid excessive sacrifice of anal mucosa during haemorrhoidectomy. He identified the cause of postoperative pain, stenosis and faecal continence disturbances as anal deformity due to three factors: excessive scarring of the anal canal, the positioning of endoanal tubes, and the inclusion of fibres from the internal anal sphincter in the ligature of the pedicle. This operation didn't become popular because of its duration, the quite complicated technique, and the possible occurrence of bleeding during and after the operation. But in our opinion, this procedure still remains a great therapeutic option for the treatment of prolapsed haemorrhoids (third or fourth degree) or recurrences. The principles of a correct technique are accurate preparation and the high ligature of each single pedicle, minimal excision of the anodermal and anal mucosae, and accurate reconstruction of the anal mucosal layer.

Indications

This procedure is indicated for third- and fourth-degree haemorrhoids as well as all kinds of recurrences after surgical treatment, rubber band ligation, cryotherapy and sclerotherapy.

Preoperative Preparation

Mechanical

The necessity of an early post-operative bowel movement in order to remodel the anal canal makes the patient's bowel preparation very simple. Two enemas are administered to the patient four and two hours before operation. Preparation with a laxative for a complete bowel cleaning is contraindicated since it delays restarting of defecation. Diagnostic procedures (e.g., colonoscopy, rectosigmoidoscopy) should not be performed at this same time.

Pharmacological

Antibiotics are not strictly indicated. We however prefer a double administration of metronidazole (500 mg) intravenously two hours before and after the operation respectively to prevent both local and/or systemic diffusion of faeces and bacterial flora. Patients affected by heart, kidney or pulmonary diseases require heavier antibiotics coverage. Anticoagulant therapy, as low molecular weight heparin (LMWH) is administered in high-risk patients to avoid deep-vein thrombosis or compartmental syndrome. Both can arise after adopting the lithotomy position. Suspension of anticoagulant therapy in subjects affected by cardiac valve diseases, atria fibrillation, coronary or other bypasses is not mandatory but more perfect haemostasis is required of the operator.

Technique

The patient is placed in standard (St Marks) lithotomy position. Disinfections must be applied to the perineum and both buttocks. The operative field is centred on the anus. In women, a white sterile swab is put inside the vagina to prevent contamination. A urinary catheter is placed in older or incontinent women or men.

The anaesthesiologic procedures are always discussed by the anaesthesiologist with the patient and are modulated by age, psychological habit, and medical indications. In our opinion, general anaesthesia with laryngeal mask is the best option. This procedure avoids all problems related to the spinal anaesthesia technique (more frequent and dangerous bleedings, urinary dysfunction).

An accurate inspection of the anal canal with mapping of the pedicles using an Eisenhammer retractor is the first step of the operation. Haemorrhoidectomy is performed using a Parks' retractor, which is left in situ during the operation. A saline solution with 1:250,000 adrenaline is injected just under the mucosal plane to make the dissection of mucosa–submucosal haemorrhoids more comfortable and bloodless. The incision is performed around a haemostat raising the squamous mucosa over the external part of the piles. A Y-incision (Fig. 13.1) is made 3–5 cm from the mucocutaneous junction between the mucosa of the upper canal and the anorectal junction. The vascular pedicle is completely freed from the mucosa on each side (Fig. 13.2) and the muscle plane beneath, ligated at its uppermost ends and excised (Fig. 13.3). The reconstruction of the mucosa is achieved by suturing the mucosal flaps down to close the wound. A small perianal area is left bare to allow spontaneous drainage (Fig. 13.4). The procedure is then repeated for all the remaining piles.

In patients with four-quadrant haemorrhoidal involvement, the flap advancement technique, described by Hawley (1973), is used to avoid extensive baring of the anal canal, which leads to slower healing rates and severe postoperative pain.

Lateral sphincterotomy can easily be performed in order to reduce postoperative pain or treat co-existing anal fissure.

In order to avoid postoperative pain, we sometimes infiltrate the internal anal sphincter with ketorolac as described by many authors. Another useful technique is infiltration of the pudendal nerve with ropivacaine. None of these procedures is applied to patients operated using a peripheral anaesthesia regimen. An Anal Spongostan® is left in the anal canal after accurate control of haemostasis.

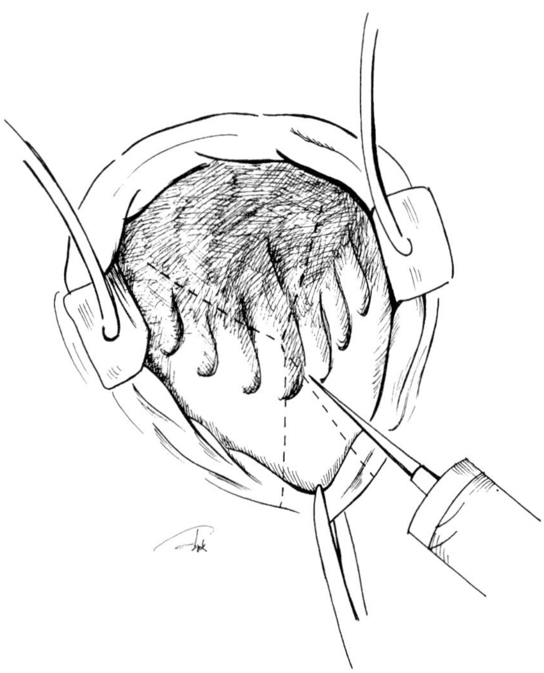

Figure 13.1. Local injection and incision.

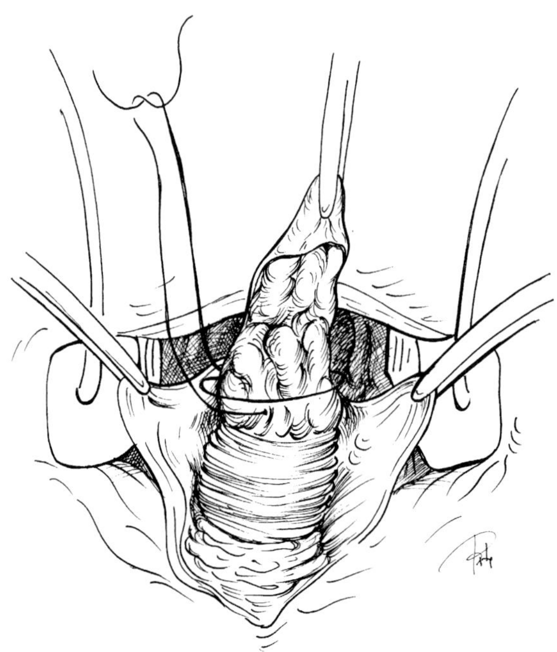

Figure 13.2. Preparation of the pedicle.

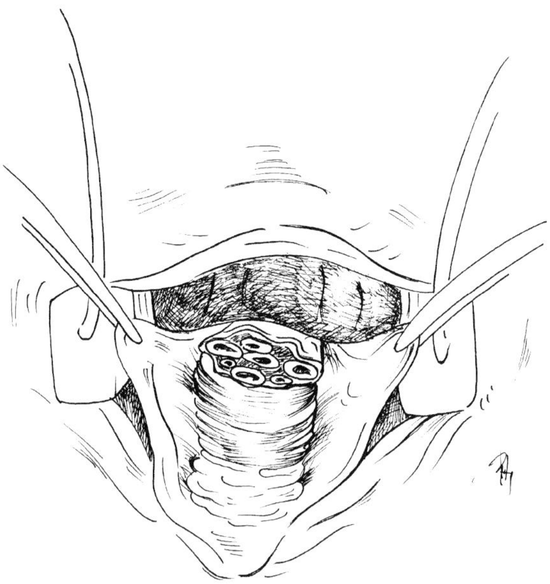

Figure 13.3. The pedicle excised. Note the internal anal sphincter below. The ligature is not shown.

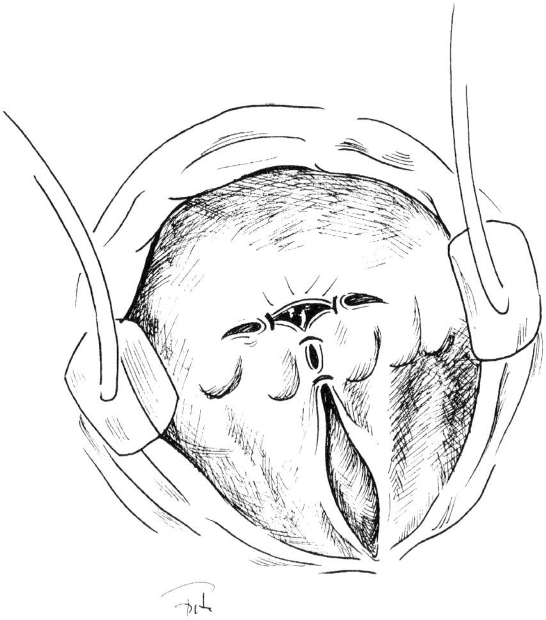

Figure 13.4. The final results after reconstruction of the mucosal plane.

Postoperative Management

Postoperative management focuses on administration of not more than 1,000 ml of fluids. A small, single dose of betamethasone is administered to reduce local oedema, together with a ketorolac or ketoprofen bolus.

From the first postoperative day, therapy consists of: (i) a high-fibre diet, (ii) stool softener (mineral oil), and (iii) ketoprofen or ketorolac tablets twice daily. This ensures early evacuation and the reduction of pain and local inflammation. Warm sitz baths are also recommended to keep the wounds clean. The patient is discharged as soon as possible with the telephone numbers of the surgeons. The first bowel movement must occur not later than 60 hours after the operation. In adverse situations, a mild laxative or an enema is administered, always by the surgeons themselves, using a soft Foley catheter.

Follow-up Regimen

A visit is made on the seventh postoperative day to evaluate sphincter tone and wound healing. Sometimes a digital exploration can be required to eliminate the internal sphincter spasm that may follow the healing process. If this spasm is found to be particularly persistent, the patient is invited to return every second day to repeat the same manoeuvre until the spasm resolves.

Results

Despite haemorrhoidectomy being described as one of the most painful operations, postoperative pain, assessed subjectively in our experience with 1,315 patients treated by Parks operation, was reported as mild in 1,023 cases (77.7%), moderate in 253 (19%) and severe in 39 (2.9%). Bleeding was observed in 25 patients. Eighteen were treated with simple tampons while seven required surgical haemostasis. Only one patient needed a single whole blood transfusion. Primary wound healing occurred within a mean time of four weeks in 94.5% of patients. Early complications were submucosal abscess in three patients and submucosal haematomas in another four. The abscesses were treated with antibiotics and surgical incision was required only in one case of haematoma. One patient developed a massive mucosal oedema that required surgical excision.

Urinary dysfunction developed in 242 patients (18.4%) and required catheterisation in 106 of these for at least 24 hours. These complications were more frequent (71.5%) after peripheral as opposed to general anaesthesia (28.5%), and in male patients (76.8%) as opposed to female ones (23.2%). Faecal impaction occurred in 46 patients (3.4%) and was always resolved with two enemas.

During long-term follow up, 82 patients (7%) developed a recurrence, 75 (6.5%) suffered from skin tags, while anal stenosis occurred in 19 cases (1.6%). Recurrences were surgically treated in five cases, while 73 required rubber band ligation and four were resolved by means of infrared coagulation. Stenoses required six surgical corrections (two lateral anal sphincterotomy, four anoplasties) and 13 balloon dilatations.

In 36 patients (3.2%) minor flatus incontinence arose. None of them required another operation because of the minimal social impact of the inconvenience.

EDITORIAL COMMENT

This was the first serious attempt to remove haemorrhoidal tissue while conserving the mucosa. After removal of the submucosal pile elements, the technique allowed resuture of the mucosa (which became a feature of the Ferguson operation; Ch. 12).

The technique has not been widely adopted in the UK, not even at St Marks Hospital where Sir Alan Parks worked: the five other staff surgeons continued to use the Milligan–Morgan operation. The principal disadvantage of the operation was that it was time consuming, and was not superior in its results, despite claims that it was less painful. A further criticism was that the suture lines broke down as soon as postoperative defecation took place, converting the wounds to an open type.

When Hamish Thompson showed that haemorrhoids were not a single-tissue – venous – structure but were modified anal cushions with substantial elements of connective tissue and mucosa/submucosa, the theoretical basis for the Parks operation was undermined, although good results were recorded. There are few reports of comparisons between submucosal and closed haemorrhoidectomy techniques. As a matter of general observation, one would conclude that the method has been superseded by the Ferguson technique, to which it gave support.

References and Further Reading

Hawley PR (1973) Haemorrhoids. Adv Surg 8:235–40

Henry MM, Swash M (1992) Coloproctology and the Pelvic Floor. Second Ed. Butterworths, London

Hosch SB, Knoefel WT, Pichlmaier U, et al. (1998) Surgical treatment of piles. Dis Colon Rectum 41:159–64

Ibrahim S, Tsang C, Lee YL, Eu KW, Seow-Choen F (1998) Prospective, randomized trial comparing pain and complications between diathermy and scissors for closed haemorrhoidectomy. Dis Colon Rectum 41:1418–20

Mann CV, Glass RE (1997) Surgical Treatment of Anal Incontinence. Second Ed. Springer, London, pp 147–60

Milito G, Cortese F, Brancaleone C, Casciani CU (1997) Submucosal haemorrhoidectomy: surgical results and complications in 1,315 patients. Techniques in Coloproctology 1:128–32

Mortensen N, Romanos J (1997) Haemorrhoids. In: Nicholls RJ, Dozois RR (eds) Surgery of the Colon and Rectum. Churchill Livingstone, New York, pp 209–31

Parks AG (1956) The surgical treatment of haemorrhoids. Br J Surg 43:337–51

Sielezneff I, Salle E, Lécenyer J, Brunet CH, Sarles J Cl, Sastre B (1998) Morbidité post-opératoire précoce aprés hémorroidectomie selon la technique de Milligan e Morgan. J Chir (Paris) 134:243–7

Thomson WHF (1975) The nature of haemorrhoids. Br J Surg 62:542–52

Zaheer S, Reilly WT, Pemberton JH, Ilstrup D (1998) Urinary retention after operations for benign ano-rectal diseases. Dis Colon Rectum 41:696–704

14 Circular Stapler Anopexy For Prolapsing Haemorrhoids

Per-Olof Nyström and Rune Sjödahl

Summary

The current use of the circular stapler for treatment of prolapsing haemorrhoids originated in Italy by Dr Antonio Longo in 1993. The technique was fully developed and released by 1997. More than 55,000 operations have been completed to date, mainly across Europe but also in South America, Japan, Singapore, and recently in the US. Many case series have been reported at various meetings during the last few years but only two publications are available that scientifically compare the technique with traditional operations. In the near future there will be published several more randomised clinical trials that aim to determine the result in the intermediate term (up to one year) in comparison with excision (Milligan–Morgan).

Introduction

Haemorrhoidectomy by means of a stapler device has previously been attempted. Both the linear cutting staplers (TLC or GIA) and the linear non-cutting staplers (TL or TA) were used (O'Bichere et al., 1998; Abbasakoor et al., 2000). These attempts have not been embraced, perhaps because it does not make sense to excise the haemorrhoid with its overlying anoderm with a stapler and leave the staples in situ in the anal canal and the wound outside the anus, i.e., a completely closed excision. But if the haemorrhoids are dissected free from the internal sphincter, it is only the stalk of the haemorrhoid that is transected with the stapler, and this can be done with a simple ligature while it is not necessary in diathermy haemorrhoidectomy.

The situation is different with the recently proposed circular stapler haemorrhoidectomy (ILS or CEEA) (Longo, 1998; Pescatori et al., 1997; Altomare et al., 1999). It is not really an excision of the haemorrhoids but a method to correct the mucosa prolapse that is associated with the haemorrhoids. It is, therefore, better described as an "anopexy". It is important to understand this distinction between excision of the haemorrhoids and the reduction and fixation of the prolapse of the anal canal and lower rectal mucosa. Technically, a circumferential submucosal purse-string suture is applied above the ano-rectal ring and a column of the mucosa is excised with the circular stapler. The resulting scar will fix the mucosa at the level of the ano-rectal ring (about two cm above the dentate line) and prevent the prolapse. The principle is not entirely new but it is the same idea as the rubber band technique and sclerosing injections. Both are applied just above the haemorrhoid and produce submucosal scarring that prevents the prolapse and shrinks the haemorrhoid. Because the scar is induced at this level, there is minimal pain.

Indications for the Stapled Anopexy

Why should circular stapler anopexy be performed if rubber banding is the same principle? It is all a matter of degree of the prolapse. For a minor or

Table 14.1. Sample of questions for self-reported symptoms with regard to the haemorrhoids. From the patient questionnaire of the STOPP trial (the acronym for the multicentre trial conducted in Sweden, Denmark and the UK. The trial compares stapled anopexy with Milligan–Morgan with one-year follow-up). Statistical analysis is done on a nominal scale: never = 0, less than once a week = 1, etc.

The following questions deal with haemorrhoids. Your answers should reflect the latest two-week period.

25. How often do you have pain from the haemorrhoids?	☐ Never	☐ Less than once a week	☐ 1–6 times weekly	☐ Every day (always)
26. How often do you have itching or discomfort of the anus?	☐ Never	☐ Less than once a week	☐ 1–6 times weekly	☐ Every day (always)
27. How often do you have bleeding when passing a motion?	☐ Never	☐ Less than once a week	☐ 1–6 times weekly	☐ Every day (always)
28. How often do you soil your underclothes (soiling from the anus)?	☐ Never	☐ Less than once a week	☐ 1–6 times weekly	☐ Every day (always)
29. How often do you reduce a prolapsing haemorrhoid with your hand when passing a motion?	☐ Never	☐ Less than once a week	☐ 1–6 times weekly	☐ Every day (always)
30. How often do you have a prolapse of the haemorrhoid when walking or sitting during the day?	☐ Never	☐ Less than once a week	☐ 1–6 times weekly	☐ Every day (always)

intermittent prolapse, rubber banding may be just as adequate. Most colorectal surgeons apply only one or two ligatures per session, which poses a limit to what can be treated easily with rubber banding. When the prolapse is major or involves all three haemorrhoids, it becomes difficult to treat with rubber banding and most surgeons propose an excision.

The typical patient who needs a formal operation for haemorrhoids will complain of prolapse of the anal canal upon every bowel motion and the prolapse needs to be manually reduced. This information unequivocally identifies a group of patients that are suitable for the stapled anopexy (see Table 14.1). They would be rated as grade 3 haemorrhoids. The ligaments that anchor the anal mucosa to the internal sphincter have been extended or torn allowing the anal canal to slide along with the haemorrhoids (Thompson, 1975). Whether patients that have an intact anal canal with haemorrhoids but no need to manually reduce them should also be candidates for an operation is a matter for debate. Patients with even lesser degrees of haemorrhoids should be treated medically with dietary fibre, or have rubber band ligation.

We suggest that prolapse is the key indication for stapled anopexy, while bleeding in the absence of prolapse is usually not an indication. This statement does not disregard that most patients that seek attention for haemorrhoids suffer from bleeding. However, the bleeding is most often experienced as stains on the paper, while major bleeding that drips into the toilet is much less common. In the former case, medical treatment with fibre should be attempted for a period, possibly followed by rubber band ligation.

In fixed external prolapse that cannot be reduced (Grade 4), the stapled anopexy has no place as its success is entirely dependent on the reduction of the prolapse. Also, for those with a large external component with hard fibrosed skin tags, this operation is less suitable because the external component will need additional excision. The Milligan–Morgan operation is then a better choice. Minor soft skin tags are acceptable because they can be excised after the anopexy has been completed. Such residual skin tags are then excised as they occur outside the anus, which does not cause a lot more pain. Haemorrhoids that are acutely thrombosed, swollen and prolapsed are no indication for the stapled anopexy. Again, the Milligan–Morgan excision is the better operation for such patients.

The Stapled Anopexy Operation

Preoperatively, the rectum is evacuated with an enema. A urinary catheter is not necessary. We do not use prophylactic antibiotics for anal procedures. The patient is preferably placed prone but the lithotomy or left-lateral positions are also suitable. We prefer a general anaesthesia because it takes longer for the patient to recover from an epidural or spinal block. A sacral block is excellent when available. The operation can also be done with a perianal block with a local anaesthetic agent but this will not be sufficient for the actual cutting of the mucosa with the stapler. This needs additional blockage of the mucosa with local anaesthetic or an intravenous anaesthetic.

The kit provided by Ethicon Endo-Surgery (HCS 33 kit) is designed for this procedure and provides the means for a highly standardised operation (see Fig. 14.1). The anus is relaxed and dilated with the dilator of the kit after which the anoscope is introduced and its rim is sutured to the perianal skin with four stitches. The prolapse must be properly reduced by the anoscope and the stitches keep it in place. The anoscope is 3 cm long; just sufficient to pass the dentate line that is seen covered by the distal rim of the anoscope. Having observed this, the surgeon has complete control of the anatomy. The speculum of the kit is introduced, which will stretch the mucosa of the lower rectum and allow the surgeon to place the purse-string suture 4 cm above the dentate line using a 2/0 Prolene. The suture should begin at the site of the most prominent prolapse because the excision tends to be larger at this site for reasons that are explained below. The suture is carried a full circle taking care to stay submucosal at 4 cm above the dentate line. Care is also taken to begin the next bite precisely where the previous stitch exited so there are no gaps that will give an incomplete excision or even allow the stapler anvil to pass outside the suture when introduced. It must be emphasised that proper reduction of the prolapse with the anoscope and the precise positioning of the purse-string suture are the keys to making this operation simple and successful.

The stapler, maximally opened, is introduced through the anoscope so the anvil reaches beyond the purse-string suture. Traction on the suture confirms that it closes around the shaft of the stapler. Tie the suture with one throw only and bring the loose ends of the suture through the channels of the stapler casing. Again, by slight traction on the suture, more mucosa will be pulled into the chamber of the casing and hence a wider excision. However, the main pull will be at the site of the knot and this site will be the widest excision.

Introduce the stapler through the anoscope into the anal canal while closing it maximally. The stapler casing has a scale that shows when the stapler, with no effort, has been introduced 4 cm. In women, always palpate the posterior vaginal wall to ensure that it is not entrapped by the stapler. Then fire and retract the stapler. Inspect the stapler line that should be about 2 cm above the dentate line. Bleeding spots will be seen in 20–40% of instances. They are picked up with forceps and cauterised, or a stitch may be used for haemostasis. Complete the operation by infiltrating the staple line with a local anaesthetic (without adrenalin), which will produce a totally pain-free patient in the immediate postoperative hours. There is no indication for a transanal drain or a Spongostan tamponade. The operation will take about 15 minutes but the variation is large (Table 14.2). In our experience, and that of others, the surgeon is well advised to spend a few extra minutes to ensure that haemostasis is satisfactory.

The excised doughnut should be opened and inspected for any inadvertent excision of the muscular wall. This will be seen quite often, especially at the site of the knot, but the piece should be small. The proper excision will be a circumferential 2–3 cm column of mucosa with no anoderm. As mentioned, it is important to understand that the operation is a prolapsectomy and anopexy, not an excision of the haemorrhoids, which partly remain in situ below the staple line. By pulling a piece of gauze through the anus after the stapling, the resolution of the prolapse can be tested.

Postoperative Course

Stapled anopexy is eminently suitable for day-case surgery. With a general anaesthetic supplemented with local anaesthetic of the staple line, the patient will suffer no pain in the first hours. While this is easily achieved also for a conventional excision, the total pain experience after stapled anopexy is distinctly different from that of the Milligan–Morgan operation. About 80% of the patients with the stapled procedure will experience minor pain (VAS $\leq$ 5) in the following days and the pain is usually over within the week according to early Italian experiences (unpublished manuscripts by A. Longo and A. Capomagi). Morphine is not needed

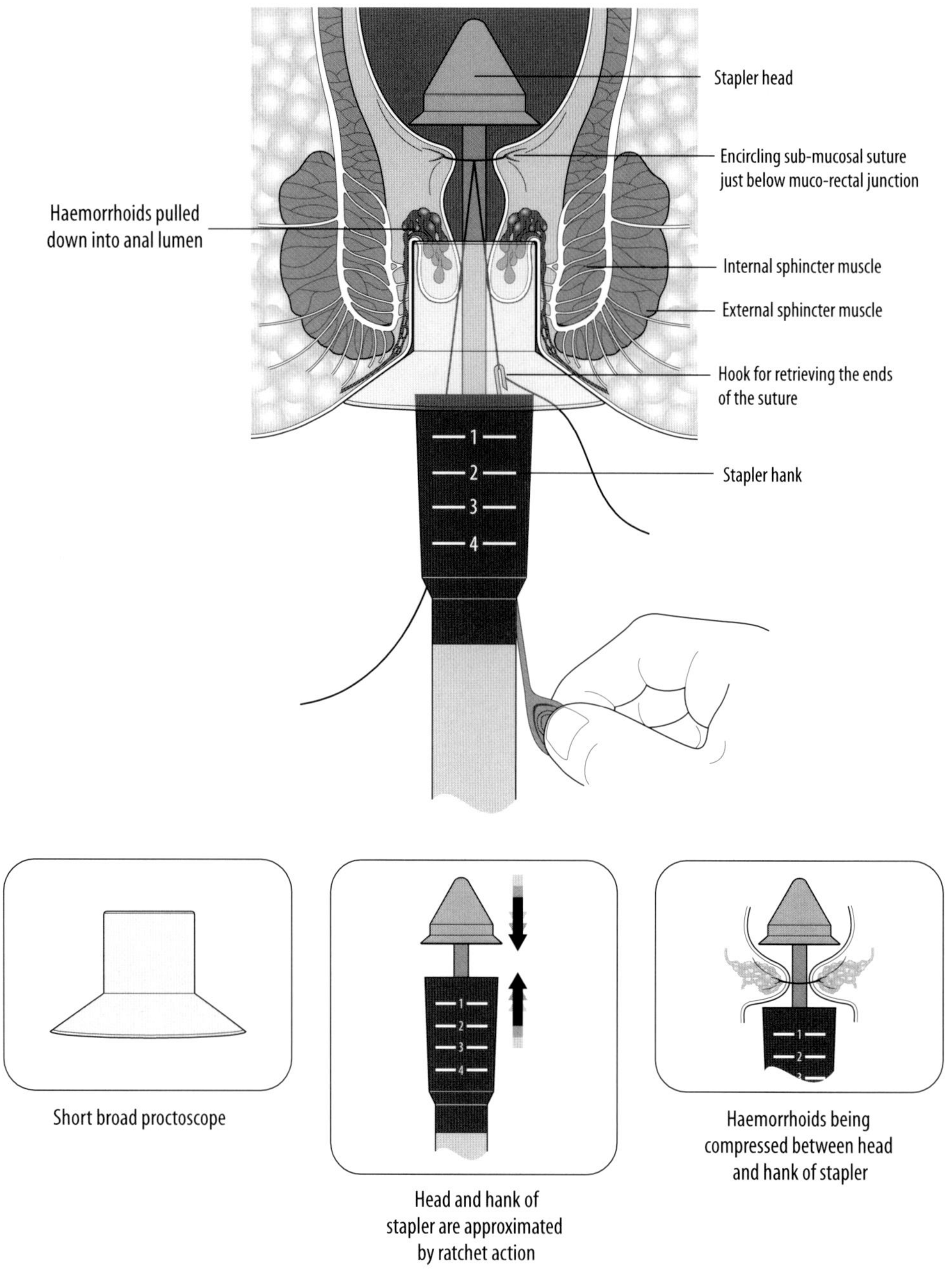

Figure 14.1. Principle of the stapled anopexy for prolapsing haemorrhoids. 1) The prolapse has been reduced with the anoscope, which is 3 cm long and its distal rim just covers the dentate line. 2) The submucosal purse-string suture is 4 cm above the dentate line. 3) The stapler when closed and fired will produce a muco–mucosal stapled suture 2 cm above the dentate line.

in the postoperative course but diclofenac or even paracetamol usually relieves pain for the few days it is needed. There are patients in our experience who avoided pain medication entirely. One in five patients, however, will experience significant pain that may last for as long as 14 days.

Recent studies that compared stapled anopexy with Milligan–Morgan excision substantiated the lesser pain of stapled anopexy. One randomised study with pain as the primary end-point showed an average pain score over the first ten days of 2.1 versus 6.5 on a 10-grade scale ($p < 0.0001$) (Mehigan

Table 14.2. Operation time for the stapled anopexy

Author	Mean operating time (minutes)	Range
Longo (1998)	8	6–21
Capomagi§	11	6–35
Rowsell (2000)	14	–
Savian§	16	5–60
Milito§	16	12–45
Arbman§	16	10–45
Mehigan [2000]*	18	9–25
Smedh§	25	15–40
Nystrom§	25	12–60

Notes:
§ Unpublished manuscript.
* Anaesthesia time.

Table 14.3. Postoperative pain and resumption of work in 25 patients each of stapled anopexy and Milligan–Morgan haemorrhoid excision (interim result from the STOPP trial)

	Anopexy	Milligan	
Relief of daily average pain within 14 days	100%	60%	P = 0.001
Relief of defaecatory pain within 14 days	84%	40%	P = 0.003
Resumed work within 14 days (of 19 vs. 22 employed)	74%	41%	P = 0.06

et al., 2000). Pain relative to the expectation of patients was also much less with the stapled procedure. Another randomised study found very similar scores and difference of pain to the advantage of anopexy (Rowsell et al., 2000). An interim analysis of the first 25 patients of each procedure (anopexy or Milligan–Morgan) of the STOPP trial showed that all with stapled anopexy had an average daily pain score of two or less within 14 days but almost 20% still had defaecatory pain at that time (Table 14.3).

Stapled anopexy is not a pain-free operation as was sometimes claimed in the early period of its introduction. Indeed, all patients experience some pain but usually much less than with the conventional haemorrhoid excision. While the pain peaks on day four to seven after a Milligan–Morgan operation, the anopexy patients usually do not need pain medication at that time. More intense pain is associated with stapling near the dentate line and possibly with excision into the muscle wall (A. Longo, personal communication). Some patients state that it is not really pain but a sensation of discomfort and cramp that may be associated with an urge to defaecate. We have, as have others, seen patients in whom the operation provoked profound urgency, multiple daily visits to the toilet, and partial incontinence lasting from weeks to several months in the absence of pain. Perhaps as many as 5% of the patients will have disturbing symptoms of this sort.

In-hospital stay is not required unless for social reasons or associated medical conditions. The majority of patients will also manage with sick leave for just a few days but some need more than a week (Table 14.3). Hospital stay and sick leave are both heavily dependent on local traditions. The Milligan–Morgan operation is increasingly done by day surgery and surgeons with this practice will find it easier to discharge patients with the stapled anopexy (Carapeti et al., 1999; Hunt et al., 1999). One recent randomised study with in-hospital stay as the primary endpoint found significantly shorter hospital stay with the anopexy, 1.1 days versus 2.8 days for the Milligan–Morgan (Rowsell et al., 2000). Another randomised study found the length of stay to be no different as most patients were discharged within 24 hours regardless of the type of operation (Mehigan et al., 2000).

Postoperative Complications

The most important immediate complication is bleeding from the staple line (Table 14.4). The staple line must be carefully inspected and any bleeding spots taken care of. In our experience, as well as that of others (A. Herold, personal communication), postoperative bleeding is mainly seen during the learning curve. Inflammation or thrombosis of a residual haemorrhoid below the staple line is a procedure-specific complication that is probably due to severing the proximal blood drainage of the haemorrhoids. We have seen two such cases; one was re-operated with excision the following day and the other after two weeks. Others have similar experience. Oedema and haematoma of the anus as reported by some surgeons are probably also consequences of severing the proximal blood drainage of the residual haemorrhoids.

Stenosis at the site of the staple line is uncommon contrary to expectations. Of our three instances, we have seen none that was important. One was easily dilated under anaesthesia while two disappeared spontaneously.

Table 14.4. Postoperative complication rate after circular stapler anopexy in 804 operations. Source: Unpublished manuscripts, same as in Table 14.1

Complication	Per cent
Urine retention	6.7
Postoperative bleed	2.1
Anal oedema or haematoma	1.5
Acute inflammation of residual haemorrhoid	1.2
Stenosis	0.5
Total immediate complications	97/804 12.1%

Urinary retention is reported in rates between 5% and 10%. It seems to be related to postoperative pain, the amount of intravenous fluid, and the use of epidural anaesthesia. Several surgeons maintain that this complication is avoidable by local anaesthetic injections of the staple line to control postoperative pain.

Serious Complications of the Stapled Procedure

A case of pelvic sepsis was recently described (Molloy and Kingsmore, 2000). This patient had had a standard stapled anopexy with intact staple line 2 cm above the dentate line. The patient was discharged two hours after the operation but was readmitted the same evening with a temperature of 38.5°C. Computed tomography showed extensive retroperitoneal gas of the pelvis extending to the pancreas. At reoperation, the pararectal tissues were inflamed and a small pocket of pus was identified outside the rectum although the staple line was intact. Culture of the pus showed growth of coliforms, Bacteroides fragilis and a clostridum species. After drainage and an end colostomy the condition settled. A second case has been seen, again with retroperitoneal gas, but this patient was treated with antibiotics alone (G. Sunderland, personal communication). It is unusual that fermenting bacteria produce gas along fascia planes to this extent when there is no necrosis of the tissues. Also, it is almost inconceivable that intraluminal gas should penetrate the staple line and an intact rectal wall. However, it is known that emphysema of the thorax can occur without an identified source of leak from the airways. Perhaps the intraluminal pressure can be increased postoperatively by contraction of the rectum to produce this phenomenon.

There are verbal accounts of more than one rectovaginal fistula and at least one rectal perforation. It is quite conceivable that the vaginal wall can be included in the staple line if the purse-string suture is made too deep. This possibility may serve as a momentum to ensure proper placement of the suture and to digitally ascertain that the vaginal wall is not engaged before firing the stapler. The mechanism for perforation of the rectal wall is more difficult to understand unless introduction of the stapler is forced. Possibly, there was a gap in the submucosal suture so the stapler head, with some force, was introduced between the suture and the rectal wall. The stapler must be introduced to its proper length without undue force, or the stapler should be removed to check that the purse-string suture is properly placed. Because of redundant rectal mucosa, it can be difficult to view the entire rectal circumference when applying the suture.

Stapled anopexy can occasionally be associated with persistent anal pain. This circumstance was recently described from St Marks Hospital and caused the suspension of their comparative trial (Cheetham et al., 2000). They encountered five patients (out of 22 operated) who were characterized by pain and defaecatory urgency that had lasted for several months (and more than a year in one patient). An external review including interview and physical examination of the patients provided no obvious explanation nor did the operation notes, histology of the specimens, ano-rectal manometry and endoanal ultrasound examination. Since this complication became known, several surgeons involved in trials have audited their operations but no further case was identified. One more case is known, however, and there are two surgeons who may have encountered one further case each.

Long-term Results with Stapled Anopexy

There is, to date, little published about the final result with the stapled anopexy (Longo, 1998). Our own experience, corroborated by verbal reports of others, suggests that the large majority of the patients do very well. Some Italian surgeons, especially Longo, have a vast experience that dates back

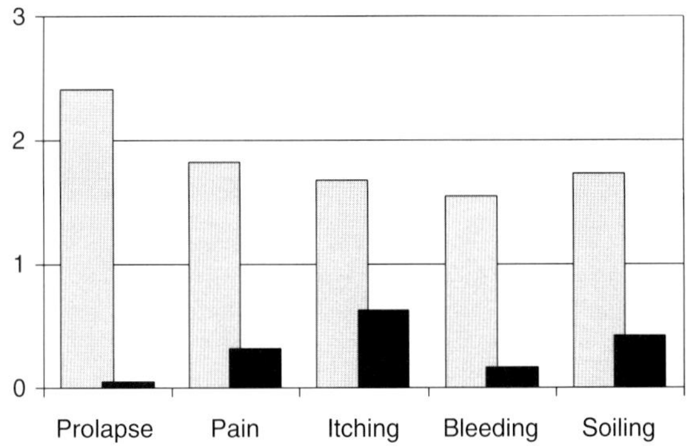

Figure 14.2. Resolution of symptom 3–6 months after stapled anopexy determined by symptom questionnaire in 22 preoperative and 19 postoperative patients. Maximum score is 3 for each symptom (see Table 14.2). All comparisons are statistically significant $p < 0.001$.

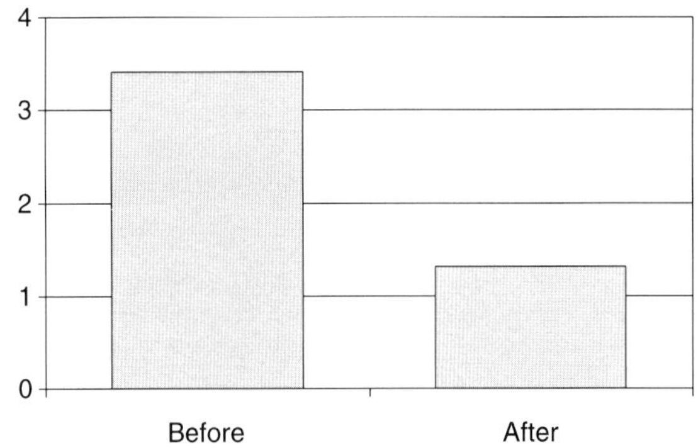

Figure 14.3. Pre- and postoperative scores of disability and social inconvenience from symptom questionnaire in 22 preoperative and 19 postoperative patients operated for prolapsing haemorrhoids with the stapled anopexy. Sum of two questions, maximum score 6 points, $p = 0.001$.

to 1993. Manuscripts by Italian surgeons that we were kindly allowed to review stated that the recurrence rate is less than 5% after one or more years of follow-up. However, comparisons with the traditional excision in the long perspective are not available.

In determining the final result, it is appropriate to consider the indication for the operation. If, as we propose, the indication for stapled anopexy is the correction of an anal prolapse associated with the haemorrhoids, then most patients (in excess of 90%) will report that the prolapse that needed manual reduction has disappeared (Fig. 14.2 and 14.3). It is a pleasure to see patients after some months and hear them say how content they are to be relieved of this major discomfort. Most patients will also report that bleeding is much less common or has ceased entirely, as have other associated complaints (Fig. 14.2). Because we have not used other indications for the stapled procedure (e.g., non-prolapsing haemorrhoids), we are unable to tell from personal experience what such results would be.

The haemorrhoids are not entirely excised by the stapled anopexy because the staple line is targeted 2 cm above the dentate line. It is, therefore, not unusual to see haemorrhoids in their normal position although the haemorrhoid is rarely large. Any external haemorrhoids are also not excised and will therefore remain although they are usually reduced in size. This is also true of skin tags that were not excised separately at the time of the stapled anopexy. In short, the external component will remain although it is usually smaller secondary to the permanent reduction of the prolapse.

There are patients who are not completely relieved of the prolapse but will display partial prolapse with a residual haemorrhoid. Whether this result is a consequence of the learning curve or is inherent in the technique remains to be determined. As long as it is no longer needed to reduce the prolapse manually, the few patients with minor residual prolapse appear to be relatively content. It is likely, though, that some patients having had the stapled anopexy will eventually need supplementary excision to remove a residual haemorrhoid or external component. On one occasion, we have submitted such a patient to a second stapled anopexy with good result.

EDITORIAL COMMENT

The Editor has no experience of this method of treatment. He has reservations about unnecessary sacrifice of normal tissues, especially sensory mucosa, as well as the potential for sphincter damage, septic complications, bleeding, and anal stenosis.

Because the operation requires special equipment, including disposable staples, costs are higher. Therefore, the results will need to be markedly superior if the technique is to replace current surgical operations that already yield excellent short- and long-term sequelae.

References

Abbasakoor F, Nelson M, Patel B, Morgan A, Carr N, Woodward A, et al. (2000) Linear stapler haemorrhoidectomy: an alternative to standard haemorrhoidectomy? Int J Colorectal Dis 2:22–5

Altomare D, Rinaldo M, Chiumarolo C (1999) Treatment of external ano-rectal mucosal prolapse with circular stapler; an easy and effective new surgical treatment. Dis Colon Rectum 42:1102–05

Carapeti EA, Kamm MA, McDonald PJ, Chadwick SJ, Phillips RK (1999) Randomised trial of open versus closed day-case haemorrhoidectomy. Br J Surg 86(5):612–3

Cheetham M, Mortensen N, Nystrom P, Kamm M, Phillips R (2000) Persistent pain and faecal urgency after stapled haemorrhoidectomy. Lancet, submitted manuscript

Hunt L, Luck A, Rudkin G, Hewitt P(1999) Day-case haemorrhoidectomy. Br J Surg 86:255–8

Longo A (1998) Treatment of haemorrhoid disease by reduction of mucosa and haemorrhoidal prolapse with a circular suturing device: new procedure. In: Sixth World Congress of Endoscopic Surgery; Rome, Italy 3–6 June, pp 777–90

Mehigan B, Monson J, Hartley J (2000) Stapling procedure for haemorrhoids versus Milligan–Morgan haemorrhoidectomy: randomised controlled trial. Lancet 355:782–5

Molloy R, Kingsmore D (2000) Life-threatening pelvic sepsis after stapled haemorrhoidectomy. Lancet 355:810

O'Bichere A, Laniado M, Sellu D (1998) Stapled haemorrhoidectomy: a feasible day-case procedure. Br J Surg 85:377–8

Pescatori M, Favetta U, Dedola S, Orsini S (1997) Transanal stapled excision of rectal mucosa prolapse. Techniques in Coloproctology 1:96–8

Rowsell M, Bello M, Hemingway D (2000) Circumferential mucosectomy (stapled haemorrhoidectomy) versus conventional haemorrhoidectomy: randomised controlled trial. Lancet 355:779–81

Thompson W (1975) The nature of haemorrhoids. Br J Surg 62:542–52

15 "Total" Hemorrhoidectomy

Julius C. Bonello

In 1882, Walter Whitehead introduced his technique for the radical cure of hemorrhoids. In this paper, he describes an almost circumferential incision around the rectum leaving only strips of mucous membrane continuous with the skin. Five years later, in 1887, Whitehead presented 300 consecutive cases of symptomatic hemorrhoids that had been cured using a new technique. In this article, he discusses using exclusively a circumferential incision, thereby modifying his own original procedure. This modified procedure is known today as the Whitehead or complete hemorrhoidectomy.

In the decade following the publication of this paper, large series utilizing this 360-degree incision were reported with results ranging from very good to excellent. Despite these favorable reports, general surgical and colon and rectal textbooks of the early twentieth century treated the Whitehead hemorrhoidectomy rather perfunctorily. Matthews, in 1893, asserted that the Whitehead procedure was seldom indicated, while Decosta, in his 1894 textbook, stated that "only a surgeon who can master violent hemorrhage should venture to perform the Whitehead hemorrhoidectomy". By 1923, even Lockhart-Mummery, because of his disdain for the original procedure, spoke of a modified Whitehead hemorrhoidectomy.

The 1930s marked the beginning of the thirty-year period during which the term Whitehead hemorrhoidectomy almost disappeared from the literature as various authors shunned the name Whitehead and presented their own radical procedures. Buie (1932), Fansler (1933), and others utilized the circumferential technique with certain modifications, the most common being the use of sliding skin grafts to prevent the two most dreaded complications: mucosal ectropion and ano-rectal stricture. Anatomic studies by such seminal physicians as Goligher, Parks, and Morgan and Thompson in the 1950s, and the development of colon and rectal fellowships in the United States culminated in the 1970s with a renaissance in colon and rectal surgery. Highly specialized surgeons began to reintroduce good-to-glowing reports of the Whitehead hemorrhoidectomy. What, then, is the reason for the demise of the Whitehead hemorrhoidectomy during the early part of the century? I believe it was secondary to the confusing and oftentimes misleading terminology of the anatomy presented in the general surgical and colon and rectal textbooks.

Mr Whitehead stressed that the incision be made at the mucocutaneous junction. Although, today, we take for granted that this is the dentate line, this was not always the case. Textbooks of general surgery published in the mid-1800s to the 1950s differ in the nomenclature and the anatomic terms used to describe the area of the ano-rectum. Keen's general surgical textbook published in 1908 spoke of the white line of Hilton as the mucocutaneous junction. This error was echoed by authors Andrews, Bodkin, Gant and Lockhart-Mummery. Although Buie described the correct anatomy accurately and succinctly in 1932, the picture portraying the anatomy during his amputative hemorrhoidectomy is thought by some to be misleading.

In his original description, Hilton stated that his white line was the mucocutaneous junction. The accompanying figures showed the line to be the caudal edge of the internal sphincters seen through the anoderm. In an informal study by the author, the distance between the dentate line and the white line of Hilton was measured in thirty consecutive patients undergoing ano-rectal surgery. The distances range from 0.3–2.0 cm with a mean of 1.3 cm. Therefore, mistaking the white line of Hilton for the mucocutaneous junction would mean the difference between good results and an ectropion.

Indications

Patients with circumferential prolapsing mixed hemorrhoids are candidates for the complete hemorrhoidectomy or one of its many modifications. Certain preoperative precautions should be taken when employing this hemorrhoidectomy. Contraindications to complete hemorrhoidectomy are as follows.

1. Minimal hemorrhoids.
2. Excess scar from previous disease or operation.
3. Unusually thin, tight anoderm.
4. Severe irritable bowel syndrome.
5. Any pre-existing disease or operation which results in chronic diarrhea.
6. Patient with anal incontinence.
7. Patient with incarceration, strangulation, or both who presents 24 hours or more after onset (relative contraindication).

Preoperative Preparation

All patients undergoing hemorrhoidectomy undergo preoperative flexible sigmoidoscopy and, if older than 45 years, should undergo a colon x-ray or colonoscopy to rule out an occult cause of bleeding. Special consideration is given to patients who have diarrhea to rule out the possibility of undiagnosed inflammatory bowel disease.

The patient is advised that he will be in the hospital for 1–2 days and will be able to return to work in 2–4 weeks.

Preoperative preparation includes two enemas given prior to surgery. Oral preoperative preparation is not indicated for this technique. No laxatives or antibiotics are used before or after the procedure.

Technique

Most of the procedures are performed under either general anesthesia or low spinal or saddle block. Occasionally, some women may undergo this procedure under local anesthesia supplemented by IV sedation.

All patients are placed in the jackknife position with two pillows under the hips and a pillow under the ankles assuring the patient is comfortable. The advantage to this position is that during the procedure, all bleeding that occurs will fall away from the operating field affording better visualization during the sometimes difficult dissection. No attempt is made to sterilize the skin other than using Betadine spray. The operative area is not shaved and usually the buttocks are separated by adhesive tape. In all patients undergoing this procedure, local infiltration with local anesthetic with epinephrine is used. Bupivacaine (0.25%) with 1:200,000 adrenaline is used to infiltrate both the submucosal area of the hemorrhoid and into the muscle to afford postoperative relaxation. Intravenous fluids are kept to a minimum to prevent postoperative urinary problems. No hyaluronidase (Wydase) is used.

After infiltration with local anesthetic to relax the sphincter, the anal canal is examined digitally and a Pratt bivalve speculum or Smith–Buie retractor is placed in the patient's rectum. With curved, double-pointed operating scissors, dissection is begun at the dentate line and continued along this line for a third-to-half the circumference of the anal canal. Sometimes, because of severe prolapse and/or trauma secondary to prolapse, the dentate line is difficult to identify. In this case, one must err on the conservative side and make the incision in rectal mucosa. Utilizing Allis clamps, the cut edge of the hemorrhoid-bearing rectal mucosa and associated mucosal prolapse is then gently elevated by sharp dissection from the underlying internal sphincter muscle throughout the length of the initial incision along the dentate line. The hemorrhoidal mass is then transected. The distal cut edge of anoderm is elevated and its undersurface debrided (undermined) of external varices. (Fig. 15.1). The skin tags from previous external thrombosed hemorrhoids can be removed. However, over diligence at this point can and has created flap necrosis resulting in healing by secondary intention. The same procedure is then repeated to complete the remaining circum-

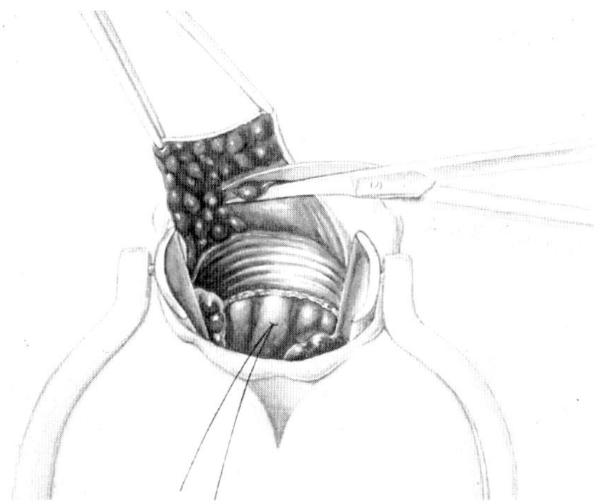

Figure 15.1. Removal of the haemorrhoids from beneath the anoderm; the haemorrhoid-bearing rectal mucosa has been transected prior to this.

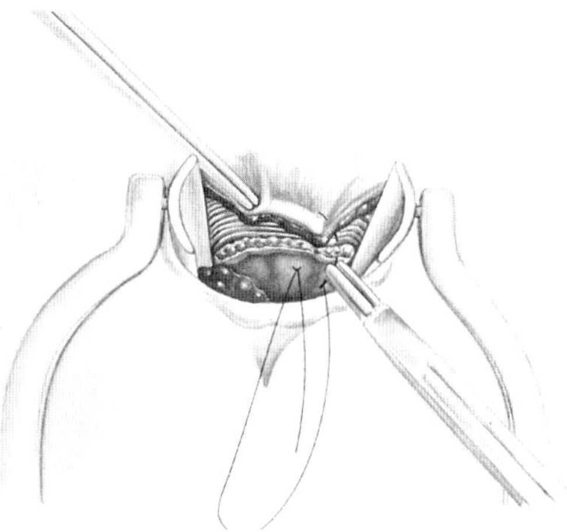

Figure 15.2. Resuture of the cut edges. Note the sutures include a portion of internal sphincter (see text).

ference. Starting posteriorly, a 3-0 Vicryl is used to perform the anastomosis between the anoderm and the rectal mucosa. It must be stressed that the suture must pass from the mucosa into the internal sphincter *at least 1 cm proximal to its distal edge* (Fig. 15.2). This maneuver is facilitated by using a retractor that stretches the internal sphincter so that its distal end is not only visualized but also palpated. This suture then catches the anoderm, which is *pulled down* (cranial) to the neodentate line (Table 15.2). This is performed from posterior (12 o'clock position) to the lateral (3 and 9 o'clock) positions. This can be done using running or interrupted sutures: I prefer interrupted. The same is then repeated from the 6 o'clock position around to both lateral aspects. When placing these sutures into the anoderm, the anoderm is pulled away from the previously placed suture. This results in a redundancy of anoderm at the lateral (3 and 9 o'clock) positions. By tenting this redundant skin upward, a lateral excision can be made perpendicular to the neodentate line as in a closed hemorrhoidectomy incision. This incision is then closed with a running 3-0 Vicryl from the dentate line out to the periphery. When the anastomosis is finished, a neomucocutaneous junction has been created. A piece of rolled gel-foam is then placed in the patient's rectum. Fluff gauze is left in place at the anal opening and is taped in place. The following are surgical imperatives:

1. The initial incision must be made either proximal to or exactly at the dentate line.
2. To recreate the mucocutaneous junction, one must approximate mucosa to the anoderm, incorporating the internal sphincter at least one centimeter proximal to its caudal edge.

Post-Operative Care

After the operation, patients are encouraged to limit their fluids until such time as they void spontaneously. The rate of catheterization after a complete hemorrhoidectomy in our hands remains between 25% and 30%. Once spontaneous voiding has taken place, patients are allowed fluid and food ad lib. During the hospitalization, IM Meperidine on demand is given routinely and is switched to oral analgesics on the day they are to be discharged. Ice packs are applied to the perineal area for the first 12 hours, followed by warm packs for the rest of their hospitalization. Patients are encouraged to take as many sitz baths as required for cleanliness and comfort throughout their postoperative period. Patients must be kept on a bulking agent to maintain an adequate anal canal diameter. Stimulant laxatives and mineral oil are not allowed, as diarrhea must be prevented. Neither rectal nor self-dilations should be necessary if a proper bowel program is established. Anti-diarrheal (Lomotil and Imodium) or narcotic analgesics may be used to promote slight constipation in patients with loose stools. If the patient does not have a bowel movement by the third postoperative day, a one-ounce dose (30 cc) of Milk of Magnesia is prescribed.

Patients return to the clinic three weeks after surgery and undergo a digital examination. If it is apparent that the patient is beginning to form a contracture, the patient is placed on an anti-diarrheal medication such as Lomotil or possibly even Codeine.

Complications

The most common complications in our series of 356 complete hemorrhoidectomies have been urinary retention as mentioned above, followed by wound complications in 9% and fecal impactions in 2%. Our rate of symptomatic contracture was five patients out of 356 complete hemorrhoidectomies. Three of these patients required a simple internal lateral sphincterotomy. There were no cases of mucosal ectropion in our series. However, if a patient does have a mucosal ectropion, he must return to the operating room for excision of the ectropion with or without a sliding skin graft.

EDITORIAL COMMENT

This may be regarded as the operation that refuses to die. As far back as the early part of the twentieth century, anxieties were evident regarding the dangers of "total hemorrhoidectomy". Anal stenosis and mucosal ectropion were especially feared. These complications were manifest to a degree that the search for safer alternatives became imperative. These consisted of sub-total removal with preservation of skin bridges, of which the Milligan–Morgan technique became a prominent example.

But sub-total hemorrhoidectomies demand excellent judgment of the amount of hemorrhoid tissue that can be removed, while at the same time, satisfactory preservation of skin bridges is achieved. This problem can become overwhelming when hemorrhoids surround the entire circumference of the anal canal. Historical reports of large series and modern papers on the results of total hemorrhoidectomies both strongly suggest that the procedure is much safer than was feared, and that the Whitehead-type procedure performed by a good technique does not have an unacceptable degree of risk.

The Editor believes that total hemorrhoidectomy is not needed for any case of hemorrhoids other than that which presents with circumferential extension that is too pronounced to be handled by filleting or skin bridge division, as described in Ch. 11. If needed, however, total hemorrhoidectomy can be used as an ethical treatment.

Summary

Although the number of surgical hemorrhoidectomies is decreasing secondary to timely office procedures in early hemorrhoidal disease, an occasional patient with circumferential prolapsing mixed hemorrhoids will present to your office. If no contraindications are present, a complete hemorrhoidectomy or one of its modifications is a viable treatment option for these patients. However, I believe that this procedure should be performed only by surgeons who are thoroughly familiar with this technique.

References

Bonello JC (1988) Who's afraid of the dentate line? The Whitehead hemorrhoidectomy. Am J Surg 156:182–6

Whitehead W (1882) The surgical treatment of hemorrhoids. BMJ 1:148–50

Whitehead W (1887) Three hundred consecutive cases of hemorrhoids cured by excision. BMJ 1:449

Wolff BG, Culp, CE (1988) The Whitehead hemorrhoidectomy. An unjustly maligned procedure. Dis Colon Rectum 31:587–90

16 Pre-, Peri- and Postoperative Management

Charles V. Mann

Preoperative Workup

Assessment

General Precautions

Although haemorrhoid operations are generally classified as minor or intermediate procedures, they often involve a general anaesthetic and are not altogether risk-free; some complications can be serious, although they are fortunately rare. For these reasons, proper attention must be paid to preoperative care. Because haemorrhoids themselves are not life threatening, if a patient suffers from a preventable complication from the operation, it is a serious reproach to his surgeon, with possible medico-legal consequences.

General areas for preoperative care may be considered under various headings, as follows.

(i) *Age.* If the patient is elderly (i.e., more than 70 years of age), serious consideration should be given as to the necessity for surgery. If the patient also suffers from age-related infirmities, an operation should be considered unduly risky unless special circumstances are operative.

(ii) *Cardio-vascular problems.* Minor degrees of hypertension can be accepted (although consideration should be given to any medications used). Significant high-blood-pressure problems, a history of cardiac failure or myocardial infarction, or any other serious pathological condition of the cardiovascular system must always involve consultation with medical colleagues as to the advisability of surgery, as well as their involvement in the patient's care over the operation period. A recent history of myocardial infarction or cerebro-vascular incident are contraindications to surgery. In all cases, the anaesthetist should be warned about potential problems arising from cardiovascular sources, so that he can take the necessary precautions (e.g., as to whether an adrenaline infiltration should be used at operation). A preoperative ECG should be arranged in all cases where cardiovascular disease may lead to problems, and should be assessed by a competent expert.

If the patient has a history of heart-valve abnormality, prophylactic antibiotics must be given to cover the operation to prevent infective endocarditis.

(iii) *Pulmonary diseases.* To reduce postoperative chest infections, cigarette smoking should be stopped at least two weeks preoperatively (although many patients may clandestinely ignore this advice). Treatment by physiotherapy and preoperative antibiotics may be required for patients who suffer from chronic bronchitis. If chronic obstructive airway disease were present, a haemorrhoidectomy would be considered an extremely risky treatment to advise, unless the condition was extremely mild; however, even a mild case might require specialised care postoperatively in an intensive care unit.

A chest x-ray is regarded as a necessary part of preoperative workup for all patients about to undergo an operation under general anaesthesia. Lung-function tests are indicated for all patients with obstructive airway problems, and their results must be taken into careful consideration before operation is advised.

(iv) *Diabetes*. This should have an expert planned programme for control over the entire operation period, especially the 24 hours of surgery and postoperative recovery. Blood sugar levels should be properly monitored, and a medical colleague may assist with treatment, although the anaesthetist should have primary responsibility.

(v) *Renal diseases*. Unless renal failure is present, haemorrhoidectomy can be advised, but renal disease may affect choice of drugs which may be given to the patient, as well as their dosage.

(vi) *Prostate enlargement*. The risk of postoperative retention if the patient has an enlarged prostate is quite high, and is increased further by epidural or spinal anaesthesia (which should be avoided whenever possible). The patient should be aware of this possibility, and of any treatments which may be required, e.g., an indwelling catheter, or even a prostatectomy. Emptying the bladder immediately prior to surgery, by a catheter if necessary, reduces the chance of retention, and should be done in all patients considered to be at particular risk.

(vii) *Urine infection*. Any urinary infection, from whatever cause, should be cleared up preoperatively.

(viii) *Porphyria*. Because an attack of acute porphyria can be precipitated by anaesthetic drugs (e.g., alcuronium, barbiturates, enflurane, etomidate, halothane, thiopentone and many others) and by many drugs that may be needed for postoperative care (e.g., analgesics, antibiotics), any history of this rare condition should figure prominently in the patient's records so that suitable precautions can be taken (the list of "unsafe" drugs to use should be consulted).

(ix) *Drugs*. The drug history is an important part of preoperative workup. Particular note should be made of the following preparations, for the reasons given: (a) Contraceptive drugs, because of increased risk for postoperative thrombo-embolic phenomena. (b) Monoamine oxidase antidepressants, because of potential anaesthetic complications (e.g., large rise in blood pressure). (c) Fenfluramine (appetite suppression) because of interactions with anaesthetic agents. (d) Tranquillisers and other drugs for disorders of the CNS, which may cause intra-operative control of the blood pressure difficult. (e) Anticoagulants, which includes liberal use of aspirin, as these may promote haemorrhage. All medications used by the patient, with their doses, need to be recorded and many need to be stopped for at least two weeks prior to surgery, e.g., the contraceptive pill.

(x) *Anaesthetics*. Enquiry should be made about previous anaesthetics, and especially if any untoward reactions were experienced. A history of a recent halogen-based anaesthetic should be sought (as for dental extraction, for example) because there is evidence that early exposure to further use of such agents may be associated with dangerous side effects, including liver damage. Note should be made of any episode of post-anaesthetic respiratory depression, which may indicate an abnormal response to muscle relaxants.

(xi) *Obesity*. Pronounced obesity, but short of morbid obesity, may cause difficulties, such as anaesthetic problems (especially in the prone face-down position); increased intra-operative bleeding (from engorgement of the anal veins due to pressure on the abdominal veins, especially in the lithotomy position); satisfactory access to the operative field may be impeded. Morbid obesity is a contraindication to operation.

In most clinics, preoperative assessment includes some routine screening tests as follows.

(a) Profile of normal blood values. The haemoglobin level is particularly important, but all can be of value for a diagnostic overview.

(b) Sickle cell test. The sickle cell trait, and sickle cell disease, are no longer confined to particular groups, and should be excluded by routine testing.

(c) Blood group (and Save serum). Although a blood transfusion is hardly ever needed, if one becomes necessary it is usually in the context of an unexpected severe haemorrhage.

(d) Chest x-ray. Although the need for a routine preoperative chest x-ray is not universally agreed, the author believes this simple, cheap precaution is wise to obtain, especially if a general anaesthetic is planned.

(e) Urinalysis for protein and sugar. *It needs to be emphasised that if preoperative screening tests are ordered, they must be looked at.* There is no defence in law if misdiagnosis occasions complications which could have been avoided if the tests had been examined: for example, if the presence of diabetes or sickle cell disease has not been picked up.

The possibility of HIV presence cannot be tested for in the UK without the patient's permission. In other countries, this rule does not apply. If the presence of HIV (let alone AIDS) is suspected but is not proven (or excluded beyond all doubt by a negative test) the patient should be treated as if he was infected: in almost all circumstances, surgery should be avoided (see Ch. 23 for further information) and office treatments preferred.

Perineal and Anal Problems

Many of the local problems which can influence surgical management are dealt with in the chapters describing individual operations. However, many of them apply to all procedures, and those which deserve additional discussion are as follows.

(i) *Skin infections.* The moist environment of the perineum and anal regions provide ideal conditions for growth of bacteria and fungi. Spread of fungal infections from the vagina to the perianal skin is not uncommon. Sexually transmitted diseases can be transferred to the anus in both hetero-and homosexual individuals. Surgery in the face of active infections affecting the skin in and around the anorectum is contraindicated, not only because of the obvious risk of surgical complications, but also because of the hazards to medical staff. The special problem of HIV infection is discussed in Ch. 23.

Fungal infections (e.g., candidiasis) can almost always be eliminated by appropriate treatment in the waiting period for surgery.

Warts (papilloma virus infection) may respond to applications of topical medicaments (e.g., Podophyllin ointment). Florid manifestations of warts usually require surgical intervention for their elimination (e.g., by "scissor excision" technique), and it is wise not to combine this with any treatment for haemorrhoids unless only a few isolated warts are present. If warts have been treated but haemorrhoids are still causing symptoms that justify intervention, it is best to carry out their treatment expeditiously, as mucus discharge from the piles can encourage recurrence of the warts.

(ii) *Skin diseases.* The squamous epithelium of the lower anal canal, as well as the perianal skin itself, can be affected by any dermatological condition. Eczema and psoriasis are not infrequently present.

Every effort should be made to clear up any skin disease prior to surgery, but non-operative treatments are not contraindicated. The patient should be warned that treatment for the piles will not affect any symptoms that are caused by their skin ailment, e.g., pruritus.

Anal malignancies can cause serious difficulties for diagnosis and management in a patient who presents with haemorrhoids (Bowen's intra-epithelial carcinoma can be overlooked quite easily). If the patient suffers from thrombosis of their haemorrhoids, a small anal carcinoma can be disguised; if a malignant ulcer is present, this can be ascribed to the thrombosis unless a high index of suspicion (which should be aroused by *any* ulcer of the ano-rectum) prompts immediate recourse to a biopsy of the ulcer.

Leukaemia infiltrates may occur in the anal region, and have a characteristic bluish-red colour in many instances, which is combined with firmness on digital pressure. Leukaemia and polycythaemia rubra vera can both promote thrombosis in haemorrhoids.

(iii) *Skin sensitivity manifestations.* Longstanding applications of steroid-containing preparations can cause thinning and depigmentation of the perianal skin. *Atopy* causes eczematoid manifestations and blistering of the anal skin, which can lie behind chronic use of topical steroids. The consequences of steroid use include delayed or faulty healing of wounds, so that, despite the difficulties posed for the relief of the patient's symptoms, such topical applications should be discontinued for several months before a surgical operation. Steroids may also be an important factor for promoting anal infections, another reason for their discontinuance.

Before they ever consult a proctologist, many patients have used over-the-counter remedies, often for many years. Considerable numbers of them develop sensitivity to these preparations and suffer from an inflamed, soggy anal skin. Even such "simple" preparations as zinc oxide cream can cause an allergic response, and preparations containing local anaesthetic are notorious for causing such sudden severe reactions that they precipitate an emergency consultation. For any patient in whom there is any reason to believe that a sensitivity reaction is responsible for skin damage around the anus, the wise decision must be to postpone any surgical treatment until stopping the antigen stimulus has allowed the skin to recover. If the patient is allergic to local anaesthetics, these must not be used during any haemorrhoid operation.

(iv) *Other local conditions*. Dermatitis resulting from mucus leakage can be severe, and the inflamed fissured skin which characterises the condition can cause considerable operative difficulties, as well as interfere with wound healing after a haemorrhoidectomy. In most cases, preoperative treatment based on avoidance of overexposure to water (i.e., too many baths or swabbings) and the use of barrier creams (E45; Vasogen; zinc and castor oil) will lead to improvement that is sufficient to permit surgery; non-operative treatments (e.g., banding) are not contraindicated by dermatitis, and as efficient treatment of the mucus leakage problem depends upon elimination of its haemorrhoidal (or other) cause, these should be offered at the same time as other treatments of the skin.

Bowel Regulation

Although special precautions regarding bowel regulation are described for many of the individual procedures described in the appropriate chapters, certain general principles apply to surgical treatment, and these can be usefully applied to a patient's preoperative assessment.

No patient should be admitted for an elective haemorrhoidectomy without previous instruction for achieving regular unforced defaecation, preferably on a daily basis. The stools should have soft consistency ("putty-like" is a frequent description) and be of reasonable size ("sausage (not chipolata) shaped"). If bowel movements are irregular (both too few or too often are equally undesirable); or the stools are too hard; or straining defaecation is uncorrected, the circumstances are in place for postoperative problems, and it is usually too late for their correction when the patient is admitted. The best ways to optimise defaecatory actions are described in Ch. 6, with the mainstays of treatment being plentiful fluids, extra roughage in the diet, and increased exercise. The patient should always come to surgery weaned off any reliance on laxatives or other stimulating preparations. The emphasis on increased fluid intake, which is the keystone of the anti-constipation arch, is convincingly justified when it is remembered that small bowel "enemas" (i.e., a fluid overload) can be used as a means to evacuate the colon.

In the first 24–48 hours after haemorrhoidectomy, the advisability of early passage of a formed stool, however soft, may need to be modified for some procedures. If a closed haemorrhoidectomy has been performed, for instance, early stretching of the anal wounds is undesirable. For such cases, the stools may need to be loose for the first few days, and a twice-daily dose of magnesium sulphate (5–10 gm) or Lactulose (15 ml) are good preparations to use for this purpose. It is the author's practise to advise such medication after a Milligan–Morgan open haemorrhoidectomy in order to reduce pain and to encourage early defaecation postoperatively.

Once the early postoperative period is over, and defaecation has been established, the rules for each patient's bowel regulation, which have been delineated by the preoperative assessment, should be reverted to.

Antibiotic Policies

Prophylactic antibiotics are not required for haemorrhoid operations except for special indications, to be discussed. However, no patient should come to surgery without an enquiry as to any known, or possible, allergy to antibiotics. Certain problems require the use of antibiotics as part of preparations for surgery, as follows:

(i) *Heart-valve disorders and prostheses*. If a patient has a heart-valve disorder, or has undergone valve-replacement surgery, any haemorrhoid procedure must be covered by prophylactic antibiotics to prevent infective endocarditis.

(ii) *Chronic bronchitis and smoking.* Cigarette smoking should be discontinued for two weeks prior to haemorrhoid surgery. Chronic bronchitis, especially if purulent sputum is manifest, should be treated preoperatively by physiotherapy and a course of antibiotics to eliminate bacterial presence. Acute upper respiratory tract infection is a contraindication to surgical intervention. Immune deficiency, either known or suspected, is an indication for prophylactic antibiotic cover of haemorrhoid surgery if there is justification by powerful arguments to permit surgical intervention in such a situation. The special circumstance of haemorrhoid interventions in patients with HIV infection is discussed in Ch. 23. Urinary tract infections should be eliminated before admission for operation, and a male patient with an enlarged prostate causing symptoms of prostatism should have their operation covered by a single IV prophylactic dose of a suitable antibiotic, e.g., Ampicillin 1.0 gm IV.

(iii) *Anal sepsis.* In the special circumstances of an emergency operation, e.g., for strangulated piles, the severity and risks of any anal sepsis must be assessed preoperatively. If any infectious risk is suspected, antibiotic cover should be given, which should include an antibiotic active against anaerobic bacteria (e.g., Metronidazole 400 mg daily for five days).

Anxiety Management

Almost every patient approaches haemorrhoid surgery with anxiety, and often with dread. Most patients anticipate severe pain, and view any reassurances by their surgeon with scepticism. Anxiety can aggravate problems of management after surgery, especially for achieving early defaecation, and some patients of especially nervous disposition may deserve preoperative treatment if this is recognised either by their demeanour or by their medical history. If a patient who is advised to have a haemorrhoidectomy exhibits an unusual degree of anxiety, he/she should be given a course of the appropriate anxiolytic or tranquilliser (Diazepam 10–15 mg daily in divided doses is often a good choice). It should be remembered that constipation is a side effect of such drugs, and may need preventive measures.

When the patient is admitted, it may be necessary to treat an acutely anxious subject, with the caution that this must not increase anaesthetic risks. It is desirable that the patient should be calmed, as overanxiety may increase the need for postoperative opiates, make bowel regulation difficult and increase risk for postoperative retention of faeces. Judicious use of a tranquiliser can resolve this difficulty.

Regulation of Food and Drink

It has been stressed elsewhere that all haemorrhoid patients should be given active management of their diet, and encouraged to take plenty of liquids (water, principally). Once the patient is admitted, he/she should be encouraged to take plenty of fluids, as a temporary fluid excess will mitigate the inevitable tendency to dehydration (associated with an operation under a general anaesthetic), which promotes, in turn, a hard stool. Intake of coffee and tea should be reduced to a minimum as caffeine can be constipating.

Food intake should be restricted to small quantities of easily digested, non-spicy, products. Bulking agents and laxatives should be discontinued preoperatively.

Prevention of Deep-vein Thrombosis

Female patients should have been advised to stop the contraceptive pill at least 10 days before they are admitted for operation. Sometimes, however, patients are admitted who are at increased risk of deep-vein thrombosis (e.g., a past history of thrombosis; prominent varicose veins; have not stopped the Pill; have mobility problems) and require this risk to be diminished by specific therapy. This should include anti-thrombosis stockings, and can occasionally require the operation to be covered by low-dose subcutaneous injection of anti-coagulant at the time of surgery (e.g., Minihep Calcium 0.2 ml is often suitable, but the dose must be determined by the patient's weight so as not to increase surgical haemorrhage). It is always better to cancel the operation than to take an unjustified risk of thromboembolism.

Haemorrhage Risks

Some patients present risks of increased surgical blood loss. In many cases, all that is required is for them to stop taking large doses of aspirin or other NSAID 24–48 hours before the operation. If a patient is admitted who is taking anti-coagulants for a serious health hazard (cardiac or cerebral vascular incident), it is urgently necessary to consider the justification for surgery; in most cases, it is clearly imperative to cancel the operation, and since the operation could only be performed after planned reversal of the anti-coagulant therapy, the author has never been able to defend this in the context of haemorrhoid surgery.

Perioperative Precautions

This section outlines simple precautions taken at the time of surgery that can make haemorrhoid operations cleaner, simpler and more comfortable, as well as shortening healing time. Added together, they can make the difference between a grateful patient and a critical one. The period covered is from the final hours in the ward to the twelfth postoperative hour, after which, full recovery from anaesthesia can be anticipated.

(i) *Preoperative rectal evacuation.* The patient should be told to have a satisfactory defaecation within six hours of surgery. If this does not occur, a stimulatory mini (Fleet) enema should be given shortly before pre-medication. If the surgeon finds delegation of these decisions is unsatisfactory (and patients appear in the operation room with significant faecal presence in the rectum), it is best to make a preoperative enema (or even two) a routine requirement.

(ii) *Pre-medication.* Although many surgeons and anaesthetists would disagree, the author is in favour of pre-medication. A premedication not only lessens preoperative anxiety but also reduces the need for anaesthetic drugs and gases; postoperative recovery is often smoother, and the doses of pain-killing drugs, especially opiates, are reduced. For day-case surgery, a premedication is usually omitted as the prime consideration must be for early recovery from the anaesthetic.

(iii) *Low-spinal, epidural and caudal anaesthesia.* All three techniques (low spinal, epidural, caudal) are used to provide anaesthesia for the anal region, as well as local infiltration nerve blocking procedures. They can be used to substitute for a general anaesthetic (as for many day-case procedures) or to supplement a general anaesthetic. In the case of epidural anaesthesia, the line can be left in place to facilitate postoperative pain control if this is judged desirable. Where the surgeon is able to influence the decision as to the use of these techniques, he should recall their well-known tendency to increase the incidence of postoperative retention of urine. The author has only used local and regional anaesthetic techniques for day-case surgery, and caudal (sacral) anaesthesia has been favoured.

(iv) *Rectal cleansing.* After the patient has been positioned for the operation, digital examination should be performed to check for rectal faecal content. If, despite every precaution (see (i) above), a significant degree of faecal presence is discovered, this should be evacuated, either using moist finger swabs or a low rectal washout through a proctoscope. Care must be taken to evacuate all liquid residues before proceeding.

(v) *Skin preparation.* Use of a coloured antiseptic solution is desirable, so that all areas are treated, and that excessive amounts are not applied. Certain features are very important: (a) the solution should not be chemically damaging (e.g., mercury-containing solutions should not be used), (b) the solution should be hypoallergenic (e.g., iodine-containing solutions should be avoided), and (c) the solution should be non-flammable (e.g., spirit-based antiseptics should be shunned). Too-liberal application of *any* solution, however carefully chosen, can lead to pooling around the operation field, with consequent risk of damage to the skin. A fire hazard is a serious possibility if the solution can be ignited, for example by a diathermy spark. Skin preparation should proceed from the periphery inwards, finishing with the anus itself. Intra-anal cleansing is not required.

(vi) *Application of drapes.* Drapes should be securely fastened, and there should be a good margin between their edges and the anal region. Nothing is more disturbing than insecure drapes moving across the operation field during surgery, or skin clips falling over the anus. Drapes with preformed windows are often unsatisfactory because a standard-sized window is often either too large or too small. After years of trial and error, the author found that fastening the corners of the drapes with atraumatic silk skin sutures provided the most satisfactory solution for secure skin draping in the right positions for the individual patient.

(vii) *Local infiltration.* In most anal operations this is very desirable; the solution used should be a combination of weak adrenaline or epinephrine (1:200,000) with local anaesthetic (1% Lignocaine or Bupivacaine), and the amount used should not be more than 15 ml. The use of such infiltration is described for each operation in the requisite chapters, but their use confers the following advantages (a) a dry operation field (b) reduced intra-operative pain stimulation (c) lessened immediate postoperation pain. Many anaesthetists are reluctant to allow use of such infiltrations for fear of anaesthetic complications (e.g. cardiac irregularity if a halogen type anaesthetic is used) but such fears are misplaced if due care is taken; in particular, accidental intravenous injection must be avoided by extreme care during the infiltration.

(viii) *Anal dilation.* Anal dilatation with the fingers is usually unnecessary, especially if the surgeon uses a dilator-retractor of the Parks or Eisenhammer pattern: it may also increase problems of incontinence postoperatively. In the few patients who come to surgery with high anal tone, mild anal dilation can facilitate access to the anal canal and the bases of the haemorrhoids. "Two-finger" dilatation is usually sufficient. It is the author's view that sphincterotomy is also usually unnecessary as an adjunct to haemorrhoid surgery, but, if anal dilatation is required, it is possible that sphincterotomy should be considered as a better choice.

(ix) *Catheter use.* This has been discussed elsewhere (see preoperative workup above). In general, a catheter is not required for haemorrhoid surgery. However, all patients should have an empty bladder when they enter the operation room, and, if this not the case (or not known), a catheter should be used to empty the bladder before the patient is positioned for surgery.

(x) *Positioning.* Whether the prone or lithotomy position is employed, the end-result should be provision of: (a) excellent access to the operation field, (b) unimpeded space for the surgeon (and an assistant if one is required), (c) perfect lighting, which should be focussed on the anal region, (d) maximum comfort for surgeon, assistant and scrub nurse, who should be seated whenever possible, (e) easy availability for any surgical instruments and (f) maximal opportunities for team participation.

Postoperative Care

This section deals only with broad general principles of postoperative care, the details of which may need to be adapted for particular techniques.

(i) *Pain relief.* Relief of postoperative pain is a priority for postoperative management; there is never any justification for allowing an excessive degree of suffering. It is claimed (although trials have not fully substantiated this) that closed wounds are less painful than open ones, but in both cases defaecation can be extremely painful for the first few days; after five days, pain diminishes rapidly.

The first defaecation. When a patient realises that his/her first defaecation is imminent, a timely injection of pethidine (100 mg) can be extremely helpful. However, in most cases this is not practical. It has already been advised that an over-anxious patient should be calmed with an anxiolytic or tranquilliser (p. 113), and, other than this, most pain relief must concentrate on adequate control of post-defaecation pain. For this, the use of opiates is the best remedy; a small immediate intravenous dose of pethidine (25 mg) is very effective, which can be prolonged by a synchronous, more slowly acting, subcutaneous or intramuscular injection (75–100 mg) of the same drug.

Subsequent defaecations. Although opiates should be used freely when indicated for initial defaecation, they should not be employed for subsequent episodes, as the patient may come to rely on them. For later defaecations, non-constipating oral analgesics are usually sufficient (e.g., sublingual buprenorphine, 400 mg is a useful drug, but others are available), and after the fourth or fifth postoperative day, mild analgesics, such as paracetamol tablets, are all that are required.

Some evidence has been produced that oral Metronidazole (400 mg daily for five days) reduces postoperative pain. If this accords with a surgeon's own experience (and this is not always the case) there seems to be no contraindication to prescribing this antibiotic, as it is remarkably free from side effects. Patients must be warned strongly against alcoholic drinks, however, as Metronidazole has Antabuse-like properties.

In addition to drugs, post-defaecation pain responds to immediate hot soaks, which is in any case an essential element of cleansing the anal wounds from faecal contamination (see next).

(ii) *Wound Care.* As with other anal wounds, post-haemorrhoidectomy wounds should be kept clean by regular hot baths, which also get rid of blood and other debris. If the anal wound is an *open* one, lengthy immersion is an advantage, and there is no evidence that this damages the tissues or delays healing; for *closed* wounds, prolonged immersion is not only unnecessary but may cause early separation of the suture line, and should therefore be avoided. Crystals of salt or an antiseptic solution (e.g., Ster-Zac) can be added to the bathwater at the surgeon's discretion but there is no evidence for their efficaciousness.

If adherent blood or debris does not come away with hot bathing, wound irrigations with a detergent solution or a desloughing agent (e.g., hydrogen peroxide, benzoic acid) can be helpful. If a syringe and nozzle are used, the solutions can be directed at particular areas needing special attention.

Local dressings that are applied to anal wounds tend to adhere, and removal can be painful; they also retain faecal particles, as well as smelly discharges, thus exposing the wounds to extra risks of contamination and delayed healing. For these reasons, they should not be used. Instead, frequent bathing, with in-between applications of a light cream or ointment, and the anal wounds protected by a soft absorbent pad, are all that are required. If anal wounds are kept clean, they are extremely resistant to septic complications and heal rapidly. The author is prepared to state categorically that frequent baths with applications of ointments do not interfere with the speed or the strength of wound healing.

If a dressing has been placed in the anal canal to control postoperative oozing, or if a pack has been required (which should be a very rare occurrence), it should always be removed early, at the latest by the first postoperative day. In most cases, removal in the ward can be achieved without difficulty, and is made bearable for the patient by a preliminary hot soak and the use of intravenous morphine (5–10 mg) at the moment that the dressing is pulled free. If a small residual piece of gauze or cotton wool remains behind, this can be left to separate of its own accord at subsequent defaecations, without impairing healing. If it is found that a dressing or pack will need considerable force to remove, with attendant danger for starting bleeding, it is best to arrange a brief anaesthetic, rather than cause an agonising episode that is also potentially risky. Replacement of an anal dressing or pack is rarely required.

Patients need to be warned that loss of *small* amounts of bright red blood is not unusual during the healing period after a haemorrhoidectomy and may be experienced for several weeks. *Large* blood loss is *not* usual and generally accompanies a complication, such as secondary haemorrhage. Immediate recourse to medical help is indicated, with hospital admission a necessity in almost all cases.

(iii) *Bowel Management.* This has been alluded to earlier (p. 112). The principles that underlie proper bowel regulation post-haemorrhoidectomy are: (a) early defaecation, to start postoperatively before the third or fourth day, and preferably within the first 48 hours, (b) rapid transformation of early abnormal ("watery") postoperative stools to the desirable normal shape and consistency, and (c) establishment of regular (once daily is ideal) non-straining defaecation. The means to achieve these ends are described in Ch. 6).

(iv) *Digital Examination.* The necessity for finger examination after haemorrhoid surgery is controversial. Many surgeons believe it is unnecessary, especially after a closed haemorrhoidectomy when they fear that it may cause disruption of the suture lines. For those surgeons who do not recommend digital examination as a routine, there remains the problem of ensuring that it is carried out when it is necessary.

After an open haemorrhoidectomy, provided satisfactory skin bridges are preserved and passage of formed stools is established within a few days, digital examination is not mandatory. *After a closed haemorrhoidectomy*, provided near-normal defaecation is taking place by the end of the first week, digital examination is never required until the final check-up is carried out after several weeks; it is to be noted that watery stools are desirable for the first postoperative week to minimise disruption of suture lines by faecal trauma.

Indications for digital examination after open haemorrhoidectomy include: (a) doubts concerning the skin bridges, (b) failure to pass stool by the end of the fourth postoperation day, and (c) unusually severe postoperative pain.

After all haemorrhoid operations, if digital examination reveals any degree of narrowing, remedial action is called for. This consists of daily passage of a finger until the patient has been trained to use a dilator (e.g., medium-size St. Marks pattern anal dilator) once or twice daily. *Anal stenosis* should never occur but if, despite every precaution, this does happen, operative measures may be needed, as described under complications (Ch. 20); early anal stenosis that is free from dense fibrosis can respond to anal dilation under anaesthesia, followed by regular dilatations for at least several months, until the fibrous tissue has matured.

Some simple precautions can make a postoperative digital examination less painful: (a) a pain-killing injection can be given prior to the procedure, (b) the patient should be reassured that the examination will not be done without sensitivity to their discomfort, (c) the finger should be covered in a *smooth* rubber finger stall (not a crinkly plastic sheath) and be well lubricated; a local anaesthetic gel (Lidothesin; 1% Xylocaine gel) may add some topical analgesic effect to supplement their lubricant properties, (d) the anal verge should be generously smeared with gel prior to finger insertion, (e) the finger should be inserted very slowly and gently with a slight rotary motion, (f) once inserted to its full extent it should be kept still for a short while before completing the examination; this allows any anal spasm to subside, and the anaesthetic properties of the gel to take effect, (f) the anal examination, once started, should be unhurried but thorough, and conducted with constant verbal reassurance, and (g) once the examination is complete, the finger should be withdrawn as slowly and gently as it was inserted; rapid digital extraction produces sphincter spasm, and further pain. These "rules" may seem obvious, but on too many occasions postoperative digital examination is carried out abruptly at the bedside without any thought for the inevitable pain it produces; "do as you would done by" should be the guiding principle to prevent intense pain, which can lead to an unsatisfactory examination.

If an attempt at postoperative digital examination proves impossible because of patients' resistance or anal narrowing, an immediate examination under anaesthesia should be arranged. Under anaesthesia, a narrowed anus can be dilated and/or any faecal retention can be relieved by an immediate rectal washout. If the anal narrowing is slight and superficial, once it has been dilated, it should not require any further treatment (although the usual need to establish early normal defaecation must be satisfied). If there is any doubt that the narrowing down could recur, use of a dilator (see next) is indicated.

(v) *Use of a dilator.* Use of an anal dilator is only necessary for rare and specific indications. Nevertheless, its employment should be skilful, which indicates the necessity for discussion. The most important indication is to assist in the correction of postoperative anal stenosis that is not so severe that operative correction is necessary.

The medium-size St. Marks dilator, or a Hegar dilator of equivalent diameter, are both suitable for the correction of minor degrees of anal narrowing, and patients are easily trained in their use. In almost all cases, the dilator is employed after the anus has been dilated digitally (see previous section), but in rare instances it can be used to prevent the anus narrowing down after a difficult haemorrhoidectomy, especially if skin bridges are deficient in any way.

The dilator should be well lubricated with a light gel (e.g., K-Y jelly); local anaesthetic gels should not be used as there is a risk of sensitisation with long-term, frequent applications, and ointments are both sticky and less effective. The dilator should be inserted slowly to the required length (to the shoulder of the St. Marks dilator) and held in place for several minutes, before being removed equally slowly.

If a patient has difficulty in establishing normal defaecation postoperatively, and if the surgeon suspects that they may revert to bad defaecatory patterns when they leave hospital (food fads, laxative use, curry diets, etc.), it is sometimes wise to insist on daily passage of a dilator until healing is complete. It should be stressed that development of postoperative anal stenosis is virtually impossible if a dilator is used properly for the four to six weeks that the anal wounds take to heal post-haemorrhoidectomy; this can be a valuable defence against an accusation of negligent surgery, which is more likely from eccentric or mentally unstable patients. But, it must be stressed that it is the responsibility of the surgeon to ensure that the patient is trained to use the dilator correctly, preferably by personal observation or, at least, by delegation to suitably trained staff.

(vi) *Discharge policy.* Only when the surgeon is satisfied by the provisions for proper outpatient care, and that all precautions are in place for the prevention and management of any complications, is a patient's discharge from hospital advisable.

The patient should be provided with any necessary supplies of medicines (e.g., analgesics, local applications) and dressings until alternative sources are available. A discharge note should be provided giving details of treatment, and the date for return to the hospital. The aftercare of day-case operations needs special arrangements (see Ch. 24). If the patient does not have access to medical help from a community doctor, or receive visits from a designated nurse, they must know how they can contact the hospital in the event that an emergency situation arises; the possibility of ambulance transport is desirable.

Summation

A technically proficient operation is the essential basis for the best possible result of a haemorrhoidectomy. However, a good operation can be ruined by incorrect or ill-judged management. Therefore, attention to the details of pre-, peri- and postoperative care are very important; sadly, these are areas which are often ignored by surgeons, who are happy to leave them to juniors or nurses until a problem arises. One of the great colo-rectal surgeons of the past, W.B. Gabriel, dressed the wounds of his patients personally; we should learn from his example that careful focus on key elements of peri-operative care can pay rich dividends for a successful result. For this reason, even "trivial" subjects, such as digital examination, have been given a prominent position in this chapter.

EDITORIAL COMMENT

The degree of care exercised by a surgeon in the peri-operative management of his haemorrhoid cases will be rewarded in equal measure by the gratitude of his patients. All surgeons should exhibit an equal amount of skill in ward bedside matters as that which they devote to the operation itself. Only if they do so can they consider themselves masters of their craft. Pain relief after haemorrhoidectomy is made difficult by peaking during defecation, which makes analgesia liable to over- or under-treatment. Over-treatment is better than under-treatment, and if pain is effectively relieved by timely resort to opiates (NSAIDs and buprenorphine), many other complications (urinary and faecal retention, for example) can be prevented.

17 The Operative Treatment by, and Results of, Diathermy Haemorrhoidectomy

F. Seow-Choen and K.S. Ho

Introduction

Although most patients with symptomatic haemorrhoids may be successfully managed without the need for surgery, there are still a large number of patients who require surgical excision of haemorrhoids. In our department from April 1989 to May 1998, a total of 9,693 haemorrhoidectomies were performed.

Surgical excision of haemorrhoids is notorious for severe postoperative pain. The amount of postoperative pain is highly variable, and depends on factors such as individual pain threshold, racial and cultural differences, quality and type of anaesthesia, postoperative analgesia, and the surgical technique. Some of these factors are more important than others in decreasing postoperative pain. For the surgeon, it is attractive that certain surgical techniques result in fewer postoperative complications and cause less pain than other techniques.

There have been many modifications of surgical technique in attempts to reduce pain. The use of anal dilatation has been shown to reduce post-haemorrhoidectomy pain (Watts et al., 1964; Goligher et al., 1969). However, this was associated with an increased risk of severe sphincter damage and anal incontinence. Laser haemorrhoidectomy was also believed to be less painful and bloody. However, expensive and cumbersome equipment as well as lengthy training has limited its widespread use (Wang et al., 1991).

Milligan–Morgan's open haemorrhoidectomy, in which the wound is left open, is commonly used in some parts of the world, while others believe in Ferguson's closed haemorrhoidectomy in which the mucosa and skin are closed after removal of the haemorrhoids. Whitehead described a radical method for treatment of circumferential haemorrhoids. In all of these techniques, the haemorrhoidal tissues were dissected using scissors and the vascular pedicles were ligated. The use of diathermy in the past was frowned upon as it was thought to result in increased postoperative pain. The converse, however, is nearer the truth, and diathermy haemorrhoidectomy results in less pain postoperatively.

We use diathermy alone, without scissors, for the dissection and division of the haemorrhoidal tissues. This may be adapted for all the different techniques of haemorrhoidectomy that have been described. Diathermy (Valley-Lab, Boulder, CO) is set in pure coagulation mode, with a high value of between seven and eight.

Patients are normally placed in the lithotomy position and can be operated under general, regional, or even local anaesthesia. There is no need to infiltrate the area with adrenaline prior to the procedure although this can be used if desired. Anal dilatation is not performed as it may cause uncontrolled fragmentation of the anal sphincter and anal incontinence. The anus is not packed as it contributes to anal spasm and increases postoperative pain.

Postoperative care includes oral analgesics, topical 2% lignocaine jelly and dietary fibre additives. A laxative may also be given for the first two or three postoperative days. A micronized flavonidic frac-tion is usually given as well to reduce the risk of post-haemorrhoidectomy haemorrhage (Ho et al., 1995). In addition, local perineal hygiene is maintained by regular cleaning with tap water from a shower spray. Sitz baths are more cumbersome but may be used if desired.

Open Haemorrhoidectomy

This is an adaptation of the Milligan–Morgan method of open haemorrhoidectomy. After displaying the haemorrhoidal tissue, the mucocutaneous junction is cut with diathermy. Each pedicle is dissected with diathermy in coagulation mode to its apex above the dentate line, and excess haemorrhoidal tissue is amputated by diathermy without transfixion suture or ligature. Adequate mucosal bridges must be preserved. Local 0.5% bupivacaine infiltration is used at the end of the procedure for postoperative anaesthesia.

We compared the results of using scissors and diathermy for open haemorrhoidectomy (Seow-Choen et al., 1992). Forty-nine consecutive patients with symptomatic prolapsed piles that were unsuitable for or had failed non-excisional treatment were recruited into the study. They were randomised prospectively for conventional scissors excision with ligation or for diathermy excision. A randomisation ratio of one conventional scissors haemorrhoidectomy to two diathermy haemorrhoidectomies was chosen. This was because diathermy haemorrhoidectomy was a new technique then, and its numbers were increased to enhance any difference that may result from this technique.

Sixteen patients in the scissors group underwent conventional scissors haemorrhoidectomy. After local infiltration with 1:20,000 adrenaline in 0.5% bupivacaine, each haemorrhoid was dissected free with scissors. The pedicle was isolated and transfixed, after which excess haemorrhoidal tissue was amputated. Haemostasis was completed with coagulation diathermy. Thirty-three patients had diathermy haemorrhoidectomy as described above.

The median time for the surgery was 20 minutes (range 10–40 minutes) and 10 minutes (range 5–35 minutes) for scissors excision and diathermy groups, respectively ($p < 0.05$). Both groups stayed a median of three days (range two to five days) for the surgery. Each patient was given a chart to document the average amount of pain for eight postoperative days. This was done using a linear analogue scale of 0 to 10, with 0 being no pain and 10 being the most severe pain ever experienced by the patient. The amount of analgesics required and the number of bowel movements were also documented.

There was no statistical difference in the severity of postoperative pain between the two groups. However, the use of oral analgesics was significantly lower in the diathermy group ($p < 0.02$). There was no significant difference between the two groups in terms of intramuscular pethidine or topical analgesic requirement.

The median length of follow-up was 35 weeks in both groups (range 20–50 weeks in the scissors group and 20–51 weeks in the diathermy group). Three patients in the scissors group and one patient in the diathermy group developed mild anal stricture, which were adequately treated by bulk laxatives alone. All wounds in both groups healed completely. There was no incidence of post-haemorrhoidectomy bleeding or incontinence in either group.

We concluded that diathermy excision of haemorrhoids was a significantly faster procedure than scissors excision; there was no need for ligation of the vascular pedicles, and there was a significant reduction in the oral analgesic requirements. The diathermy method does not cause any increase in early or late postoperative complications.

Bassi and Bergami (1996) also arrived at the same conclusion when they compared the results of closed haemorrhoidectomy, open scissors (Milligan–Morgan) haemorrhoidectomy and open diathermy haemorrhoidectomy without ligature of the pedicle. They studied 135 patients and found that open haemorrhoidectomy was associated with less postoperative pain, and patients in the diathermy group used less analgesic. There was also no increased risk of postoperative haemorrhage in the group without pedicle ligation.

Andrews et al. (1993), using a smaller group of only 20 patients, found that there was no difference in the duration of stay or postoperative pain. This, however, may be due to the small sample size of the study.

Closed Haemorrhoidectomy

The technique of using diathermy for dissection of haemorrhoids is also applicable to closed haemorrhoidectomy. We use a modified version of closed haemorrhoidectomy.

Following adequate anaesthesia, the haemorrhoidal columns are displayed. The haemorrhoidal tissues are then dissected free using diathermy. The vascular pedicle is isolated individually and transfixed with an absorbable suture. The pedicle is then buried under the mucosa as the latter is closed. We do not perform anal dilatation or anal packing. The reason for ligating the pedicle in closed haemorrhoidectomy is not to decrease postoperative haemorrhage but to establish the first stitch for closing the mucosa.

We compared prospectively in a randomised trial this technique against closed haemorrhoidectomy using scissors dissection (Ibrahim et al., 1998). Both groups had 20 ml of 1:20,000 adrenaline in 0.5% bupivacaine infiltrated before surgery. Both groups had identical surgery with the exception of the method of dissection of the haemorrhoidal tissues. All patients had three haemorrhoids removed.

Forty-four patients underwent diathermy closed haemorrhoidectomy, while 47 underwent closed haemorrhoidectomy using scissors excision.

There was no statistical difference in the operating time between both groups. Pain score was assessed with a linear analogue scale by a blinded investigator. The median pain scores were similar between the two groups for all seven days. There was no statistical difference in the severity of postoperative pain. Those in the diathermy group required less oral analgesic over seven days ($p < 0.001$). However, intramuscular pethidine use was higher in the first 24 hours after surgery in the diathermy group. There was no statistical difference in the use of lignocaine jelly or in the number of days to the first bowel movement.

There were no differences in early or late postoperative complications including that of post-haemorrhoidectomy bleeding, wound dehiscence or anal stricture. We postulated that the pain from diathermy in the first day postoperatively may be due to oedema from diathermy, but this improved rapidly. Overall, there was less pain compared to scissors excision.

We also conducted a study between closed and open haemorrhoidectomy using diathermy in a prospective randomised trial (Ho et al., 1997b). Open haemorrhoidectomy was performed without ligation of the pedicle, while in closed haemorrhoidectomy, the pedicle was transfixed and the mucosal wound edges were sutured with absorbable sutures.

Thirty-three patients underwent closed haemorrhoidectomy using diathermy and 34 patients underwent open haemorrhoidectomy using diathermy. There was no significant difference in the time taken to perform closed or open diathermy haemorrhoidectomy. There were also no differences in the postoperative pain score or analgesic requirement between the two groups. Patients with open haemorrhoidectomy had earlier bowel movements ($p < 0.001$) than closed haemorrhoidectomy patients; however, the length of time of hospitalisation was not significantly different between the two groups.

There were also no differences in the incidence of postoperative bleeding or faecal impaction. However, complete wound healing took significantly longer after closed haemorrhoidectomy (mean (sem) 6.9 (0.7) weeks) compared with open haemorrhoidectomy (mean (sem) 4.9 (0.4) weeks) ($p < 0.05$). Although primary repair should lead to earlier wound healing in the closed haemorrhoidectomy group, this was not realised because of wound infection and dehiscence in eight patients after closed haemorrhoidectomy.

Parks (1956) postulated that post-haemorrhoidectomy pain might be due to exposed and denuded anal sphincter resulting in anal spasm. He thus advocated closed or submucosal haemorrhoidectomy, claiming that pain is minimal following this technique. Other studies later showed that there was no improvement in pain scores following closed haemorrhoidectomy (Watts et al., 1964; Roe et al., 1987). This also was confirmed in our study.

Special Circumstances

Circumferential Prolapsed Piles

The technique of diathermy for haemorrhoidectomy can also be used for circumferential prolapsed piles.

The two common methods of treatment for circumferential prolapsed piles are modified radical haemorrhoidectomy and the four-pile haemorrhoidectomy. Instead of using scissors dissection and ligation of the pedicles, we adapted the use of diathermy to both of these methods.

For four-piles haemorrhoidectomy (Fig. 17.1), diathermy is used for excision of all three primary

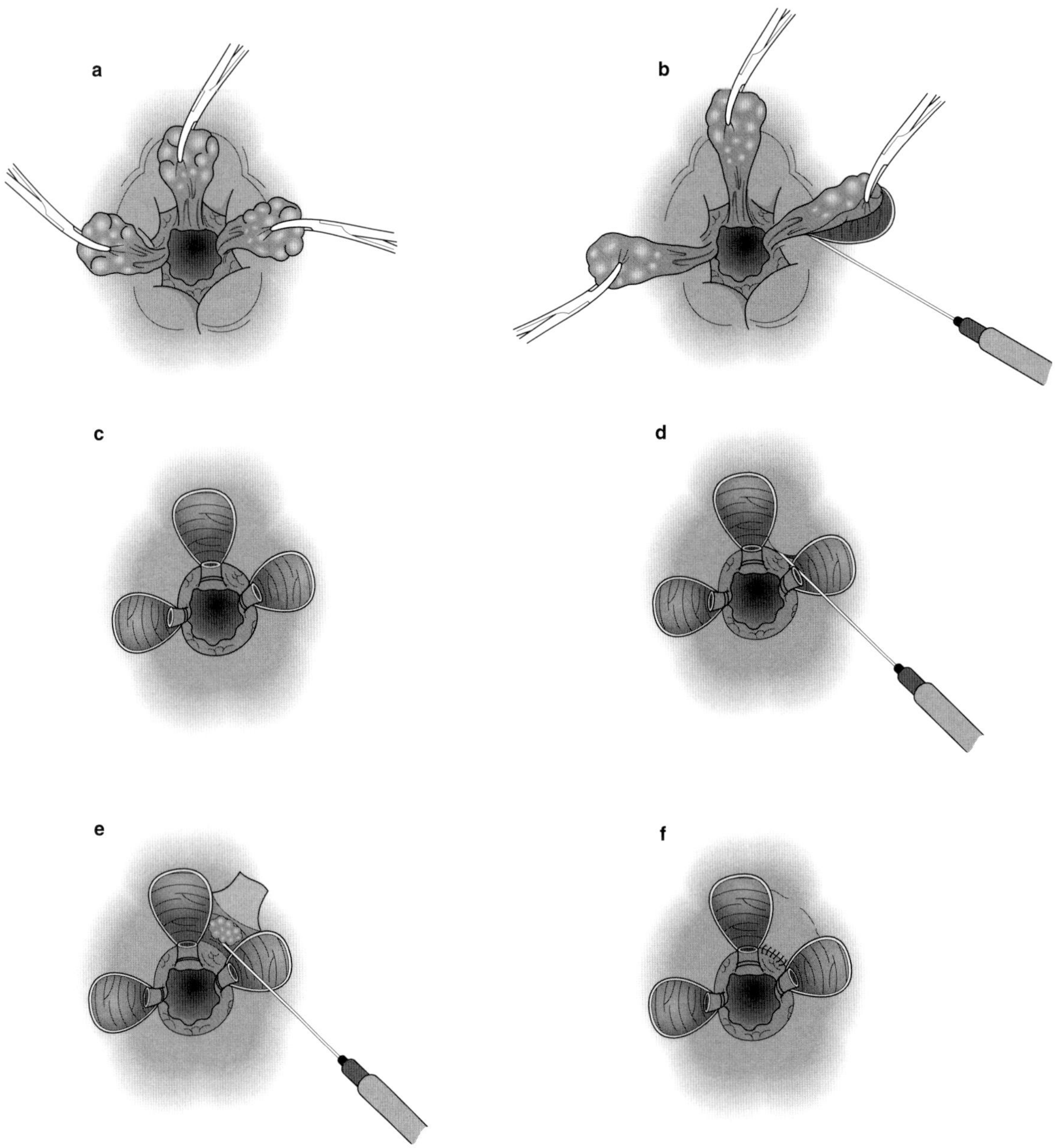

Figure 17.1. Four-piles haemorrhoidectomy. The three primary piles are displayed (a). Diathermy haemorrhoidectomy is done for each of the three primary piles (b). The three primary piles have been removed (c). The remaining largest secondary pile dissected (d) and haemorrhoids beneath the raised flap excised (e). The mucocutaneous continuity restored (f).

piles as previously described. The remaining largest secondary pile is then selected and dissected and excised using diathermy, without ligation of the pedicle. The mucocutaneous continuity of that pile is then restored using absorbable suture.

For modified radical haemorrhoidectomy (Fig. 17.2), the ano-rectal mucosa is divided into three parts circumferentially and each third dealt with individually. Artery forceps are applied to cause further prolapse of the normal rectal mucosa above the pile-bearing area and to put this third of the ano-rectal circumference on a stretch. Diathermy is used to make an incision above the dentate line. The mucosal flap is raised and freed from the underlying

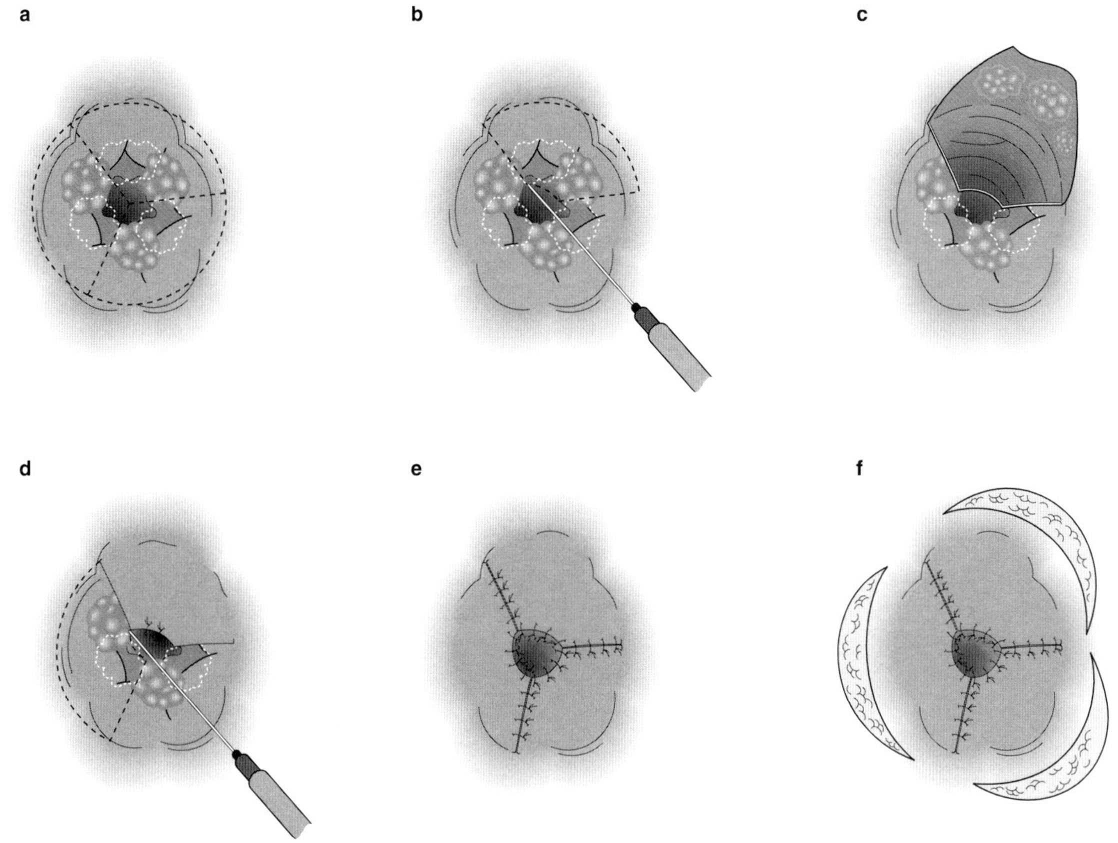

Figure 17.2. Modified radical haemorrhoidectomy. The ano-rectal mucosa was divided into three parts circumferentially (a). Incision made using diathermy above the dentate line (b). The mucosal flap was raised and freed from the underlying internal sphincter by diathermy (c) and all the haemorrhoids excised. The flap was then stitched to the proximal divided mucosal edge of the rectal mucosa and internal sphincter with absorbable suture (d) while the other parts are dissected. After completion of remaining two parts (e). Circumanal release incisions made when flap tension was excessive (f).

internal sphincter by diathermy. Grossly evident haemorrhoidal tissue and excess mucosa is then removed, taking care to avoid devascularisation of the flap. The flap is then stitched to the proximal divided mucosal edge of the rectal mucosa and internal sphincter with absorbable suture, thus pulling the anal skin and mucosa upwards into the anal canal. This level should be at or above the previous dentate line. This is repeated with the remaining two-thirds of the anal canal. On the occasions where flap tension is excessive, circumanal release incisions can be made as required (Fig 17.2f).

We compared the above two techniques in a prospective randomised trial (Seow-Choen and Lee, 1995). Twenty-eight patients with large third- or fourth-degree piles who were not suitable for the standard three-piles haemorrhoidectomy were recruited. Fourteen patients were randomised to radical haemorrhoidectomy and 14 to four-piles haemorrhoidectomy.

The median duration of surgery was 30 minutes for the radical group and 10 minutes for the four-piles haemorrhoidectomy group ($p < 0.05$). Following healing of the haemorrhoidectomy wounds, all patients in the radical group were completely continent compared to 12 of 14 (85.7%) in the four-piles group.

Two other patients (14.3%) in the four-piles group developed anal stricture requiring anal dilatation. Five patients in the radical haemorrhoidectomy group developed wound dehiscence that required secondary suture. Of these five patients, three developed anal stricture.

Two patients had remnant anal skin tags in the radical group, compared to nine patients in the four-piles group. Two of the patients in the four-piles group had residual symptomatic piles compared to none in the radical group.

At follow-up after six months, six patients in the four-piles group considered the results to be excellent, seven acceptable, and one was disappointed. In the radical group, two considered it to be excellent, ten acceptable, and two were disappointed.

Four-piles haemorrhoidectomy was much easier to perform than radical haemorrhoidectomy. Flap dehiscence was a problem with radical haemorrhoidectomy, occurring in 7.2–11.2% of cases. This resulted in a high incidence of anal stricture in the radical haemorrhoidectomy group, although there was no significant difference between the two groups in this study as far as anal stricture was concerned. Patient satisfaction was better in the four-piles haemorrhoidectomy group, and this operation is preferred for circumferential prolapsed piles.

Acute Haemorrhoids

Acutely thrombosed, ulcerated, or gangrenous prolapsed haemorrhoids cause severe pain and disability to patients. It has been said that emergency haemorrhoidectomy is associated with an increased risk of portal pyaemia, secondary haemorrhage, anal stenosis and faecal incontinence. However, several studies (Smith, 1967; Tinckler and Barathma, 1964; Howard and Pingree, 1968; Stern, 1964; Milligan et al., 1937) have shown that emergency haemorrhoidectomy is safe and is an appropriate way of treating acute haemorrhoids.

The technique of diathermy open haemorrhoidectomy can also be used in patients with acute haemorrhoids. We have been using diathermy open haemorrhoidectomy for almost all cases of emergency haemorrhoidectomy since August 1990.

We studied, retrospectively, 704 cases of haemorrhoidectomy performed over a 24-month period (Eu et al., 1994). All the cases of haemorrhoidectomy done in the last eight months of the study were by diathermy without ligation of the haemorrhoidal pedicles. Five hundred elective cases and 204 emergency cases were evaluated for complications and functional results. The two groups were matched for age, sex and race. Length of follow-up was identical (mean 24 months (range 12–36 months)).

None of the patients in this study had reactionary haemorrhage. Twenty-seven patients (5.4%) in the elective group and ten patients (4.9%) in the emergency group suffered secondary haemorrhage ($p > 0.05$). Fifteen patients (3.0%) in the elective group and 12 patients (5.9%) in the emergency group developed symptomatic anal stricture that required either anal dilatation or anoplasty ($p > 0.05$). Varying degrees of faecal incontinence developed in 26 (5%) patients in the elective group, and in 9 (4%) in the emergency group ($p > 0.05$). None of the study patients developed portal pyaemia or septicaemia. Thirty-eight (7.6%) patients in the elective group and 14 (6.9%) patients in the emergency group developed recurrent haemorrhoids ($p > 0.05$).

This study did not directly compare diathermy and scissors open haemorrhoidectomy in the emergency setting. However, the overall results for emergency haemorrhoidectomy showed no incidence of portal pyaemia and a low incidence of secondary haemorrhage, stricture or incontinence.

Emergency haemorrhoidectomy offers several advantages over conservative treatment of acute haemorrhoids. Definitive haemorrhoidectomy at the time of admission saves the patient a subsequent readmission for an elective surgery. The patient is also spared the pain and discomfort of non-surgical treatment for the acute episode, while the discomfort following emergency haemorrhoidectomy is the same as that following elective surgery. Furthermore, morbidity following emergency haemorrhoidectomy is not increased compared to that following elective haemorrhoidectomy.

Overall Results

We reviewed the combined results of all the patients who have had three-piles haemorrhoidectomy using diathermy. A total of 333 patients had either closed or open diathermy haemorrhoidectomy, with or without use of lateral sphincterotomy (Mathai et al., 1996) or trimebutine (Ho et al., 1997a).

There were a total of seven patients with post-haemorrhoidectomy haemorrhage (2.1%). Only two patients developed faecal incontinence (0.6%), of which one had a lateral sphincterotomy. The incontinent patient who did not have a sphincterotomy resolved spontaneously. There was only one case (0.3%) of anal stricture in the 333 patients. This was adequately treated by dilatation alone.

These results are comparable if not better than the reported incidence of 0.8% to 4.2% of post-haemorrhoidectomy haemorrhage, 1.0% incidence of anal stenosis, and 0.4% of incontinence in other series (Mortensen and Romanos, 1997; Goldberg et al., 1980; Johnstone and Ibister, 1992; Rosen et al., 1993).

The results of treatment of circumferential prolapsed piles by extended techniques were poorer than that of three-piles haemorrhoidectomy. Of 28 patients, one patient developed incontinence to gas and one to liquids (7.1%). Another five patients developed anal stricture, of which four (14.3%) were adequately treated with dilatation, and the last patient required flap surgery (3.6%). This is low, however, compared to complication rates of up to 34% reported in other series (Boccasanta et al., 1998).

Conclusion

Diathermy haemorrhoidectomy is safe, fast and effective for the performance of open, closed, emergency or radical haemorrhoidectomy.

EDITORIAL COMMENT

The Editor has no experience of diathermy techniques but very large series have been reported by Lentini and others, with excellent results. There is no doubt that use of diathermy for dissection instead of a scalpel diminishes intra-operative bleeding and eliminates the need for a crown ligature – at least in almost every case. Whether it is safe to omit crown ligation in every case is a doubt that continues to worry the Editor (who again emphasizes his absence of experience); there are haemorrhoid cases which have substantial pulsatile vessels supplying them for which ligation would seem to be a sensible precaution to take. Since a carefully performed ligation should be free of any risks (see p. 79), the Editor's reservations about avoiding a crown tie in all cases will not go away. This small caveat does not detract from the message that haemorrhoids can be removed safely and effectively by diathermy technique, in which crown ligation is an "optional extra".

References

Andrews BT, Layer GT, Jackson BT, Nicholls RJ (1993) Randomized trial comparing diathermy haemorrhoidectomy with the scissors dissection Milligan–Morgan operation. Dis Colon Rectum 36(6):580–3

Bassi R, Bergami G (1997) The surgical treatment of haemorrhoids: diathermocoagulation and traditional techniques. A prospective randomized study. Minerva Chir 52(4):387–91

Boccasanta P, Venturi M, Orio A, Salamina G, Reitano M, Cioffi U et al. (1998) Circular hemorrhoidectomy in advanced hemorrhoidal disease. Hepatogastroenterology 45:969–72

Eu KW, Seow-Choen F, Goh HS (1994) Comparison of emergency and elective haemorrhoidectomy. Br J Surg 81:308–10

Goldberg SM, Gordon PH, Nivatvongs S (1980) Hemorrhoids. In: Essentials of Ano-rectal Surgery. Lippingcott, Philadelphia

Goligher JC, Graham NG, Clark CG, De Domba FT, Giles G (1969) The value of stretching the anal sphincter in the relief of post-haemorrhoidectomy pain. Br J Surg 56:859–61

Ho YH, Foo CL, Seow-Choen F, Goh HS (1995) Prospective randomized controlled trial of a micronized flavonidic fraction to reduce bleeding after haemorrhoidectomy. Br J Surg 38:776–7

Ho YH, Seow-Choen F, Low JY, Tan M, Leong AFPK (1997a) Randomized controlled trial of trimebutine (anal sphincter relaxant) for pain after haemorrhoidectomy. Br J Surg 84:377–9

Ho YH, Seow-Choen F, Tan M, Leong AFPK (1997b) Randomized controlled trial of open and closed haemorrhoidectomy. Br J Surg 84:1729–30

Howard PM, Pingree JH (1968) Immediate radical surgery for hemorrhoidal disease with extensive thrombosis. Am J Surg 116:777–8

Ibrahim S, Tsang C, Lee YL, Seow-Choen F, Ho YH, Leong AFPK et al. (1998) Prospective randomized trial comparing pain and clinical function between diathermy versus scissors closed hemorrhoidectomy. Dis Colon Rectum 41:1418–20

Johnstone CS, Ibister WH (1992) Inpatient management of piles: a surgical audit. Aust N Z J Surg 62:720–4

Mathai V, Ong BC, Ho YH (1996) Randomized controlled trial of lateral internal sphincterotomy with haemorrhoidectomy. Br J Surg 83:380–2

Milligan ETC, Morgan CN, Jones LE, Officer R (1937) Surgical anatomy of the anal canal and the operative treatment of haemorrhoids. Lancet ii:119–24

Mortensen N, Romanos J (1997) Hemorrhoids. In: Nicholls RJ, Dozois RR (ed) Surgery of the Colon and Rectum. Churchill Livingston, New York, pp 224–9

Parks AG (1956) The surgical treatment of haemorrhoids. Br J Surg 43:337–51

Roe AM, Bartolo DC, Velacott KD, Locke-Edmunds J, Mortenen NJ (1987) Submucosal versus ligation haemorrhoidectomy: a comparison of anal sensation, anal sphincter manometry and postoperative pain and function. Br J Surg 74:948–51

Rosen L, Sipe P, Stasik JJ, Riether RD, Trimpi HD (1993) Outcome of delayed hemorrhage following surgical hemorrhoidectomy. Dis Colon Rectum 36:743–6

Seow-Choen F, Ho YH, Ang HG, Goh HS (1992) Prospective, randomized trial comparing pain and clinical function after conventional scissors excision/ligation vs. diathermy excision without ligation for symptomatic prolapsed hemorrhoids. Dis Colon Rectum 34:1165–9

Seow-Choen F, Lee HC (1995) Prospective randomized study of radical versus four-pile haemorrhoidectomy for symptomatic large circumferential prolapsed piles. Br J Surg 82:188–9

Smith M (1967) Early operation for acute haemorrhoids. Br J Surg 54:141–4

Stern W (1964) Thrombosed haemorrhoids: immediate surgical treatment. Med J Aust 2:635

Tinckler LF, Barathma G (1964) Immediate haemorrhoidectomy for prolapsed piles. Lancet 141:810–2

Wang JY, Chang-Chien CR, Chen JS, Lai CR, Tang R (1991) The role of lasers in hemorrhoidectomy. Dis Colon Rectum 34:78–82

Watts JM, Bennett RC, Duthie HL, Goligher JC (1964) Healing and pain after haemorrhoidectomy. Br J Surg 51:808–17

18 Laser Haemorrhoidectomy

Charles V. Mann

Lasers destroy tissue by concentrating the energy of electromagnetic radiation. The energy can be deployed over an area or can be focussed into a narrow beam. If diffused over the operative field, a laser can be used to ablate a mass of tissue (as with an adenomatous polyp or a haemorrhoid), or if it is concentrated into a narrow beam, it can be used as a cutting tool; in both cases it has a coagulative haemostatic effect which allows a dry operation field and obviates the need for ligation or diathermy. The tissue destruction is achieved without much smoke or steam emission to obscure vision. When the laser is used instead of a diathermy cutting needle, its line of dissection is narrower, with very little damage to the tissue alongside. This, together with its freedom from smoke or sparking, aids considerably in the precision of the dissection, as well as diminishing the residues of dead or damaged cells. This last point is important, as there is less interference with healing by necrotic tissue than is associated with the use of diathermy, at least in theory. Most experts who employ laser instruments for surgical purposes have settled for the nd-YAG laser (nd-YAG laser is an abbreviation for *ne*o*d*ymium-*Y*ttrium-*a*luminium-*g*arnet laser to distinguish it from other types (argon, CO_2) as the best type of laser tool, but it is expensive.

The disadvantages or otherwise of using a laser may be listed, as follows:

(i) The equipment is expensive, both to purchase and to employ.
(ii) The energy beam is invisible and extremely powerful. Special goggles must be used by the surgeon and all other staff in the operating theatre.
(iii) Compared to a conventional closed haemorrhoidectomy, no appreciable differences can be demonstrated for early results, and some disadvantages were reported (Senagore et al., 1993).
(iv) Apart from abolishing the need for haemostatic measures, particularly pedicle ligation, the use of a laser does not alter the requirements of the procedure, which are to achieve removal of all haemorrhoid tissue together with preservation of adequate skin bridges.
(v) Haemostasis can be catered for by cheaper and easier methods, for example, by infiltration of 1:200,000 adrenaline solution and/or the use of diathermy (Lentini, 1990).
(vi) Providing pedicle ligation (when it is necessary) is performed with due appreciation of the fine details of technique (see p. 79), it does not cause complications (or, at least, so rarely that it is a very weak reason for preferring laser use).

Overall, when these disadvantages are put in context, the laser instrument begins to appear more a fashion accessory than a necessity.

There are some general drawbacks which are inseparable from instruments which rely on physical methods of tissue destruction (e.g., diathermy, laser). All of them leave an unavoidable residue of necrotic tissue that can delay healing, but, although this has been noted for the laser (Senagore et al., 1993), it must be said that there have been no clinical consequences from this effect. Perhaps more importantly, suture of the wound edges (as for a closed technique) becomes less secure than after scalpel dissection, with early dehiscence and possible haemorrhage as associated complications. Both diathermy and laser instruments increase the hazards of physical injury to staff, and of fires and explosions.

Justification for the extra expense and trouble which is caused by choosing a laser-based technique needs to be provided by evidence of less pain, earlier discharge, fewer complications and speedier return to work; marginal benefits, especially if they are unproven, are not sufficient. Even at a basic level of critical analysis, substantial improvements when compared to cheaper alternatives must be demonstrated. To date, none of the advantages claimed for the laser have been substantiated by a properly constructed large-scale randomised clinical trial.

As with using the diathermy technique (Ch. 17) – which is a much cheaper method – using the laser for dissection obviates the need for a crown ligature; otherwise, the operative techniques are not altered.

EDITORIAL COMMENT

Lasers are an expensive addition to those haemorrhoidectomy techniques which have in-built haemostatic advantages. For purposes of dissection, lasers seem to have little or no advantages over simpler and cheaper alternatives (e.g., diathermy, scalpel). When used to ablate the haemorrhoids in-situ, delayed wound healing is observed. In addition to their cost, use of lasers requires additional precautions that make it unattractive, at least to the Editor (e.g., the need for goggles by all theatre personnel). Since haemostasis is achievable by simple measures in properly executed scalpel dissections, or can be obtained by using a diathermy loop, this technique is unlikely to be widely adopted.

References and Further Reading

Iwagaki H, Higuchi Y, Fuchimoto S, Orita K (1989) The laser treatment of haemorrhoids: results of a study on 1,816 patients. Japan J Surg 19:658–61

Leff EI (1992) Haemorrhoidectomy – laser vs. non-laser: outpatient surgical experience. Dis Colon Rectum 35:743–6

Lentini J, Leveroni JT, Aure C (1990) Twenty-five years experience with the high-frequency transistorised loop, with special reference to haemorrhoidectomy without suture. Coloproctology 4:239–49

Senagore A, Mazier PW, Luchterfeld MA et al. (1993) Treatment of advanced haemorrhoidal disease; a prospective randomised comparison of cold scalpel vs. contact nd–YAG laser. Dis Colon Rectum 36:1042–9

Wang JY, Chang-Chien CR, Chen JS, Lai CR, Tang RP (1991) The role of lasers in haemorrhoidectomy. Dis Colon Rectum 34:78–82

19 Cryotherapy

Charles V. Mann

Despite early enthusiasm, and the persisting advocacy of some surgeons, cryotherapy has not established itself as a mainstream procedure for treating haemorrhoids. Therefore, the Editor does not feel justified in providing space for a detailed description of the technique, although those who wish for this information can consult the references given at the end. The early hopes (and claims) that cryotherapy is a painless and effective method for ambulant treatment of haemorrhoids have not been sustained by experience. The "best" results are obtained with a liquid nitrogen probe (Fig. 19.1).

The drawbacks of the technique include:

1. In many, if not most, cases, a general anaesthetic is required so that an anal dilatation can be carried out to allow the haemorrhoids to be properly exposed for application of the cryoprobe. In those patients where a general anaesthetic is inadvisable or not chosen, a caudal can be used, but still adds to the demands of the technique.
2. The extent of freezing, both in depth and area, cannot be defined accurately, so that either under- or over-treatment is common. If the circumferential extent of freezing is excessive, normal tissue is sacrificed, with consequent risks for anal stenosis. If too little haemorrhoid tissue is frozen, early recurrence and return of symptoms is inevitable. The larger the haemorrhoids requiring treatment, the greater the chance of under- or over-freezing.
3. Cryotherapy is safest and most effective when used for small- or moderate-sized haemorrhoids. However, for such first- or second-degree haemorrhoids, excellent alternative treatments are available (e.g., by rubber band ligation, Ch. 9) for which neither an anaesthetic nor expensive equipment is needed, and which pose no problems for ambulant treatment.

Efforts have been made to improve the accuracy and effectiveness of cryotechniques, principally by substituting liquid nitrogen for carbon dioxide instruments; the deeper and more rapidly freezing machines are more expensive to buy and to operate, and have not eliminated the fundamental problem of ensuring a predictable result.

If, on the other hand, a solution is sought by resorting to repeated applications, this has the associated risk of multiple anaesthetics, as well as continuing episodes of unpleasant symptoms during the post-freezing periods.

If a large mass of haemorrhoid tissue is treated by cryotherapy, attempts to overcome the problem of freezing such a large amount of tissue by increasing the time and/or depth of cooling brings with it an aggravated risk for destruction of anoderm and deep structures, including larger vessels and sphincter muscle. Anal stenosis, secondary haemorrhage and incontinence have all been reported. Cryotherapy frequently produces unpleasant after-effects, both immediate and longer term.

Immediate after effects include pain (which can affect two thirds of patients, and be severe in some cases); profuse discharge of watery mucus, which occurs in almost all cases, and may persist for several weeks; bleeding, which is not uncommon during the first two or three weeks (it is usually minor, but can be serious in some patients and life-threatening in a few); faecal soiling; pruritus and an

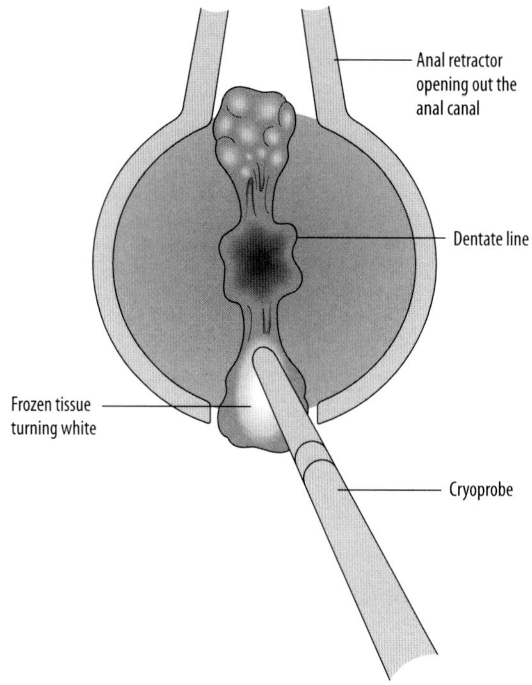

Note the following:-

1. The frozen tissue becomes a white solid mass (ice-ball).
2. While the circumferential limits of freezing may be reasonably clear cut, the depth of freezing is not apparent.
3. An anal retractor has been needed to display the haemorrhoid(s) to be frozen: this is true for virtually all cases.
4. Application of jelly to surfaces that are not to be frozen can protect these areas very effectively.
5. The probe needs to be reheated before it can be separated.

Figure 19.1. Cryoprobe applied to a prolapsing haemorrhoid.

offensive odour (which is also a reflection of wound contamination by anaerobic bacteria).

Longer-term after effects include prolonged wound-healing time. Because effective cryodestruction depends upon instant production of intracellular ice crystals (hence the preference for liquid nitrogen probes), there is always a thin intermediate layer of incompletely frozen cells between the frozen (dead) and warm (alive) tissues. The more abrupt the freezing, the less the extent of partially frozen tissue, but it is never entirely absent even when a liquid nitrogen probe is used. These partially damaged fringes hold back healing, which may take up to six weeks to be completed. Such prolonged delays in wound healing are a major inconvenience to the patients, especially when there has been substantial destruction of anoderm.

Long-term results (years rather than weeks) have been reported as showing that more than two-thirds of patients suffer from a return of symptomatic haemorrhoids within ten years of cryotherapy. This is much worse than the results of surgical haemorrhoidectomy, for which five per cent would be a generally accepted figure. Taken together with the short-term disadvantages described above, the conclusion that treatment of haemorrhoids by cryotherapy is inconsistent with the expected standards of modern treatment would appear reasonable.

EDITORIAL COMMENTS

The Editor had a tiny experience of cryotherapy for haemorrhoids when he was able to adapt a machine purchased for another use. Although none of his patients expressed displeasure with the results, the Editor found the technique unreliable, and that healing took a long time – two or three times longer than after scalpel haemorrhoidectomy. Cryotherapy is used by only a few surgeons at the present time, as it was found that patients hated the unpleasant after-effects (mainly, the profuse unsocial discharge from the wounds). The treatment is now regarded as unneeded and outdated by coloproctologists.

References and Further Reading

Ferguson EF Jr. (1988) Alternatives in the treatment of haemorrhoidal disease. South Med J 81:606–10

Goh Hak-Su (1993) Management of uncomplicated haemorrhoids. In: Fielding LP, Goldberg SM (eds) Operative Surgery, Fifth Edition. Surgery of the Colon, Rectum and Anus. Butterworth-Heinemann, Oxford Boston, pp 784–8

Goligher JC (1976) Cryosurgery for haemorrhoids. Dis Colon Rectum 19:223

Irving AD, Walker MA (1987) Cryosurgery for haemorrhoids: six years' review of "cured" patients. J R Coll Surg Edinb 32:267–9

Kaufman HD (1978) Haemorrhoids: an "outpatient package". J R Coll Surg Edinb 23:40–43

Lloyd-Williams K, Haq IU, Elem B (1973) Cryodestruction of haemorrhoids. BMJ 1:666

O'Connor JJ (1975) The role of cryosurgery in management of ano-rectal diseases: a study of cryosurgical techniques. Dis Colon Rectum 18:301

Oh C (1981) One thousand cryohaemorrhoidectomies: an overview. Dis Colon Rectum 24:613–7

Smith LE, Goodreau JJ, Fouty WJ (1979) Operative haemorrhoidectomy versus cryodestruction. Dis Colon Rectum 22:10

20 Complications of Surgical Hemorrhoidectomy

Marvin L. Corman and Stephen I. Allison

Treatment of hemorrhoids can be by sclerotherapy, rubber band ligation, cryotherapy, infrared coagulation, ultroid therapy,* bipolar diathermy (BICAP), or surgical excision by various techniques. One should employ the most appropriate treatment option according to the indications that have already been described. This chapter will focus on the complications of surgical hemorrhoidectomy.

To avoid the pitfalls of hemorrhoid surgery, conscientious effort is required – not only with respect to meticulous surgical technique, but also with regard to a compulsive approach to postoperative management. One must also consider other disease states such as inflammatory bowel disease, and the HIV-positive patient when considering surgical intervention. Also, the pregnant patient poses a difficult management problem. The following is a partial list of the potential problems of surgical hemorrhoidectomy:

- Pain
- Urinary retention
- Urinary tract infection
- Constipation
- Fecal impaction
- Hemorrhage
- Infection
- Anal tags
- Mucosal prolapse
- Mucosal ectropion
- Rectal stricture
- Anal fissure
- Pseudopolyps
- Epidermal cysts
- Anal fistula
- Pruritus ani
- Fecal incontinence
- Recurrent hemorrhoids

Pain

Although pain is not actually a complication of surgery, it is nonetheless the single most important reason why patients avoid hemorrhoidectomy.

Although epidural morphine has been employed for analgesia after hemorrhoidectomy at some centers, in our opinion, the appropriate prevention of pain is narcotic analgesic medication administered in adequate doses and given frequently (e.g., 75 to 125 mg of Demerol every two-to-three hours). Unfortunately, this is not an option in the discharged patient.

A great deal of emphasis has been applied to the management of pain in the hemorrhoidectomy patient, not only because of the pain itself, but because of the role it plays in urinary symptoms (see the following section). The literature abounds with alternatives in the management of discomfort. Goldstein and colleagues employed a subcutaneous morphine pump in postoperative pain management. Although this was not a controlled study in the true sense, the authors concluded that the combination of *outpatient hemorrhoidectomy* and the pump was cost-effective when compared with the inpatient stay. Toradol (ketorolac tromethamine) has also been advocated in ano-rectal surgery. Gen-

* Ultroid therapy is the application of direct (d.c) electrocoagulation to treat bleeding associated with haemorrhoids.

erally, 60 mg (2 ml) is injected directly into the anal sphincter musculature at the time of its exposure during ano-rectal procedures, especially hemorrhoidectomy. Studies suggest that there is a much-reduced incidence not only of pain, but also of urinary retention.

Another pain management option that has recently been published is the application of transdermal fentanyl (Duragesic). The authors concluded that fentanyl provides an effective analgesic alternative that essentially improves the transition to outpatient management by a non-narcotic pain medication. In a subsequent letter to the editor, however, criticism was expressed for encouraging the use of a contraindicated medication. It was felt that there is an unacceptably high incidence of hypoventilation with possible respiratory depression. In fact, recommendations against this use have been included with the package insert by the manufacturer.

Urinary Retention

Urinary retention is the most common complication following hemorrhoidectomy. Bleday and co-workers reported a 20 percent incidence of postoperative urinary complications. Factors often held responsible include the following:

- Spinal anesthesia
- Rectal pain and spasm
- High ligation of the hemorrhoidal pedicle
- Rough handling of tissue
- Heavy suture material
- Numerous sutures
- Fluid overload
- Rectal packing
- Tight, bulky dressings
- Anticholinergics
- Narcotics

Pain and fluid overload are the primary factors that cause urinary retention. If pain medication is inadequate, the patient cannot relax the sphincter mechanism sufficiently to urinate – it simply hurts too much. One must limit fluids. This requires education of the anesthesiologist, the nurses, and the house officers. Frightening the patient with a catheter or leaving standing orders for catheterization is a self-fulfilling prophesy for its subsequent insertion. The minimal intravenous infusion necessary is given during the operation, and the infusion is terminated in the recovery room. If hospital regulations require that an intravenous line be maintained, a heparin lock will suffice. Oral fluids are restricted until the following morning. Finally, patients are not routinely catheterized; this is carried out only when the bladder is distended or the patient complains, and then only after examination by a physician. In the morning, with the commencement of sitz baths, most patients will void who have not already done so. Once the nursing service has been educated not even to inquire about voiding, the incidence of retention and the associated complication of urinary tract infection will be significantly reduced.

If catheterization is necessary, it should be performed with a balloon catheter. If the residual urine is determined to be greater than 500 ml, the catheter should be left in place for 24 hours, because it is unlikely that the patient will be able to void subsequently. Conversely, with a residual of less than 500 ml, the catheter can be removed with a reasonable expectation that spontaneous urination will occur.

Despite the discussion on the methods for preventing urinary retention, the subject today may be moot. It has become so onerous to obtain permission for hospitalization for hemorrhoidectomy that more patients are being forced to deal with this concern on their own. It is interesting to note that reports suggest that the incidence of outpatient retention may not be different from the in-hospital rate, perhaps even less. Local anesthesia is associated with a significantly lower incidence of urinary retention when compared with spinal anesthesia.

Urinary Tract Infection

Urinary tract infection is usually a direct consequence of catheterization for urinary retention. The most common offending organisms are coliform bacteria. Appropriate antibiotics and catheter removal usually result in rapid resolution, but chronic infection, cystitis, and pyelonephritis can be late sequelae. Here again, the value of avoiding urinary retention cannot be overestimated.

Constipation

Patients who undergo hemorrhoidectomy await their postoperative bowel evacuation less than enthusiastically and often view the enema intended to facilitate this function with apprehension. The enema is gladly forfeited by most individuals if it can be replaced by some more acceptable method.

Constipation after ano-rectal surgery must be either relieved effectively or prevented, because if it is untreated, it may lead to fecal impaction – a matter of special concern in this group of patients. Despite this concern, as long as 72 hours may elapse after operation before a laxative agent is first administered. Factors that contribute to this lag include the effects of analgesic medications given before or after the operation, the effects of anesthesia, and local physiologic dysfunction resulting from surgical manipulation, bed rest, and the patient's fear of painful defecation. A history of irregular bowel function and colonic hypomotility may complicate the problem further.

We believe that a stimulant laxative should be given on the evening of the operation and continued in increasing doses until defecation occurs. This should be in conjunction with fiber supplementation to act as a bulk laxative. After the first evening after surgery, the patient should be encouraged to drink five or six glasses of water per day to aid the action of the fiber. One should expect defecation by the second or third postoperative day. After the third postoperative day with no bowel action, a gentle tap-water enema should be considered.

As with the management of urinary retention, few individuals can be permitted the luxury of remaining in the hospital to await the first bowel action. Whereas this is the optimal approach, both for patient comfort and for reassurance, appropriate discharge instructions can and should include a bowel-management program conducive to satisfactory bowel evacuation (e.g., a bulk laxative and a stimulant laxative).

Hemorrhage

Massive hemorrhage that occurs in the recovery room is always the result of a technical error and can usually be attributed to improper or inadequate ligation of the hemorrhoid pedicle. This most commonly occurs if the pedicle is simply hand-tied rather than suture-ligated. Such a complication requires emergency surgical intervention. This should be quite unusual when the Ferguson hemorrhoidectomy is performed, because meticulous care is taken in closing the wounds.

Management of active bleeding after hemorrhoidectomy includes submucosal injection with 1 to 2 ml of 1 : 10,000 adrenaline, direct pressure with a finger or gauze, the use of topical epinephrine, or suture ligation.

Delayed hemorrhage (i.e., 7–14 days postoperatively) is probably the result of sepsis in the pedicle. This occurs in approximately 2 percent of hemorrhoidectomies. Patients may experience renewed slight bleeding, the passage of clots, or massive hemorrhage. Bleeding one week or more following surgery when the patient has previously ceased bleeding warrants examination. Treatment varies from expectant management to in-hospital observation, transfusion, and resuture. In-hospital options include observation alone, bedside anal packing with absorbable gelatin sponge (Gelfoam), Foley catheter technique for tamponade of the bleeding point, or if these fail to control the hemorrhage, suture ligation is required. In our opinion, delayed hemorrhage usually is not a preventable complication.

Infection

It seems surprising that, as hemorrhoidectomy is carried out in a field with numerous and varied bacterial organisms present, there is not a higher incidence of septic complications following the operation. As Lal and Levitan have pointed out, it would not be surprising if hemorrhoidectomy were followed by transient bacteremia and low-grade fever as a result of the relatively constant release of bacteria into the bloodstream from a feeding focus. For example, an 8.5 percent rate of bacteremia has been reported following proctoscopic examination of patients with no evidence of lower intestinal disease. However, despite the presence of potentially virulent organisms (e.g., clostridia, anaerobic streptococci, bacteroides, Escherichia coli), septic problems are uncommon.

It has been hypothesized that the major venous drainage of the rectum, by passing through the superior hemorrhoidal veins into the portal system, is cleared of organisms by the reticuloendothelial system of the liver. This hepatic clearance, by effectively removing the bacteria released into the circulation, may be important in minimizing the impact of rectal colonic flora in the systemic circulation and may be the reason why infection is an uncommon complication after hemorrhoidectomy. Furthermore, as sitz baths are a routine part of the postoperative care, most skin problems (e.g., cellulitis, abscess) would be treated in an essentially prophylactic manner. In an experience of well over 1,000 hemorrhoidectomies, I cannot recall ever having to drain an abscess in the postoperative period.

Anal Tags

Anal tags, which can interfere with proper cleansing of the anus and thus lead to skin irritation, can usually be avoided by excising redundant skin at the time of operation. I suspect, however, that tags more often than not are the result of the manner in which the wounds heal, perhaps analogous to keloid formation in other incision sites. Bothersome tags can be excised as an office procedure if symptoms warrant.

Mucosal Prolapse

Inadequate removal of redundant or mobile rectal mucosa at the time of hemorrhoidectomy may result in mucosal prolapse. Patients may complain of a lump that requires manual reduction. Problems with mucous discharge and pruritic symptoms are common.

Treatment usually consists of rubber ring ligation of the prolapsed mucosa. If there seems to be extensive or circumferential involvement, the surgeon should conduct the examination while the patient strains on the toilet in order to look for procidentia.

Prevention of this complication requires that the surgeon remove any redundant mucosa at the time of hemorrhoidectomy.

Ectropion

Because the mucosa is more mobile than the perianal skin, the tendency for mucosal descent is greater than the likelihood of the skin ascending to reline the denuded anal canal. If redundant mucosa above the site of the excised hemorrhoid tissue is not properly anchored to the underlying internal sphincter, the mucosa can heal outside the anal verge. If the entire anal mucosa is removed, and the cut edge is sutured to the perianal skin, the characteristic Whitehead deformity may be produced. If the surgeon anchors the mucosa to the skin in one or more quadrants, a partial ectropion may result. Interestingly, Khubchandani has reported treatment of anal stenosis by doing just what has been condemned – advancing the mucosa, albeit not beyond the anal verge. Ectropion can lead to mucous discharge, skin irritation, and pruritus ani. Prevention requires excising the redundant mucosa and anchoring the cut edge as described.

As long as no stricture is present, a simple excision and transverse suture of the wound edge to the underlying internal anal sphincter will suffice. The open wound should heal without the mucosal extrusion. An alternative approach is to perform an anoplasty (discussed next).

Anal Stricture

A considerable area of mucosa and anoderm may be denuded when the physician attempts to remove extensive, encircling hemorrhoids. If hemorrhoids are present in many areas, only minimal sections of intact, elastic anal tissue may be left following excision. With progressive healing, fibrous scar tissue may proliferate and contract the ano-rectal outlet. When healing is complete, a narrow, foreshortened stenotic orifice may remain.

As with ectropion, anal stenosis is a preventable complication. If adequate skin bridges are preserved, the risk for reducing the circumference of the anal canal is minimized. However, in the presence of gangrenous hemorrhoids, distortion of the anal canal, chronic fibrosis, chronic fissure, external tags, and hypertrophied anal papillae, extensive removal of involved tissue is often necessary to accomplish an adequate hemorrhoidectomy. Under these circumstances, the surgeon has two options – either compromise on the amount of tissue removed and accept the consequences of patient complaints of residual disease, or consider the possibility of performing an anoplasty at the time of hemorrhoidectomy.

The physician must attempt to preserve skin bridges – even one bridge is better than none. If, because of sepsis, sloughing, or radical surgery (not treated by anoplasty), the potential for stricture formation becomes manifest, daily digital examination of the rectum is advisable while the patient is still in the hospital. It is probably worthwhile to advise the patient concerning insertion of a dilator twice daily after hospital discharge. Weekly office visits are also suggested. Prevention of anal stricture when there is legitimate justification for concern is, in my opinion, the only indication for frequent digital examinations and the use of a dilator. If the wound heals without a stricture, digital examination and the use of a dilator can be discontinued, usually within six to eight weeks. However, if a healed, fixed stricture develops, we prefer to perform an anoplasty rather than to have the patient use a dilator indefinitely.

Rectal Stricture

Stricture of the rectum is a rare sequela of hemorrhoidectomy and usually is misdiagnosed as an anal stricture. The complication is caused by vigorous high ligation of the hemorrhoid pedicles that strips the rectal mucosa in several areas. It is most likely to occur if the patient has an element of prolapse or a laxity of the rectal mucosa. As with virtually all complications, prevention is the best approach. Care must be taken to avoid gathering a mass of rectal lining into the ligatures.

Management of this complication may require dilatation, either with Young's dilators if the stricture is distal, or a Hegar dilator if the stricture is higher. Operative lysis may be necessary, possibly including either advancement of the rectal mucosa or proctoplasty.

Fissure or Ulcer

An anal fissure may develop in a patient who has a contracted ano-rectal outlet after hemorrhoidectomy. Usually, the fissure is situated posteriorly. Repeated trauma from defecation results in laceration of the eschar, which may become a chronic, painful anal ulcer. Such postoperative fissures may respond to conservative management (e.g., laxatives, enemas, suppositories, topical creams such as cortisone) and dilatation. However, often an additional procedure is required, most commonly an internal anal sphincterotomy. Excision of the ulcer concomitant with the sphincterotomy may be of benefit, but some form of anoplasty may ultimately be required to increase anal canal circumference.

Pseudopolyps

Hemorrhoidectomy usually requires ligation of the stump of the hemorrhoid. Tissue strangulation will take place at the site of ligation, resulting in sloughing of the stump. This leaves a defect that heals by granulation, the end result of which may be a pseudopolyp. Another possible contributing factor is a foreign-body granuloma, which may be a consequence of the prolonged presence of suture material. This may be manifested by an edematous, polypoid, or sessile tumor at the site of the suture. Pseudopolyps can be excised with a local anesthetic or be electrocoagulated.

Epidermal Cyst

In rare instances, some months after hemorrhoidectomy, asymptomatic inclusion cysts may appear in the anal canal or in the immediate perianal region. Their origin has been attributed to retention of keratin elements, hair particles, or exfoliated squamous epithelial cells in the wound. If these cysts are bothersome, they can be removed by local excision.

Anal Fistula

Anal fistula is an unusual complication of hemorrhoidectomy, occurring in approximately 1 percent of patients. It is allegedly more common after the closed operation than the open, but the incidence is so low that this observation is probably more theoretical than factual. The fistula is inevitably low and subcutaneous, not transsphincteric or even intersphincteric unless the finding is coincidental. Fistulotomy is the appropriate treatment and can often be accomplished in the office.

Pruritus Ani

Most causes of pruritus ani are related to diet or are caused by overaggressive attention to anal hygiene. However, pruritic symptoms following hemorrhoidectomy are not unusual and may actually have an anatomic basis. A mucosal ectropion or Whitehead deformity, for example, can produce mucous discharge, which can contribute to the pruritus. With a specific anatomic abnormality, anoplasty may be advisable.

Fecal Incontinence

Fecal soilage or incontinence following hemorrhoidectomy, although infrequent, is not as rare as the physician might expect. A possible explanation is the loss of anal canal sensation resulting from removal of sensory-bearing tissue and its replacement by scar. I do not subscribe to such a theory.

Almost all patients who have impairment of fecal control following hemorrhoidectomy are elderly. If the physician takes a careful history, it will probably be discovered that many of these individuals have experienced some soilage before the operation, although the procedure may have exacerbated the problem. This is often the case when the patient has some degree of mucosal or rectal prolapse, and it is a particular concern in women. Special care should be taken when performing this operation in the older age group; it is important to avoid unnecessary sphincter stretch or sphincterotomy. Many surgeons are fond of sphincterotomy, because they believe it ameliorates the postoperative pain problem. This has not been found to be true when studied in trials. When it is performed at the posterior pile site, a keyhole deformity can result. It is a potentially hazardous maneuver in an individual without a concomitant fissure and should be avoided, especially in someone older than 60 years of age.

Recurrence

Most patients who complain of recurrent hemorrhoids usually are describing skin tags or have pruritic symptoms. However, in some cases, true hemorrhoidal veins have developed that have become symptomatic after an assumed complete hemorrhoidectomy. "Doctor, I had the operation 10 years ago, and now the hemorrhoids are back", is the commonly expressed observation. However, piles that have been removed cannot recur. The "recurrence" consists of veins that, either because of their normal appearance at the time of hemorrhoidectomy or in an effort to preserve adequate mucosal bridges, were left undisturbed. With increased pressure or collateral circulation developing over the years, dilatation occurs and symptomatic hemorrhoids result.

Because of this potential problem, all hemorrhoidal veins should be removed at the time of the surgical procedure. Tunneling out minute vessels from the underlying mucosa and debriding all veins over the external sphincter are important prophylactic maneuvers. When recurrent piles become symptomatic, ideal treatment should be by an outpatient procedure, usually rubber ring ligation or office excision.

Retroperitoneal Air

A solitary case of retroperitoneal air following hemorrhoidectomy was reported by Kriss and colleagues. The patient had been receiving steroids for rheumatoid arthritis, so this medication may have played some part in its occurrence. The authors suggest that air was introduced either during the dissection or subsequently, when the patient coughed or strained. A third explanation, not offered by the authors, is the possibility that this complication was unrelated to the operation. The patient responded well to nonoperative management.

Conclusion

Despite meticulous surgical technique, complications following hemorrhoidectomy are not uncommon but can be minimized. Awareness of potential concerns leads to prevention, the best means for dealing with these issues.

EDITORIAL COMMENT

The Editor has no comments to make as Professor Corman's chapter speaks for itself. Complications after hemorrhoidectomy are few, preventable, and treatable if they occur, although fecal incontinence may present special difficulties in very exceptional cases. All complications are managed most effectively if they are diagnosed early and corrected promptly. Expeditious treatment is the best defense against a potentially aggrieved patient.

Acknowledgement

This chapter has been taken in part from Corman ML. Colon and Rectal Surgery. Lippincott, Williams and Wilkins. Philadelphia 1998.

21 Contraindications to Haemorrhoidectomy

Charles V. Mann

The title of this chapter, which restricts its considerations to *haemorrhoidectomy* rather than the whole range of haemorrhoid operations, reflects the fact that, apart from haemorrhoidectomy, the majority of them are so extremely safe that contraindications to them are virtually nonexistent. When, however, a contraindication to haemorrhoidectomy also applies, however uncommonly, to one of the other surgical options, specific reference will be made to this.

Contraindications to haemorrhoidectomy may be divided into 1) those that relate to extra-anal causes ("General Contraindications") and 2) those that arise from anal causes ("Local Contraindications").

General Contraindications

The principal general contraindications may be listed as follows.

Age Considerations

Once a patient has reached the age of 70 years, potential adverse effects of haemorrhoidectomy begin to outweigh its advantages. The operation should not be performed in older patients without taking into account the extra risks involved for any surgical operation on geriatric subjects. Anaesthetic complications are much more common in this age group, and older men are prone to postoperative retention of urine. With increasing age, anal sphincter tone declines and this adds to the possibility of faecal and/or flatus incontinence after haemorrhoidectomy. Long-term benefits will be restricted by the diminished life expectancy after 70 years of age. Therefore, while old age does not prohibit haemorrhoidectomy, it should be performed only when the indications for intervention are extremely powerful.

Haemorrhoidectomy should also be avoided in young patients, especially if they are less than 35 years of age. This is discussed elsewhere (Ch. 5, p. 38), but there is an increased likelihood of early recurrence of piles if a haemorrhoidectomy is performed on this age group.

Chronic Illness

If a patient is infirm, and most emphatically if this is associated with old age, as discussed above, haemorrhoidectomy should not be performed.

Certain specific illnesses deserve special discussion in regard to the decision to operate, as follows:

(i) Cardiac and cerebro-vascular disease. If the patient suffers from a serious heart problem, haemorrhoidectomy should not be performed; in particular, a recent (i.e., within the past six months) myocardial infarct is an absolute contraindication. However, in any patient where the surgeon believes that the subject's cardiovascular status transfers operative risk status from "no risk" to "slight risk" (or greater), haemorrhoidectomy should rarely be advised. A history of cerebro-vascular accident is also a contraindication to haemorrhoidectomy not only because of the immediate operative risk, but also because further strokes may occur at any time.

Moderate hypertension does not prohibit surgical treatment, but if the blood pressure is very high, and especially if it is difficult to control and/or requires maximum doses of drugs such as thiazides, beta-blockers or calcium antagonists, this can pose serious problems for anaesthesia, and operation should not be advised (or, at least, postponed until the blood pressure is brought under control).

(ii) Pulmonary disease. Any patient who has severe impairment of lung function should be advised against a haemorrhoidectomy under a general anaesthetic, and even under spinal or caudal anaesthesia there is some increased risk, although these should be the preferred options.

If there is doubt about the level of respiratory reserve, investigations should be arranged to ascertain its exact measurement. In addition to a (routine) chest X-ray, a forced expiratory volume test (FEV) and a forced vital capacity test (FVC) should be ordered. It should be remembered that patients with reduced lung function tolerate the lithotomy or prone on-table positions badly, and the preferred position for surgery should be the left lateral position.

Heavy smokers should be told to stop smoking prior to surgery, preferably for at least three weeks. If they have increased sputum production, especially if it is purulent, this should be cleared up before operation by appropriate measures (e.g., physiotherapy, postural exercises, antibiotics).

If the patient suffers from chronic obstructive airway disease, a general anaesthetic is contraindicated: even if the operation is planned under spinal or caudal anaesthesia, it is wise to obtain the advice of a specialist in lung diseases before proceeding. Although this should not require mention, it must be stated that patients suffering from an acute upper respiratory tract infection (URI) should not be operated on. It is an unfortunate fact that patients with a "sore throat" have been operated upon, with serious consequences, and sometimes death; intubation is especially dangerous in patients with URI.

(iii) Diabetes. Diabetes is not a contraindication to haemorrhoidectomy, but may require special management over the operative period, especially if insulin is used. The anaesthetist must be aware of its existence, and participate actively in management both during and after anaesthesia.

(iv) Spinal diseases. Acute flexion of the lower spine, as in the lithotomy position, puts extreme stress on the lumbar region. If the patient has a significant history of spinal problem (e.g., spondylolisthesis; disc protrusion; ankylosing spondylitis), this can be a contraindication to surgery, at least in the lithotomy position. If the patient has a history of acute disc protrusion (with or without sciatica), and especially if there is a history of spinal surgery (e.g., laminectomy), the patient must be aware that there is a possibility that the operation may cause spinal complications and he must give written consent that he understands this risk; special precautions should be taken to protect the lower spine during surgery.

(v) Obesity. Obesity is often present in patients with haemorrhoids. It is not a contraindication to surgery but it should be remembered that it may cause operative problems (e.g., anaesthetic difficulties (especially for the prone face down position), increased bleeding from anal venous engorgement, interference with exposure of the operative field). Morbid obesity is a contraindication to haemorrhoidectomy.

(vi) Blood diseases. It is advisable to carry out a routine *blood profile examination* to detect any abnormality of either the red or the white cell series. Although uncommon, anaemia, polycythaemia and leukaemia can all have a relationship to haemorrhoids as a result of bleeding or thrombosis. A *sickle-cell test* is also recommended because this disorder has become widely disseminated by population movements and miscegenation, so that it is no longer limited to easily defined groups. Patients with known bleeding disorders need careful appraisal before a haemorrhoidectomy is considered, although, paradoxically, they may also aggravate bleeding from piles to the point that it becomes necessary to operate. *Haemophilia* would generally be regarded as a contraindication to haemorrhoidectomy. Some patients not known to have a blood disorder may give a history of unusually severe bleeding after a dental extraction; this should always alert the surgeon that a bleeding disorder or other coagulation deficiency is present.

Aspirin (and other NSAIDS) interfere with platelet functions, and promote bleeding. Patients with rheumatic diseases or chronic arthritides often take these drugs regularly in large doses; they should be stopped a few days before the operation.

Pregnancy and Parturition

Haemorrhoids are both caused and aggravated by pregnancy and childbirth. Surgical treatment at these times must be avoided except in very exceptional circumstances. The date of a female patient's last menstrual period must be recorded routinely in her records; any possibility of pregnancy must be tested, and if there is a positive result, surgery should be cancelled. If a haemorrhoidectomy is performed on a pregnant patient, any subsequent complication or accident (e.g., miscarriage) will be attributed by the patient to the surgery and, justified or not, litigation would be the normal consequence nowadays.

Both a gravid uterus and childbirth often increase the size and degree of prolapse of haemorrhoids. Each pregnancy involves increased risks for development, progression and recurrence of haemorrhoids. Therefore, not only should a haemorrhoidectomy be avoided during and immediately after pregnancy, but surgery is contraindicated while the woman is still intending to have more children.

Childbirth, especially a difficult one (e.g., prolonged labour; forceps delivery), is known to cause permanently diminished anal sphincter tone; in some cases, direct sphincter damage may occur (e.g., third-degree tear; faulty episiotomy). If there is a history of difficult delivery, the presence of an acceptable degree of anal tone, both resting and squeeze pressures, should be established before a haemorrhoidectomy is carried out. Anal manometry is the best method to measure anal sphincter tone, but clinical examination will usually suffice.

In some socio-economic or religious groups, frequent pregnancies are the norm, sometimes almost every one or two years. Such circumstances are a contraindication to surgical management until contraceptive use or the menopause prevent further conceptions.

Gastrointestinal Diseases

If the patient suffers from a chronic gastrointestinal disease, such as Crohn's disease or colitis, this may be a contraindication to haemorrhoidectomy for two reasons: 1) the illness may be so serious that surgical intervention cannot be contemplated or 2) the consequences of the disease, direct or indirect, may lead to a poor result. Only the second reason needs further discussion.

Direct contraindications to a haemorrhoidectomy include active ulcerative colitis and florid ano-rectal Crohn's disease. Other gastrointestinal causes to prevent surgical management are considered in the next section under Local Contraindications (p. 142).

Indirect contraindications include persistent diarrhoea and chronic constipation which are unresponsive to control measures; in neither case is the contraindication absolute. Causes of persistent diarrhoea include coeliac disease, pancreatic disorders (deficiency), short-bowel syndrome and inflammatory bowel diseases. Chronic constipation may be a consequence of dietary or environmental factors or be due to psychological illness. Unless the bowel disorder can be corrected, and the symptoms alleviated, at least to cover the period of surgical treatment, a haemorrhoidectomy should be avoided.

Drug and Alcohol Abuse

A patient with a serious problem of addiction to a controlled drug (cocaine, opioid or psychotropic addiction, in particular) should not be offered a haemorrhoidectomy unless they can be helped, if not cured.

Laxative abuse and cathartic colon are contraindications to surgery pending control of their symptoms.

Drug addicts, especially those with heroin or morphine addiction, cannot be relied on to cooperate during surgical treatment and a wise surgeon should avoid any problems by not advising an operation. Even if a surgeon is persuaded that an operation is correct management, these patients are often discovered to have positive carrier status for hepatitis B or C, which is an additional reason for avoiding surgery.

Alcohol abuse, unless it is uncontrollable or in its advanced stages (e.g., liver damage) is not an absolute contraindication to haemorrhoidectomy, but the surgeon must be confident of his ability to control any peri-operative complications (e.g., drunken behaviour, delirium tremens); if he has concerns of his ability to master any alcohol-related problems which may arise, operative treatment is contraindicated.

Anal Intercourse

Anal intercourse, even if it is habitual, does not contraindicate haemorrhoidectomy unless it is associated with a patulous ("receptive") anus. However, all patients who practice anal intercourse (and other related sexual habits, such as "fisting") should be made aware of the relationship to diminished anal sphincter tone, together with the warning that a haemorrhoidectomy will not improve tone, or diminish problems of flatus or faecal control. If a surgeon suspects that the patient could develop incontinence problems, anal manometry will give measurements that can be taken into account before a haemorrhoidectomy is performed; if necessary, the measurements can be repeated postoperatively.

Immune Deficiency Disorders and Diseases

Immune deficiency is a contraindication to haemorrhoidectomy if it is severe; the most prominent cause of severe immunodeficiency is HIV infection, particularly if AIDS has become manifest. This problem is discussed in Ch. 23.

Other causes of immune deficiency include drugs (steroids, cytotoxic agents); radiation (therapeutic, accidental exposure); infection (sepsis); and congenital diseases. In most cases, any question of a haemorrhoidectomy does not arise, as it would be so obviously inappropriate.

Local Contraindications

The principal local contraindications may be listed as follows:

- weak sphincter
- deformed anus
- mucosal inflammation
- specific diseases (TB, LGV, Carcinoma).

Weak Anal Sphincter

Significant weakness of the anal sphincters is a contraindication to haemorrhoidectomy for the following reasons: (i) the operation may further weaken the sphincter muscles, risking incontinence; (ii) the haemorrhoids may be acting as a plug for the anal lumen, and their removal may increase the likelihood of incontinence, at least for flatus; and (iii) prolapse of mucosa, with or without a haemorrhoid component, is likely within a few years, with recurrence of symptoms of prolapse and bleeding. Instead of surgery, the haemorrhoids should be treated by banding, with repeated treatments as required to control symptoms. Only if the prolapse resists this treatment can surgery be considered.

Deformed Anal Canal

The normal shape of the anal canal is a short tube, which is kept closed by sphincter action except during defaecation. If the canal is deformed, the mucosal lining loses its normal support (from being pressed against the inner aspect of the lamina propria) and consequently is easily dislocated and prone to prolapse.

Some patients are born with anal deformation. One of these is called a "funnel anus" from the shape of the deformity, which has a wide external anal orifice, which narrows down to a closed upper anal canal (hence the funnel shape). These patients depend for continence on the strength of the muscles at the ano-rectal junction and around the upper one third of the anal canal. However, the mucosal folds and anal cushions are important ancillary aids to continence lower down the canal where the lumen is not compressed by the sphincter muscles; haemorrhoids make a contribution to this soft tissue luminal plug, which acts passively like a "flannel in the bath outlet". The author concludes that it is inappropriate to increase problems for anal continence in such circumstances by removal of either haemorrhoids or mucosal tissues, and that treatment should be restricted to non-operative methods, e.g., banding. Stapling would be a poor technique for haemorrhoidectomy in patients with a funnel anus.

Fistulectomy for a high fistula-in-ano often leaves a defect of the anal wall ("gutter deformity"). Prolapse of both mucosa and haemorrhoids is promoted by this defect. In addition to the likelihood of early recurrence after surgery, haemorrhoidectomy for this situation has the same drawback of diminished continence as the operation in funnel deformity, and should be avoided whenever possible. If non-operative methods fail, resort to surgery can be justified.

Mucosal Inflammation

Both ulcerative colitis and Crohn's disease can involve the anal canal. If piles develop in these patients, all treatments have greater risks. After haemorrhoidectomy, the wounds may heal slowly or, in the case of Crohn's disease, never completely. There are also increased chances of postoperative bleeding or anal stenosis. These risks are much greater if surgery is performed when the inflammation is active. If a haemorrhoidectomy is the best treatment of the haemorrhoids, the operation should be carried out when a remission is established. For further discussion of this problem, see Ch. 23.

Specific Diseases

A few ano-rectal diseases are absolute contraindications to haemorrhoidectomy.

Tuberculosis

Tuberculous anal wounds do not heal and are extremely prone to complications such as fistulae. Bloodstream dissemination from a focus elsewhere, as well as transmission of live organisms down the gastro-intestinal tract, can respectively infect the ano-rectal region or implant on open anal wounds. One such case referred to the author had developed an ano-rectal fistula following a haemorrhoidectomy in the Middle East; subsequent investigation disclosed the tuberculous cause of the fistula to be an untreated lung lesion.

Lymphogranuloma Venereum (Chlamydia Trachomatis A, Types 1–3)

Although an established infection with LGV is unlikely to be missed, care must be exercised not to overlook its early manifestations. Haemorrhoid surgery should be deferred until the infection is cured. Surgeons working in tropical zones are most likely to meet this problem.

Venereal Diseases

In addition to sexually transmitted chlamydial infections (see also above), both gonorrhoea and syphilis can affect the ano-rectum. All are contraindications to haemorrhoidectomy until the infections have been cured by suitable antibiotic treatment.

Carcinoma

If a haemorrhoidectomy is carried out in the presence of an untreated colo-rectal carcinoma (especially one that is distally sited), two disastrous consequences follow: (1) the undiagnosed carcinoma progresses and may become incurable and (2) viable tumour cells shed from the surface of the carcinoma may (and very likely will) implant in the anal wounds, making treatment by a Miles-type ano-rectal excision inevitable, whatever treatment is offered to the proximal colo-rectal growth. The closer the colo-rectal carcinoma is to the anus, the greater the chance of implantation.

While it would be excessive to advise full investigation of the entire large bowel before each haemorrhoidectomy (e.g., by total colonoscopy), it is necessary to perform full examination of the rectum and distal sigmoid colon in every case. In all other instances where symptoms suggest in any way that a proximal carcinoma may be present, total colonoscopy and/or an air contrast barium enema must be done prior to haemorrhoidectomy.

Summation

There are very few absolute contraindications to haemorrhoidectomy (e.g., recent MI, bleeding disorders, pregnancy, tuberculosis, proximal carcinoma). There are, however, many reasons to postpone surgery or to choose alternative treatments whenever possible. An ill-considered resort to surgical treatment can have dangerous consequences for both patient and surgeon. A haemorrhoid operation, like marriage, should not be entered upon lightly or inadvisably; there is no easy divorce after surgical error, only complications and medico legal settlements.

EDITORIAL COMMENT

Contraindications to haemorrhoidectomy are not given much space (if any) in textbooks of colo-rectal surgery. They are, nevertheless, of great importance since haemorrhoids are a benign condition for which the safety of any treatment is of paramount importance. Haemorrhoid surgery should be no exception to the rule that treatment for a harmless condition should be very safe, and that any risk, however small, should be considered most carefully before the decision to operate is taken. An incomplete general history which omits information on background habits (e.g., drug use), possible pregnancy, anaesthetic risks, and other health problems (e.g., heart disease) is, in the Editor's opinion, responsible for many of the serious problems which occasionally arise after haemorrhoid surgery, although bad surgery is predominant.

22 Management of Haemorrhoid Complications. Thrombosis, Fissure-in-ano, Recurrence

Charles V. Mann

Thrombosis

Thrombosis of External Haemorrhoids ("Acute Perianal Haematoma")

Unless they are associated with thrombosis of the entire internal and external haemorrhoidal venous plexus, as in strangulated piles (see next section), a thrombosed external haemorrhoid is a result of rupture/thrombosis at a single, or sometimes multiple, isolated site(s).

Aetiology

This is not proven, but is thought to be rupture of an external vein as a result of a sudden sharp rise in intraluminal pressure, possibly related to a forceful contraction or spasm of the anal sphincters. Clinical evidence to support this conjecture is that external vein thrombosis is commonest in younger patients and often occurs after forced defaecation or following an extreme exertion (e.g., weightlifting).

Presentation

Most cases present with a painful, bluish, tense lump alongside the anal orifice, more commonly in the posterior half of its circumference. It is probable that many cases do not experience pain, as skin tags are often considered to be the end-result of a thrombosed external haemorrhoid. Sometimes there are several thromboses. A few patients consult their doctor because of the lump, rather than pain, which they fear may be a tumour. If left untreated, spontaneous resolution is usual (possibly with a residual skin tag, as stated) but rarely the clot may erode through the overlying skin and discharge itself. This is associated with surface loss of both fresh and old blood, including clots, and a crater may be left that may mimic an ulcer and raise fears of malignancy. It is important to ascertain that there is a *strip of skin between the perianal lump and the anal canal*, as this is an important identifying feature for a perianal haematoma (Fig. 22.1).

In the early stages (24–48 hours), the skin over the lump is normal, but after this there is usually some oedema; in the later stages (7–10 days) spontaneous resolution begins, with gradual disappearance of the thrombosis. As stated above, in a few cases there is spontaneous discharge of the clot, leaving a temporary cavity. Features that can allow the clinician to conclude that the cavity is not a malignant ulcer are the cleanness of its sides and base; the absence of a raised everted edge; that no induration or fixation to underlying tissues is present; and the speed of healing (which should take less than three weeks). However, the normal rules apply, that if the surgeon is unsure of the true nature of the perianal lesion, it is mandatory that a biopsy should be done for tissue diagnosis.

Although most patients present in acute pain, using great care and gentleness, digital examination, proctoscopy and sigmoidoscopy (with a small-bore instrument) can be carried out, and whenever possible these should be performed prior to treatment. If this is not possible, they must all be completed before the patient is discharged from the clinic after finishing treatment.

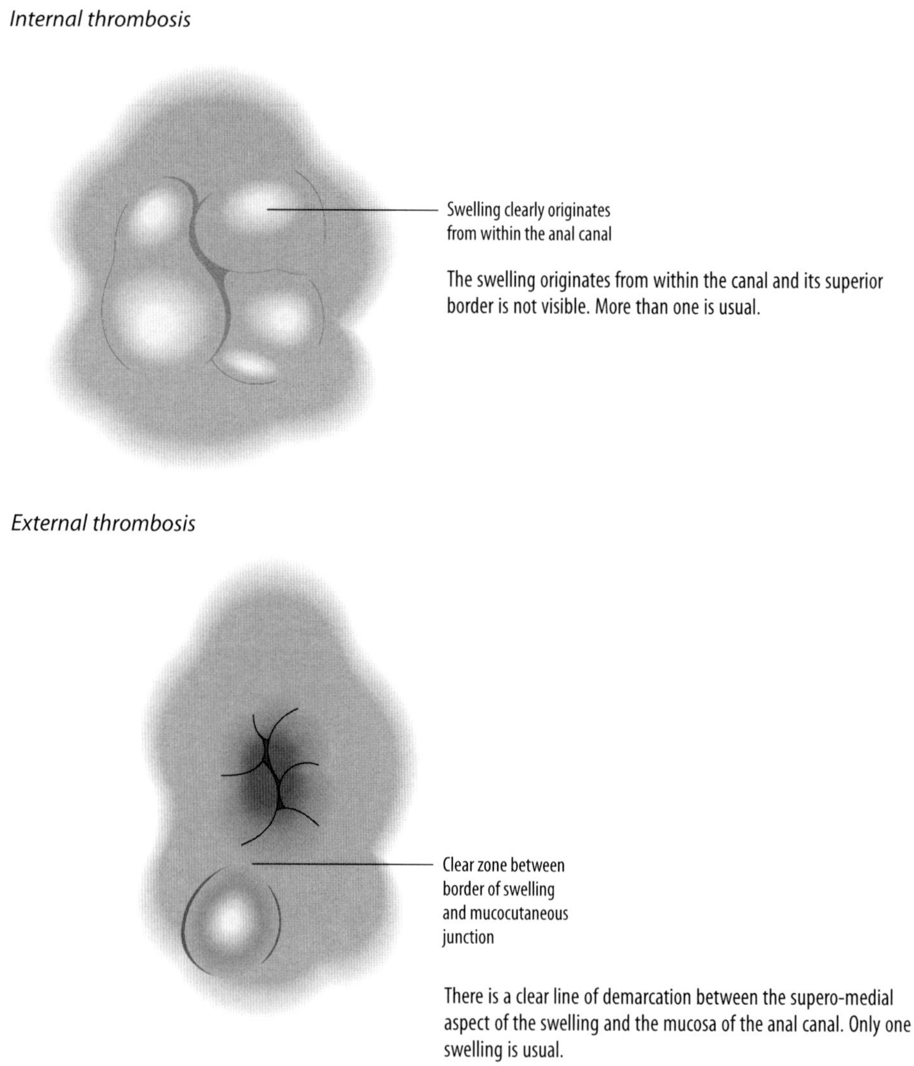

Figure 22.1. Visual sign to distinguish an external from an internal thrombosis.

Treatment (Figs. 22.2 and 22.3)

(a) *Acute presentation.* Immediate relief of pain can be obtained by evacuation of the clot under local anaesthesia. Infiltration of local anaesthetic should be done very slowly as this reduces discomfort and swelling related to the injection: the needle should be extremely fine and can be short. The solution used should be 1% lignocaine with 1:300,000 adrenaline, and the circumference, base and skin overlying the lump should be infiltrated; this not only gives complete anaesthesia but also prevents any bleeding from the wound edges and cavity surfaces (Fig. 22.2). The clot can be evacuated through a simple radial linear incision over the apex of the lump but it is important that no fragments of clot are left behind as these may delay healing or encourage wound infection. If a linear incision does not give adequate access or prevents proper healing by virtue of overhanging edges (which may also interfere with separation of clot fragments or other wound debris), a cruciform incision or cutting back excess skin can be effective (Fig. 22.3). Saucerisation of the wound is not required, and increases time for healing. After evacuation of the clot, the cavity does not need to be packed. A simple gauze pad and cotton wool dressing held in place by a "T" bandage or firm-fitting elasticated trunks are all

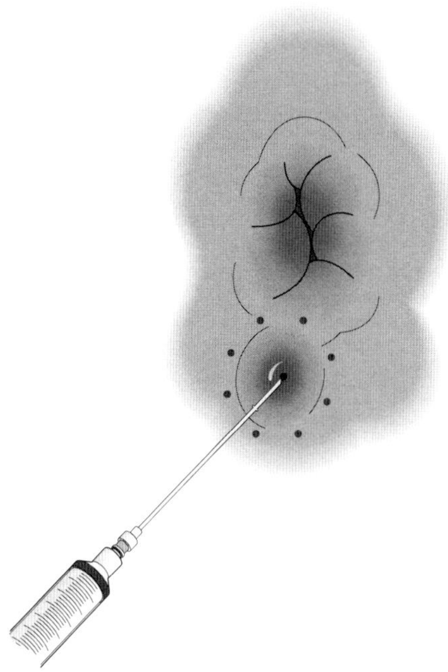

After cleaning the skin with aqueous chlorhexidine, 1% lignocaine or Bupivacaine is injected around, beneath and also over the top of the swelling.

Although bleeding from the subsequent incision is not usually troublesome, the local anaesthetic can be usefully supplemented by weak (1 : 300,000) adrenaline solution.

Figure 22.2. Injection of Local Anaesthetic.

that is necessary. The patient is advised to have frequent baths, but neither antiseptic dressings nor antibiotics are necessary. Healing is usually uneventful and speedy. The patient should return for inspection of the wound and completion of any deferred diagnostic tests after one or two weeks, and provided the surgeon is satisfied with progress, can usually be discharged.

(b) *Delayed presentation.* If the patient delays presentation for a few days, the acute pain is usually subsiding; furthermore, the clot is already undergoing natural dissolution, accompanied by invasion of blood vessels from surrounding tissues, which makes its removal more difficult and bloody. Management is therefore conservative, with reassurance and analgesia until the haematoma is reabsorbed. As for the acute case, all necessary diagnostic tests should be done before the patient is discharged. Some surgeons practise complete excision of the haematoma, and suture of the wound; although this overcomes the difficulties of clot evacuation, most surgeons regard this as overzealous management, and not entirely free from risks of septic complications; it is not advised.

Complications

There are very few complications, and they are not usually serious.

(a) *Sepsis.* In rare cases, the clot can become infected and an abscess develops. Simple lancing of the abscess, with release of pus, is curative. Even more rarely, a neglected abscess can result in a subcutaneous fistula, which will require laying open.

(b) *Skin tags.* If a skin tag results from an untreated perianal haematoma, it may need to be removed if it causes symptoms at a later date.

(c) *Recurrent attacks.* Some patients are prone to recurrent attacks of perianal thrombosis (or multiple thromboses, which are unsuitable for numerous separated incisions at a single outpatient treatment session). In both instances, high anal sphincter tone; or recurrent bouts of sphincter spasm; or activity-related episodes of maximal anal contractions may be contributory factors underlying the manifestations. For such cases, either an elective anal dilation or subcutaneous internal anal sphincterotomy may be considered, especially if anal manometry confirms that the patient has a hypertonic anal sphincter.

(d) *Multiple thromboses.* If, instead of a solitary thrombosis, the patient suffers from an acute attack of multiple thromboses, these may be unsuitable for office treatment under local anaesthesia. Conservative management is always safe and reliable, but sometimes it is possible to consider surgical removal under a general anaesthetic if the lesions are localised to one or two areas of the perianal circumference: if such treatment is justified by the symptoms, anal dilatation or an internal anal sphincterotomy can be performed at the same time (see above) but only if the surgeon is certain that there is no risk of causing incontinence.

Thrombosis of Internal Haemorrhoids ("Acute Strangulated Haemorrhoids")

Thrombosis of internal haemorrhoids may occur more frequently than can be quantified because

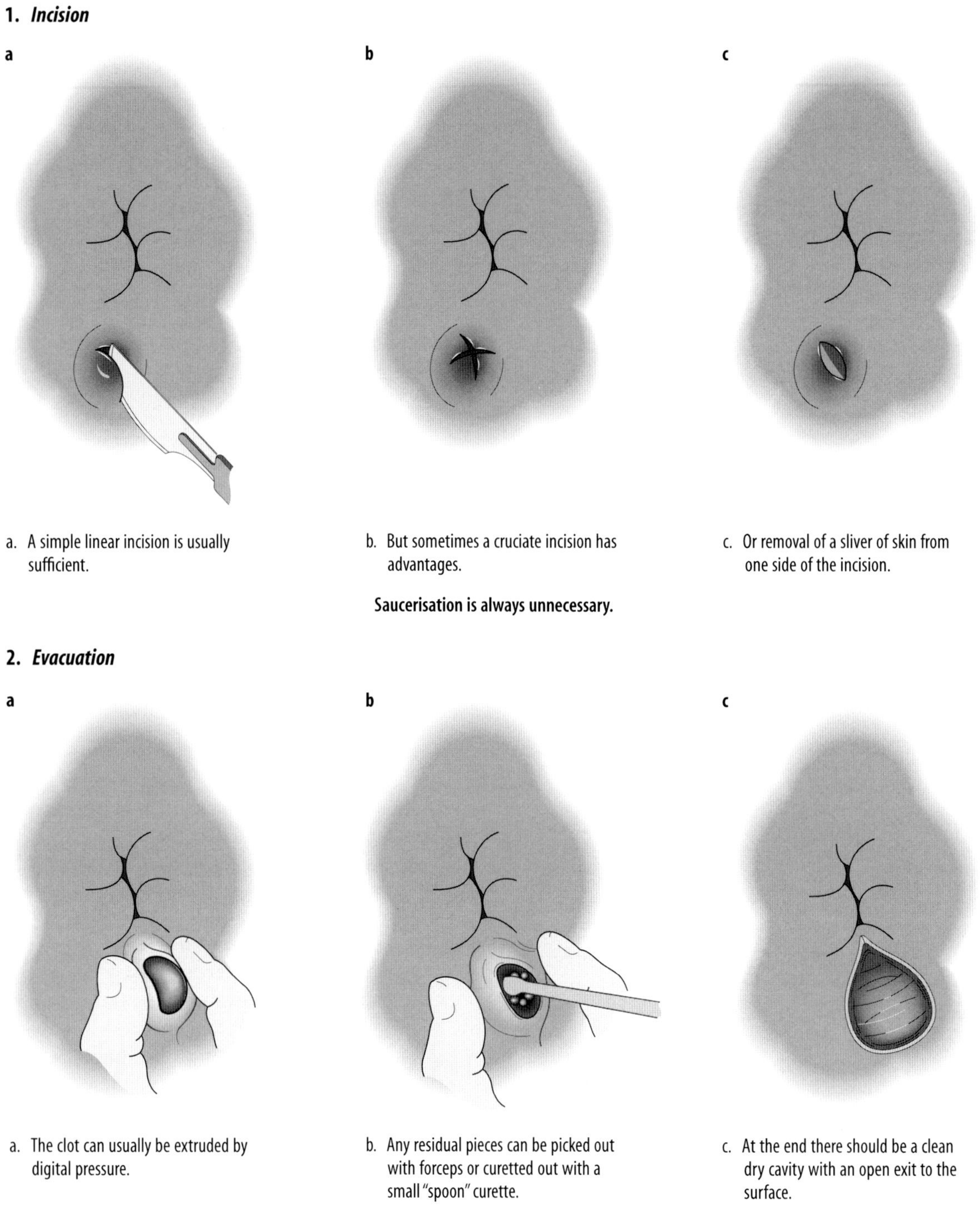

Figure 22.3. Incision and evacuation of the haematoma.

some portion of a haemorrhoid lies beneath pain-insensitive mucosa in the upper reaches of the anal canal; the rare instances of an internal submucosal anal fistula, which is presumed to arise as a result of septic complications of a thrombosed internal haemorrhoid, are partial confirmation of this supposition. In practise, however, thrombosis of internal haemorrhoids develops in piles that have been extruded from the anal canal, and is frequently accompanied by thrombosis of external haemorrhoids as well ("strangulated intero-external haemorrhoids").

Aetiology and Progress Untreated

When a ring of large haemorrhoids is pushed out, or is significantly prolapsed (i.e., large second- and third-degree piles), it can be gripped by the anal sphincters before it has returned to the anal canal. If the sphincter constriction is forceful, venous return from the extruded tissue is obstructed, and oedema and thrombosis are caused. Rapid progression of swelling and thrombosis occurs, and severe pain develops; the acute pain promotes reflex sphincter spasm, and a vicious cycle of spasm and swelling develops. The end result is a mass of engorged thrombosed veins in a matrix of oedematous mucosa, skin and soft tissue; this mass is aptly described as "strangulated piles" and can be fully established in a short time (hours). Because of its site, infection is present from the very beginning with both aerobic and anaerobic organisms, and this becomes heavy within 24–48 hours. After five days, the condition does not progress and the pain and swelling begin to subside but do not fully resolve for several weeks. Constipation is usual during the early stages, and faecal impaction is not uncommon. Paradoxically, as a result of the thrombosis, the piles may be greatly reduced in size and the patient may think he is "cured"; unfortunately, this is an illusion and, as soon as clot resorption, and later venous recanalisation, are complete, the piles gradually resume their pre-strangulation state. This means that recurrence of prolapse/thrombosis would be expected unless the haemorrhoids are treated.

Presentation

The patient presents as an emergency with severe pain. Their anguished faces and peculiar straddled gait are frequently the butt of bawdy jokes. The appearance of the turgid mass of engorged strangulated tissue surrounding the anal orifice is unmistakable. Severe spasm of the anal sphincters is usual, and reduction of the mass is impossible, not only because of the anal spasm but also because it is too large to be reaccommodated within the anal canal. After 24–48 hours, there is a characteristic strong musty odour that betokens the presence of a multitude of anaerobic bacteria. After four or five days, some parts of overstretched skin or mucosa overlying the mass may necrose and spontaneous extrusion of pieces of clot may occur.

Despite its horrific appearance and the inevitable element of infection, there are usually no systemic signs of sepsis, the temperature and pulse rate remaining normal. This may be due in part to the anal sphincter spasm, which helps to "isolate" the infected tissues from the general circulation. This point is of more than theoretical importance because it is possible for surgical treatment to relieve this barrier to bacterial spread, and allow both portal and systemic invasion by bacteria. In the pre-antibiotic era, deaths from portal pyaemia, liver abscesses and septicaemia were a serious possible risk after immediate surgical treatments, which prevented their employment. Even at the present time, the possibility of dangerous septic consequences, however rare, is enough to prevent the routine use of emergency haemorrhoidectomy for treatment, as discussed later.

At presentation, the severe pain that accompanies the condition prevents any examination other than a visual inspection, but once it is cured, all the usual routine tests for any case of haemorrhoids must be completed, including proctoscopy and sigmoidoscopy.

Treatment

Non-operative (Conservative) Management

This is the safe option, and the one that is commonly used. It does not require either a high degree of judgement or surgical expertise, and can be applied by a variety of medical practitioners, including family doctors, general surgeons, as well as proctologists. Treatment is directed at (a) relief of pain, (b) resolution of the strangulation pathology, and (c) prevention of constipation and/or faecal impaction. Once the condition has been alleviated, consideration must be directed at prevention of recurrence.

(a) *Relief of pain.* Pain may be very severe for the first few days, and resort to opiates may be necessary for many patients. Although these drugs may, in theory, increase the tendency to constipation, unless the patients' pain is effectively reduced, defaecation may be one agony too much for them, with consequent risk of faecal impaction (see below). Intramuscular injections of pethidine or morphine sulphate should be given unhesitatingly if the pain justifies their use. As soon as possible, the patient is transferred onto oral analgesics without constipating side effects. The doses of any analgesics can be reduced by simultaneous use of a tranquilliser or anxiolytic. Metronidazole has been claimed to reduce pain after a haemorrhoidectomy, and will help to reduce the anaerobic bacterial load in the strangulated tissues; for both reasons, the author advocates administration of Metronidazole (400 mg daily in divided doses) for five days, although there is no proof of its effectiveness. The patient needs to be warned to avoid alcohol while taking the drug. On the fifth day, post-strangulation pain begins to subside rapidly and ceases to be a treatment problem.

(b) *Resolution of the pathology.* Measures to reduce swelling assist greatly to diminution of pain. Such measures include 1) frequent hot soaks in a bath or sitz apparatus, 2) application of ice packs or cold compresses, and 3) recumbency.

Injections into the tissues of preparations to reduce oedema (e.g., hyaluronidase) are condemned as they are ineffective and spread infection.

(c) *Prevention of constipation and faecal impaction.* Constipation is best relieved by frequent small doses of an oral salt, such as magnesium sulphate (5 g in a tumbler of water every eight hours), which is taken until defaecation is established. Oral fluids should be increased, but food should be restricted to light, easily digested items that do not increase faecal bulk. Once defaecation has been established, the patient is transferred onto a stool softener (e.g., lactulose), but as soon as pain has disappeared and activity has been resumed, a normal diet is permissible with the optimal content of bran or a bulking agent (methylcellulose granules; isphagula). If the patient becomes severely constipated, an enema may be required: for practical reasons of delivery by a fine tube, a microenema (Fletcher's enema, Microlax) should be tried first. If this does not work, and especially if faecal impaction supervenes, a rectal evacuation under general anaesthetic is indicated. In suitable cases, this can be combined with an anal dilatation or a haemorrhoidectomy, as discussed in the next section.

Operative (Invasive) Management

One of two methods may be employed; either an immediate anal dilatation or an emergency haemorrhoidectomy. These are discussed separately.

(a) *Anal dilatation.* This is a most effective treatment for immediate relief of symptoms and rapid resolution of the condition. The risk of anal incontinence is averted by two factors: 1) the anal sphincter is usually in tight spasm before the dilatation begins, and 2) most cases of strangulation occur in patients who are not elderly. It is used most appropriately in the first few days of strangulation when pain and swelling are at their peak. The technique is described in detail in Ch. 7. No special preparation is required but the procedure should be accompanied by intra-operative antibiotic cover by a single injection intravenously of an antibiotic active against both aerobic and anaerobic bacteria. Once dilatation has been concluded, the rectum should be evacuated of all faecal content, by a washout if required, and a cold compress packed tightly against the anus. Once the patient has recovered, a light diet with plenty of fluids is started, supplemented with a daily dose of bulking agent (e.g., Isogel). Once defaecation has started, a normal diet with Bran can be resumed.

The results of dilatation can be dramatic, with immediate relief of pain and a rapid reduction of swelling, which is assisted by frequent hot baths and cold compresses. Sometimes, the swollen tissues have shrunk down to nearly normal appearances within a few days and the patient is often able to resume work in one, or at most, two weeks.

Although symptoms of piles may be relieved and their bulk considerably reduced for a few months, it is usual for the haemorrhoids to revert to their pre-dilatation size within a year. Definitive treatment is indicated at this time by an elective haemorrhoidectomy using an appropriate technique. Failure to do this will have the attached risk for a recurrence of strangulation.

(b) *Emergency haemorrhoidectomy.* An immediate haemorrhoidectomy can be considered in the first few days of strangulation, before the tissues are too infected and distorted by oedema and thrombosis. Both the decision to operate, and the technical demands of the surgery, require that the operation is performed by a senior and experienced surgeon. Combining sufficient removal of haemorrhoids with preservation of satisfactory skin bridges can be a significant challenge for the best anal surgeons. It is better to leave behind small thrombosed haemorrhoids rather than to jeopardise skin bridges, especially so as such residual elements may undergo substantial (or even total) disappearance over the months following surgery. An emergency haemorrhoidectomy would not be thought appropriate treatment in the following circumstances: 1) if there is clinical evidence of significant bacterial infection, 2) if the tissues are damaged and distorted to a degree that precludes application of the principles of haemorrhoid surgery, 3) if the process of natural resolution is imminent (or already started), 4) if symptoms are not severe, and 5) if socio-economic circumstances are unfavourable.

Certain details of the operation should be stated, as follows: 1) the operation should be covered by antibiotics active against aerobic and anaerobic bacteria; 2) infiltration of the tissues with weak adrenaline solution should be omitted; 3) the rectum should be cleansed of all faecal content before starting, if necessary by a rectal wash-out; 4) an intra-operative anal dilation (two fingers of each hand) should be performed before dissection begins; 5) the anal skin bridges to be preserved are marked out; and 6) because the mucosa is stretched, oedematous and friable, an open technique is better than a closed one as any suture line is insecure under these conditions. The infectious element also supports the preference for an open technique, which allows better protection against septic complications and retained clots and other debris.

An emergency haemorrhoidectomy can be bloodsome, both during and after surgery. The patient should be blood grouped before operation, and some cross-matched blood set aside in case it is needed. Although not required after elective haemorrhoidectomy, an anal tampon can be an additional precaution to use against the risk of early postoperative bleeding; if a tampon is used, it should be removed the next day, under a general anaesthetic in many cases.

Postoperative treatment is the same as after a standard elective open haemorrhoidectomy, but special attention needs to be paid to the increased risk of secondary haemorrhage. After the patient is discharged, he should be warned about this possibility, which can occur up to three weeks after the operation; it is important that proper arrangements are made for emergency readmission if this is necessary.

Fissure-in-ano

As might be expected, haemorrhoids are often associated with a fissure-in-ano (and the pain arising from the fissure should not be attributed to the piles).

If the haemorrhoids are small (first- or early second-degree haemorrhoids) and the fissure is a single superficial tear, treatment for the fissure should take precedence over that for the haemorrhoids. Once the fissure has been healed by appropriate treatment (use of anal dilator, dilation under general anaesthesia or an internal anal sphincterotomy may be selected as best treatment in each case), office treatment for the haemorrhoids can be carried out; if sclerotherapy is chosen for treatment, the fissure should be allowed several weeks of healing time before the injections.

If the haemorrhoids are large (bulky second-degree or third-degree), treatment for the fissure by sphincterotomy or dilation can increase their degree of prolapse, or even precipitate an attack of prolapse-thrombosis. The author recommends, therefore, that if the fissure requires one of these treatments, larger haemorrhoids should be operated upon at the same procedure; if a sphincterotomy is performed for the fissure, this can be done in the floor of one of the haemorrhoidectomy wounds, which should be left open (the sphincterotomy would create a sealed pocket beneath the suture line of a closed haemorrhoidectomy, an invitation to septic complications).

If a patient with both prolapsing haemorrhoids and a fissure is elderly or has diminished anal sphincter tone, treatment for the fissure should be cautious, and every attempt should be made to heal the fissure by conservative measures (e.g., using an anal dilator) before haemorrhoidectomy.

When a combined operation for haemorrhoids and a fissure is performed, postoperative care is the same as after a standard haemorrhoidectomy (some surgeons advocate sphincterotomy as part of their normal haemorrhoid surgery).

Recurrent Haemorrhoids

In this section, "recurrent haemorrhoids" are defined as those which recur after an operation.

Recurrence of haemorrhoids after surgical treatment is not common, although very little reliable information is available on this aspect of the haemorrhoid diathesis.

Recurrence of haemorrhoids after a definitive attempt at surgical cure is encouraged by the following factors: 1) poor selection of cases (too young), 2) bad technique (incomplete removal), and 3) faulty anal anatomy (congenital deformity, post-fistulectomy).

Poor selection. Reference has been made elsewhere to the fact that some young (often male) patients with large haemorrhoids seem to have a predisposition to develop piles, which may be genetic or environmental. If these patients are operated upon below the age of 35 years, recurrence is a distinct possibility as their predisposing factors have many more years to cause the piles to redevelop. Fortunately, in most cases, further treatment by non-operative techniques (e.g., banding) is usually possible. Pregnancy, and particularly repeated pregnancy, is a powerful cause of haemorrhoids. If a haemorrhoidectomy is performed, and further pregnancies occur, recurrence of haemorrhoids is likely. The message that should be recognised is that young fertile women should not undergo a haemorrhoidectomy until they have completed their families. If early haemorrhoids (first or second degree) are treated surgically, significant areas of the anal circumference will be untouched by the procedure. These "normal" areas contain cushion tissue that can be a site for further development of haemorrhoids.

Bad technique. Large numbers of haemorrhoidectomies are carried out by untrained and disinterested surgeons. Bad surgery is often allied to poor selection. Until this situation is corrected by extension of specialist proctological training, some recurrences from this cause must be expected: the surprising fact is that there are far fewer recurrences following bad surgery than would be expected. Technical faults which encourage recurrence include failure to display the haemorrhoids properly (which results in an incomplete haemorrhoidectomy) and incomplete removal of secondary haemorrhoids (which enlarge with time into symptomatic piles).

Faulty anal anatomy. If the anal canal is deformed ("funnel anus" or congenital deformity), weakened (atonic sphincter muscle from any cause), or damaged (post-fistulectomy, injuries), the mucosal lining of the anal canal loses its normal support. Once this happens, any mucosal-submucosal tissue that is exposed to defaecatory pressures is likely to be dislodged and develop into a haemorrhoid (a tendency that is analogous to the transformation of an anal cushion into a haemorrhoid). If a haemorrhoidectomy is carried out in a patient who has an abnormal anal canal, recurrence can be anticipated in many cases. Fortunately, anatomical or physiological anal abnormalities are uncommon, and recurrence from these causes is unusual. In many such patients, there is no practical alternative to a haemorrhoidectomy once the piles have become large, and the risk for recurrence must be accepted.

When a haemorrhoidectomy has been carried out by a good technique on a properly selected patient, it is still always necessary to carry out a programme of expert postoperative management and advice. This should take account of all the factors that have caused the patient to develop piles in the first place, such as faulty diet, sedentary life style, constipation and straining habits of defaecation. Unless this is done for each patient, a recurrence of piles will be encouraged. If recurrent haemorrhoids develop despite every precaution (or, sadly, neglect of any prophylactic measures), it is usual for them to respond to non-operative measures (sclerotherapy, banding).

Summation

Thrombosis is the commonest and most important complication of both external and internal haemorrhoids Treatment of an external thrombosis is principally by evacuation of the clot. Treatment of internal haemorrhoids presenting as prolapse/ thrombosis ("strangulation") can be by conservative measures, anal dilatation or emergency haemorrhoidectomy. Judgement is needed to select the right choice, and the procedures demand experience allied to good technique. Patients with haemorrhoids often suffer from an acute fissure-in-ano. In many patients with early (small) haemorrhoids, treatment for the fissure takes precedence over treatment of the haemorrhoids. In patients with large haemorrhoids, a combined operation for both the piles and the fissure is usually the best treatment. Recurrent haemorrhoids after surgical treatment are uncommon and iatrogenic causes include faulty selection, poor technique and deficient aftercare; a damaged or weakened anus may promote recurrence by the same mechanism that it causes haemorrhoids to develop in the first place; namely, by encouraging prolapse; but surgical removal is the only effective treatment for many cases, with banding an alternative technique for others. The need for a repeat haemorrhoidectomy is rare.

EDITORIAL COMMENT

Considering the prevalence of haemorrhoids among the general population, their presentation with a complicating condition is surprisingly uncommon, *fissure* and *thrombosis* being the most important. In most instances, any measures taken to treat the adjuvant condition can be combined with surgical treatment of the haemorrhoids. However, a haemorrhoidectomy should not be performed unless symptoms produced by the piles are enough to justify the procedure; otherwise, it is better to concentrate on curing the complicating condition, leaving treatment for the haemorrhoids for later consideration. In the Editor's practice, one exception to this rule was sphincterotomy for a fissure-in-ano; even if prolapsing haemorrhoids are symptomless in a patient with a fissure, they must be removed because of the aggravated risk of prolapse thrombosis after sphincterotomy.

References and Further Reading

Allen-Mersh TG, Mann CV (1993) In: Fielding LP, Goldberg SM (eds) Operative Surgery, Fifth Edition. Surgery of the Colon, Rectum and Anus. Butterworth-Heinemann, Oxford London Boston, pp 781–3

Goligher JC (1984) Surgery of the Anus, Rectum and Colon, Fifth Edition. Ballière Tindall, London, p 143

Mazier WP (1973) Emergency haemorrhoidectomy: a worthwhile procedure. Dis Colon Rectum 16:200

23 Treatment of Haemorrhoids Complicated by Co-morbidity

Hitesh Patel and Timothy G. Allen-Mersh

Introduction

Haemorrhoidal symptoms are common, and difficulties in management may arise when associated with other disorders. Although pain or bleeding from haemorrhoids may be troublesome, treatment of haemorrhoidal symptoms should not jeopardise the patient with co-morbidity. A team approach is necessary when managing patients with haemorrhoidal symptoms associated with other co-morbidity.

Haemorrhoids with Inflammatory Bowel Disease

Ulcerative Colitis

Inflammatory bowel disease should be excluded in all patients presenting with haemorrhoidal symptoms, since the symptoms of proctitis can initially be misdiagnosed as arising from haemorrhoids. Haemorrhoidal symptoms develop in 20% of patients with ulcerative colitis (deDombal et al., 1966; Keddie, 1980). It is thought that this may be due to the associated diarrhoea, which results in an increased anal sphincter tone (Johanson, 1997). Since drainage of the anal venous plexus occurs during relaxation of the anal sphincter, increased anal muscle tone encourages anal venous plexus engorgement leading to haemorrhoidal symptoms. It has been suggested that anal dilatation or lateral internal sphincterotomy may reduce sphincter tone and the symptoms of haemorrhoidal disease (Deutsch et al., 1987; Hancock & Smith, 1975; Creve & Hubens, 1979; Schouten & van Vroonhoven, 1986), but this approach is probably not appropriate in patients with inflammatory bowel diseases where anal sphincter tone should be retained to control loose motions. In a retrospective review of patients with ulcerative colitis who were treated for haemorrhoids, Jeffery et al. (1977) reported that haemorrhoidal treatments had low complication rates (4 complications after 58 courses of treatment). They suggested that injection sclerotherapy or rubber banding should be used where possible, and that haemorrhoidectomy should be reserved for patients with large and troublesome haemorrhoids whose colitis was in remission. Haemorrhoidectomy should probably be avoided where ileal pouch reconstruction after panproctocolectomy is likely, because haemorrhoidectomy reduces anal canal sensation.

Crohn's Disease

The anus is affected in 25% of patients with small-bowel Crohn's disease, and this rises to 47% with colonic Crohn's disease (Lockhart-Mummery, 1965; Rankin et al., 1979; Williams et al., 1981). Large oedematous external skin tags associated with Crohn's disease should not be confused with haemorrhoids. Anal Crohn's disease is usually associated with rectal Crohn's disease, and all patients with haemorrhoidal symptoms should undergo rectoscopy to avoid inadvertent haemorrhoidectomy in the presence of Crohn's disease. Occasionally, haemorrhoidal surgery is undertaken in patients without a prior history of Crohn's disease who later present with wounds that fail to heal and where the resulting ulcers have coalesced. In contrast to ulcerative colitis, anal complications such as sepsis, stenosis, ulceration and fistula occur in over 50% of patients with Crohn's disease after treatment for haemorrhoids – with up to 30% subsequently requiring proctectomy (Jeffery et al., 1977). Although a conservative approach should be followed in treating haemorrhoidal symptoms associated with Crohn's disease, selected Crohn's disease patients with severe haemorrhoidal symptoms may undergo surgery when the Crohn's disease is quiescent (Wolkomir & Luchtefeld, 1993).

Haemorrhoids with Perianal or Perineal Sepsis

Perianal Abscess or Fistula-in-ano

It is usually accepted that treatment of haemorrhoids is better avoided in the presence of ano-rectal sepsis, until the sepsis has been treated.

Perineal Infections

Haemorrhoidal surgery in patients with perineal skin conditions is said to be associated with an increased risk of developing postoperative infections (Neri et al., 1996).

Haemorrhoids with Systemic Comorbidity

Coagulopathy

Anticoagulant drugs. Conservative management of haemorrhoidal symptoms, or treatment of grade 1-to-2 haemorrhoids with infrared coagulation is preferable, as this carries a smaller risk of bleeding than phenol injection or rubber banding (Walker et al., 1990). Clotting abnormalities should be corrected prior to elective haemorrhoidectomy.

Haemophilia. Conservative management or treatment by injection sclerotherapy after factor VIII administration are the best options. Infrared coagulation may also be useful for treating haemorrhoidal symptoms in these patients, as it does not cause bleeding or tissue sloughing (Walker et al., 1990). Haemorrhoidectomy in haemophiliac patients should be reserved for those with severe bleeding necessitating frequent blood transfusions that cannot be controlled by other treatments. The availability of clotting factor VIII concentrates has made surgical procedures safer in haemophiliac patients (Rudowski, 1981). However, 10–15% of haemophiliac patients develop factor VIII inhibitors (Murali & Jager, 1987; Orangio & Lucas, 1989), and this may increase the risk of postoperative bleeding – especially from a haemorrhoidectomy wound that is healing by secondary intention.

Portal Hypertension

Ano-rectal varices are engorged rectal vessels that are present in up to 70% of patients with portal hypertension and may cause rectal bleeding (Naveau et al., 1991; Kozarek et al., 1991). They should be differentiated from bleeding haemorrhoids, either by rectoscopy or mesenteric angiography (Hsieh et al., 1986). Direct communication of haemorrhoidal vessels with the systemic venous system has not been demonstrated (Thomson, 1975; Bernstein, 1983) and, contrary to expectation, haemorrhoids do not occur more frequently in patients with portal hypertension compared to the general population (Jacobs et al., 1980; Hosking et al., 1989; Wang et al., 1991). Rectal varices should be treated by inferior mesenteric artery embolisation, transjugular intrahepatic portosystemic shunt (TIPS) or portasystemic shunt (Fantin et al., 1996). The preferred treatment of haemorrhoids in patients with portal hypertension is either injection sclerotherapy or rubber banding. Haemorrhoidectomy is better avoided in patients with portal hypertension because of the coagulopathy-associated risks of bleeding (Weinshel et al., 1986).

Immunosupression

Management of haemorrhoidal symptoms in immunodeficient patients should take account of the severity of immunodeficiency rather than its cause (Primrose & Giles, 1995). Immunosupression predisposes to postoperative infections despite antibiotic prophylaxis, and postoperative morbidity and mortality do not correlate with antibiotic use

(Moesgaard & Lykkegaard-Nielsen, 1989). Haemorrhoidal symptoms in patients with mild to moderate immunodeficiency can be treated by photocoagulation or injection sclerotherapy, but management based on conservative measures is preferable with severe immunodeficiency. Rubber band ligation may result in necrosis or even Fournier's gangrene, and immunocompromised patients who have undergone haemorrhoidal banding should be advised to seek urgent advice if they develop persistent anal pain, fever or urinary dysfunction (Scarpa et al., 1988; Shemesh et al., 1987; Buchmann & Seefeld, 1989). Haemorrhoidectomy is better avoided in immunodeficient patients, but may be justified in patients with mild immunodeficiency and severe haemorrhoidal symptoms. There is no evidence that bowel preparation prior to haemorrhoidectomy in these patients reduces complications despite suggestion that it may be advantageous (Keighley & Williams, 1999).

Leukaemia or lymphoma. Haemorrhoidal symptoms may develop in patients being treated for haematological or lymphatic malignancy, and anal lymphomatous or leukaemic lesions may be confused with haemorrhoidal disease. Conservative management of haemorrhoidal symptoms to allow treatment of the haematological disease is preferable (Musa et al., 1975). Examination under anaesthetic may be required where anal lesions are very painful. The risks of haemorrhoidectomy are poor wound healing, bleeding, and perirectal infection, which carries a high (78%) mortality in this group of patients (Barnes et al., 1984). Excision biopsy of painful nodular haemorrhoids is occasionally necessary, but where possible should be deferred until the malignancy is in remission.

HIV. Ano-rectal disease is the most frequent reason for referral of patients with HIV to the general surgeon (Miles et al., 1990), and approximately 50% of these patients require surgical treatment (Wexner et al., 1986). In a cohort of 68 AIDS patients (Allen-Mersh, 1992), the most common anal conditions were warts (37%), ulcers (25%), sepsis (10%), neoplasia (13%) and haemorrhoidal disease (15%). It should be remembered that infections such as herpes simplex virus (HSV) or warts, and neoplasms such as human papilloma virus-associated squamous cell carcinoma may produce haemorrhoidal symptoms. Anal wound healing is retarded where the CD4 count is less than 50-cells/μL (Lord, 1997), and healing is delayed after haemorrhoidectomy in patients with HIV disease (Morandi et al., 1999). The management of haemorrhoids in HIV patients is similar to that in non-infected patients and retrospective data suggest that HIV status should not alter indications for surgical management (Hewitt et al., 1996). However, HIV patients should receive anti-retroviral therapy to maximise the CD4 count and reduce viral load before haemorrhoidectomy, and haemorrhoidectomy is probably unhelpful in HIV patients with CD4 counts below 100-cells/μL. The duration of survival after surgical treatment of HIV infected patients with haemorrhoidal symptoms justifies surgical treatment (Burke et al., 1991).

Tuberculosis. Patients with active pulmonary or intestinal tuberculosis infection who develop haemorrhoidal symptoms should not be treated by haemorrhoidectomy, since tuberculous infection may spread to involve the anal wounds.

Pregnancy

Haemorrhoidal enlargement occurs after the second trimester of pregnancy because of raised intra-abdominal pressure causing pelvic venous engorgement and congestion of the anal venous plexus. This is exacerbated by constipation in up to 38% of pregnant women (Calhoun, 1992), and the general hormone-induced venous dilatation of pregnancy. Pre-existing haemorrhoidal symptoms are also likely to worsen. Preventative measures against constipation should be employed throughout the pregnancy and constipation should be treated. Topical anaesthetics can relieve pain, and the patient should be reassured that the haemorrhoids usually decrease in size in the puerperium with a reduction in discomfort. Bleeding is not usually sufficient to cause iron-deficiency anaemia. If conservative measures fail then the patient can be safely and effectively treated by injection sclerotherapy with 5% phenol in almond oil or by elastic band ligation (Simmons, 1972). Short-term treatment with flavonoids, which are pigments derived from citrus fruits that reduce inflammation and increase venous tone, has been shown to be an effective and acceptable alternative form of treatment (Buckshee et al., 1997). Infrared photocoagulation of haemorrhoids has also been reported in pregnancy without complication (Medich & Fazio, 1995). If the haemorrhoids prolapse, thrombose or become inflamed, they should be treated initially with analgesics and cold compresses. The clot in a thrombosed pile can be evacuated by incising the affected vein under local anaesthetic providing instant pain relief.

If symptoms fail to subside, haemorrhoidectomy during pregnancy may occasionally be justified. As general anaesthesia may affect the baby (Brodsky et al., 1980), local anaesthesia is preferable. Closed excisional haemorrhoidectomy under local anaesthesia (Khubchandani et al., 1972) has been reported as safe and effective (Saleeby et al., 1991). Occasionally, haemorrhoids prolapse after delivery and their immediate replacement usually fails because the stretched anal sphincter cannot hold them. The haemorrhoids then thrombose, causing discomfort in the early puerperium. Good results have been reported with haemorrhoidal surgery in the immediate post-partum period – with rapid wound healing secondary to hormonal changes and the increased elasticity within pelvic tissues (Ruiz-Moreno, 1970; Schottler et al., 1973) at this stage after childbirth. Patients should be warned that future pregnancies may cause new haemorrhoids to develop.

Haemorrhoidal Symptoms in Patients with Anal Abnormalities

Anal Fissure

Increased anal sphincter pressure is thought to have a causal role in the pathogenesis of anal fissure. Therefore, a reduction of sphincter tone by lateral sphincterotomy or topical spasmolytics such as glyceryl trinitrate (Loder et al., 1994) may constitute a simple and effective means of treating both conditions simultaneously (Delco & Sonnenberg, 1998). Haemorrhoidectomy performed at the same time as internal sphincterotomy does not increase postoperative complications (Leong et al., 1994). Direct current coagulation of haemorrhoids associated with anal fissure has been reported as effective (Machicado et al., 1997).

Abnormal Anal Sphincter Pressure, Lax Pelvic Floor or Rectocele

Patients with haemorrhoidal symptoms have higher anal sphincter pressures in comparison with no symptom controls (Arabi et al., 1977; el-Gendi & Abdel-Baky, 1986; Read et al., 1983) and these are reduced after haemorrhoidectomy (Read et al., 1982). It has been suggested that haemorrhoids in patients with high anal sphincteric pressures are best treated by anal dilatation and that in all other patients rubber-band ligation is the treatment of choice (Keighley et al., 1979).

It should be remembered that patients with abnormal perineal descent and pudendal neuropathy may have associated haemorrhoidal prolapse. Haemorrhoidectomy may exacerbate incontinence in these patients by removing haemorrhoids which act as anal cushions to close the anal canal and assist continence (Bruck et al., 1988).

Rectocele can contribute to the formation of haemorrhoids in female patients (Redding, 1973; Pitchford, 1967). Coexistent symptomatic low rectocele and haemorrhoids can be successfully treated by transrectal repair (Sullivan et al., 1968) of the rectocele and simultaneous haemorrhoidectomy (Sehapayak, 1985; Khubchandani et al., 1983). This reduces the risk of infection and recto-vaginal fistula that is encountered in the alternative combined transvaginal and anal operation. It also avoids the problem of redundant anterior rectal mucosa that remains after a transvaginal repair (Marks, 1967). However, the disadvantage of a transrectal approach is the inability to repair an associated cystocele and/or enterocele. Haemorrhoidectomy without repair of associated rectocele has a high risk of disrupting normal defecation (Heslop, 1987), precipitating the need for the patient to insert a finger in the vagina at defecation. Heslop studied a series of 15 patients with small asymptomatic rectoceles and associated haemorrhoids. Four patients underwent successful haemorrhoidectomy followed by a separate second stage colpoperineorraphy. A combined colpoperineorraphy and haemorrhoidectomy successfully treated eight patients (Heslop, 1987).

Constipation and Straining

Patients with haemorrhoids do not have constipation more frequently than control subjects without haemorrhoids (Johanson & Sonnenberg, 1994). In fact, diseases associated with diarrhoea are the most common comorbid condition in patients with haemorrhoids (Delco & Sonnenberg, 1998). Several studies have shown that straining at stool is an important precipitating factor (Burkitt, 1972; Hancock, 1977). Treatment should be directed towards correcting any irregular bowel habit before surgical treatment, because a patient who is accustomed to passing a liquid stool or habitually uses purgatives to liquefy the motions may develop anal stenosis.

Old Age

Haemorrhoidal disease may develop in elderly men secondary to abdominal straining from bladder outflow obstruction. Treatment of the bladder outflow obstruction can resolve the haemorrhoidal symptoms (Akande & Esho, 1989). As mentioned above, haemorrhoidectomy can lead to faecal soiling and incontinence where the pelvic floor is weakened, and care must be taken in elderly females to ensure that the pelvic floor is adequate before undertaking haemorrhoidectomy.

Sexual Habits

In a study of 260 homosexual men, haemorrhoids were found to occur with unusual frequency in association with other ano-rectal conditions termed the gay bowel syndrome (Kazal et al., 1976). Pre-existing anal sphincter damage from anoreceptive intercourse may be further impaired by subsequent ano-rectal surgery and therefore conservative treatment for haemorrhoidal disease is usually preferable.

EDITORIAL COMMENT

Professor Allen-Mersh has an international reputation for experience with the treatment of haemorrhoids in patients with co-morbidity from colo-rectal diseases, and has published extensively on the subject of AIDS. The Editor saw many patients with haemorrhoids who also suffered from colitis or Crohn's disease, but very few who had AIDS. In the Editor's experience, the activity of colitis of Crohn's disease was most accurately assessed by a mucosal biopsy, and that reliance on symptoms or visual appearances could be misleading. Both sclerotherapy and surgery can by risky in cases with active inflammatory bowel disease, especially phenol injections, which can result in extensive mucosal sloughing and severe secondary haemorrhage: the Editor had personal experience of two such cases. Surgeons contemplating surgical intervention should follow the guidance of experts such as Professor Allen-Mersh, but the patient's symptoms should be severe enough to justify the extra surgical risks involved, even when the patient's disease is quiescent.

References and Further Reading

Akande B, Esho JO (1989) Relationship between haemorrhoids and prostatism: results of a prospective study. Eur Urol 16(5):333–4

Allen-Mersh T (1992) Ano-rectal problems in AIDS patients. In: Cochrane J, Wastell C, (eds) The Impact of HIV on Surgical Practice. The Royal College of Surgeons of England, London, pp 48–50

Arabi Y, Alexander-Williams J, Keighley MR (1977) Anal pressures in hemorrhoids and anal fissure. Am J Surg 134(5):608–10

Barnes SG, Sattler FR, Ballard JO (1984) Perirectal infections in acute leukemia. Improved survival after incision and debridement. Ann Intern Med 100(4):515–8

Bernstein WC (1983) What are hemorrhoids and what is their relationship to the portal venous system? Dis Colon Rectum 26(12):829–34

Brodsky JB, Cohen EN, Brown BW, Jr., Wu ML, Whitcher C (1980) Surgery during pregnancy and fetal outcome. Am J Obstet Gynecol 138(8):1165–7

Bruck CE, Lubowski DZ, King DW (1988) Do patients with haemorrhoids have pelvic floor denervation? Int J Colorectal Dis 3(4):210–4

Buchmann P, Seefeld U (1989) Rubber band ligation for piles can be disastrous in HIV-positive patients. Int J Colorectal Dis 4(1):57–8

Buckshee K, Takkar D, Aggarwal N (1997) Micronized flavonoid therapy in internal hemorrhoids of pregnancy. Int J Gynaecol Obstet 57(2):145–51

Burke EC, Orloff SL, Freise CE, Macho JR, Schecter WP (1991) Wound healing after ano-rectal surgery in human immunodeficiency virus-infected patients. Arch Surg 126(10):1267–70; discussion 1270–1

Burkitt DP (1972). Varicose veins, deep vein thrombosis, and haemorrhoids: epidemiology and suggested aetiology. BMJ 2(813):556–61

Calhoun BC (1992) Gastrointestinal disorders in pregnancy. Obstet Gynecol Clin North Am 19(4):733–44

Creve U, Hubens A (1979) The effect of Lord's procedure on anal pressure. Dis Colon Rectum 22(7):483–5

de Dombal FT, Watts JM, Watkinson G, Goligher JC (1966) Incidence and management of ano-rectal abscess, fistula and fissure, in patients with ulcerative colitis. Dis Colon Rectum 9(3):201–6

Delco F, Sonnenberg A (1998) Associations between hemorrhoids and other diagnoses. Dis Colon Rectum 41(12):1534–41; discussion 1541–2

Deutsch AA, Moshkovitz M, Nudelman I, Dinari G, Reiss R (1987) Anal pressure measurements in the study of hemorrhoid etiology and their relation to treatment. Dis Colon Rectum 30(11):855–7

el-Gendi MA, Abdel-Baky N (1986) Ano-rectal pressure in patients with symptomatic hemorrhoids. Dis Colon Rectum 29(6):388–91

Fantin AC, Zala G, Risti B, Debatin JF, Schopke W, Meyenberger C (1996) Bleeding ano-rectal varices: successful treatment with transjugular intrahepatic portosystemic shunting (TIPS). Gut 38(6):932–5

Hancock BD (1977) Internal sphincter and the nature of haemorrhoids. Gut 18(8):651–5

Hancock BD, Smith K (1975) The internal sphincter and Lord's procedure for haemorrhoids. Br J Surg 62(10):833–6

Heslop JH (1987) Piles and rectoceles. Aust N Z J Surg 57(12):935–8

Hewitt WR, Sokol TP, Fleshner PR (1996) Should HIV status alter indications for hemorrhoidectomy? Dis Colon Rectum 39(6): 615–8

Hosking SW, Smart HL, Johnson AG, Triger DR (1989) Ano-rectal varices, haemorrhoids, and portal hypertension. Lancet 1(8634):349–52

Hsieh JS, Huang CJ, Huang YS, Huang TJ (1986) Demonstration of rectal varices by transhepatic inferior mesenteric venography. Dis Colon Rectum 29(7):459–61

Jacobs DM, Bubrick MP, Onstad GR, Hitchcock CR (1980) The relationship of hemorrhoids to portal hypertension. Dis Colon Rectum 23(8):567–9

Jeffery PJ, Parks AG, Ritchie JK (1977) Treatment of haemorrhoids in patients with inflammatory bowel disease. Lancet 1(8021): 1084–5

Johanson JF (1997) Association of hemorrhoidal disease with diarrheal disorders: potential pathogenic relationship? Dis Colon Rectum 40(2):215–9; discussion 219–21

Johanson JF, Sonnenberg A (1994). Constipation is not a risk factor for hemorrhoids: a case-control study of potential etiological agents. Am J Gastroenterol 89(11):1981–6

Kazal HL, Sohn N, Carrasco JI, Robilotti JG, Delaney WE (1976). The gay bowel syndrome: clinico-pathologic correlation in 260 cases. Ann Clin Lab Sci 6(2):184–92

Keddie N (1980) Ano-rectal manifestations of inflammatory bowel disease. Hosp Med 24(4):294, 296–7

Keighley M, Williams N (1999) Haemorrhoidal disease. In: Keighley M, Williams N, (eds). Surgery of the Anus, Rectum and Colon. Second Ed. W.B. Saunders, London, pp 351–427

Keighley MR, Buchmann P, Minervini S, Arabi Y, Alexander-Williams J (1979) Prospective trials of minor surgical procedures and high-fibre diet for haemorrhoids. BMJ 2(6196):967–9

Khubchandani IT, Sheets JA, Stasik JJ, Hakki AR (1983) Endorectal repair of rectocele. Dis Colon Rectum 26(12):792–6

Khubchandani IT, Trimpi HD, Sheets JA (1972) Closed hemorrhoidectomy with local anesthesia. Surg Gynecol Obstet 135(6):955–7

Kozarek RA, Botoman VA, Bredfeldt JE, Roach JM, Patterson DJ, Ball TJ (1991) Portal colopathy: prospective study of colonoscopy in patients with portal hypertension. Gastroenterology 101(5):1192–7

Leong AF, Husain MJ, Seow-Choen F, Goh HS (1994) Performing internal sphincterotomy with other ano-rectal procedures. Dis Colon Rectum 37(11):1130–2

Lockhart-Mummery HE (1965) Pathologic lesions of the anal region associated in Crohn's disease. Dis Colon Rectum 8(6):399–401

Loder PB, Kamm MA, Nicholls RJ, Phillips RK (1994) "Reversible chemical sphincterotomy" by local application of glyceryl trinitrate. Br J Surg 81(9):1386–9

Lord RV (1997) Ano-rectal surgery in patients infected with human immunodeficiency virus: factors associated with delayed wound healing. Ann Surg 226(1):92–9

Machicado GA, Cheng S, Jensen DM (1997) Resolution of chronic anal fissures after treatment of contiguous internal hemorrhoids with direct current probe [see comments]. Gastrointest Endosc 45(2):157–62

Marks MM (1967) The rectal side of the rectocele. Dis Colon Rectum 10(5):387–8

Medich DS, Fazio VW (1995) Hemorrhoids, anal fissure, and carcinoma of the colon, rectum, and anus during pregnancy. Surg Clin North Am 75(1):77–88

Miles AJ, Mellor CH, Gazzard B, Allen-Mersh TG, Wastell C (1990) Surgical management of ano-rectal disease in HIV-positive homosexuals. Br J Surg 77(8):869–71

Moesgaard F, Lykkegaard-Nielsen M (1989) Preoperative cell-mediated immunity and duration of antibiotic prophylaxis in relation to postoperative infectious complications. A controlled trial in biliary, gastroduodenal and colorectal surgery. Acta Chir Scand 155(4-5):281–6

Morandi E, Merlini D, Salvaggio A, Foschi D, Trabucchi E (1999) Prospective study of healing time after hemorrhoidectomy: influence of HIV infection, acquired immunodeficiency syndrome, and anal wound infection. Dis Colon Rectum 42(9):1140–4

Murali MS, Jager RM (1987) Hemorrhoidectomy in a hemophiliac with factor VIII inhibitors. Indiana Med 80(4):332–3

Musa MB, Katakkar SB, Khaliq A (1975) Ano-rectal and perianal complications of hematologic malignant neoplasms. Can J Surg 18(6):579–83

Naveau S, Bedossa P, Poynard T, Mory B, Chaput JC (1991) Portal hypertensive colopathy. A new entity. Dig Dis Sci 36(12): 1774–81

Neri I, Bardazzi F, Marzaduri S, Patrizi A (1996) Perianal streptococcal dermatitis in adults. Br J Dermatol 135(5): 796–8

Orangio GR, Lucas GW (1989) Management of hemophilia in colon and rectal surgery. Report of a patient with factor VIII inhibitors and review of the literature. Dis Colon Rectum 32(10):878–83

Pitchford CA (1967) Rectocele: a cause of ano-rectal pathologic changes in women. Dis Colon Rectum 10(6):464–6

Primrose J, Giles G (1995) Surgical immunology and organ transplantation. In: Cuchieri A, Giles G, Moossa A, (eds) Essential Surgical Practice. Third Ed. Butterworth-Heinemann, Oxford, pp 132–4

Rankin GB, Watts HD, Melnyk CS, Kelley ML, Jr (1979) National cooperative Crohn's disease study: extraintestinal manifestations and perianal complications. Gastroenterology 77(4 Pt 2):914–20

Read MG, Read NW, Haynes WG, Donnelly TC, Johnson AG (1982) A prospective study of the effect of haemorrhoidectomy on sphincter function and faecal continence. Br J Surg 69(7): 396–8

Read NW, Bartolo DC, Read MG, Hall J, Haynes WG, Johnson AG (1983) Differences in ano-rectal manometry between patients with haemorrhoids and patients with descending perineum syndrome: implications for management. Br J Surg 70(11): 656–9

Redding MD (1973) The relaxed perineum and ano-rectal disease revisited. Dis Colon Rectum 16(1):56–8

Rudowski WJ (1981) Blood transfusion today – "artificial blood" tomorrow. Aust N Z J Surg 51(6):618–22

Ruiz-Moreno F (1970) Surgery in the puerperium for painful ano-rectal disorders. Proc R Soc Med 63(Suppl):102–3

Saleeby RG, Jr., Rosen L, Stasik JJ, Riether RD, Sheets J, Khubchandani IT (1991) Hemorrhoidectomy during pregnancy: risk or relief? Dis Colon Rectum 34(3):260–1

Scarpa FJ, Hillis W, Sabetta JR (1988) Pelvic cellulitis: a life-threatening complication of hemorrhoidal banding. Surgery 103(3):383–5

Schottler JL, Balcos EG, Goldberg SM (1973) Postpartum hemorrhoidectomy. Dis Colon Rectum 16(5):395–6

Schouten WR, van Vroonhoven TJ (1986) Lateral internal sphincterotomy in the treatment of hemorrhoids. A clinical and manometric study. Dis Colon Rectum 29(12):869–72

Sehapayak S (1985). Transrectal repair of rectocele: an extended armamentarium of colorectal surgeons. A report of 355 cases. Dis Colon Rectum 28(6):422–33

Shemesh EI, Kodner IJ, Fry RD, Neufeld DM (1987) Severe complication of rubber band ligation of internal hemorrhoids. Dis Colon Rectum 30(3):199–200

Simmons SC (1972) Ano-rectal disorders in pregnancy. Proc R Soc Med 65(3):286

Sullivan ES, Leaverton GH, Hardwick CE (1968) Transrectal perineal repair: an adjunct to improved function after ano-rectal surgery. Dis Colon Rectum 11(2):106–14

Thomson WH (1975) The nature of haemorrhoids. Br J Surg 62(7):542–52

Walker AJ, Leicester RJ, Nicholls RJ, Mann CV (1990) A prospective study of infrared coagulation, injection and rubber band ligation in the treatment of haemorrhoids. Int J Colorectal Dis 5(2):113–6

Wang TF, Lee FY, Tsai YT, Lee SD, Wang SS, Hsia HC, et al. (1992) Relationship of portal pressure, ano-rectal varices and hemorrhoids in cirrhotic patients. J Hepatol 15(1-2): 170–3

Weinshel E, Chen W, Falkenstein DB, Kessler R, Raicht RF (1986) Hemorrhoids or rectal varices: defining the cause of massive rectal hemorrhage in patients with portal hypertension. Gastroenterology 90(3):744–7

Wexner SD, Smithy WB, Milsom JW, Dailey TH (1986) The surgical management of ano-rectal diseases in AIDS and pre-AIDS patients. Dis Colon Rectum 29(11):719–23

Williams DR, Coller JA, Corman ML, Nugent FW, Veidenheimer MC (1981) Anal complications in Crohn's disease. Dis Colon Rectum 24(1):22–4

Wolkomir AF, Luchtefeld MA (1993) Surgery for symptomatic hemorrhoids and anal fissures in Crohn's disease. Dis Colon Rectum 36(6):545–7

24 Day Case Haemorrhoidectomy

Charles V. Mann (Surgery) and M.C. Berthoud (Anaesthesia)

Surgical Considerations

General Background

The desirability of day case haemorrhoidectomy is not universally agreed. It has strong advocates, not least *governments and hospital managers*, who wish to reduce costs, and *insurance companies*, who wish to decrease payments and increase profit margins. But such agencies do not have to face reproachful patients or endure litigation, nor do they have to be available on a 24-hour basis in case complications develop in the home. Apart from the economic benefits, it is not possible to show that haemorrhoidectomies performed as day cases have significant advantages over in-hospital operations, and the risks may be greater. However, in some societies and for some individuals the costs of surgery are so high, or the pressures on hospital beds are so great, that the demand for day case surgery becomes overwhelming. The problem then becomes one of providing the best circumstances for its employment. Probably the most important consideration is the provision of safe anaesthesia and this is given particular attention in this chapter. However, other factors are also relevant, as follows.

Social Considerations

Day case surgery is limited to major towns and cities that generate enough patients to justify the provision of special units and other necessary facilities.

It is unwise to offer day case haemorrhoidectomy to a patient who lives more than a short journey (e.g., one hour) away, and ambulance transport should be available if it is necessary. The possibility for private transportation by car or taxi is a great advantage, and it is not by chance that day case surgery has its maximum provision in advanced societies in which home facilities, including a car, are generally good.

Other requirements that are so desirable that they are virtual necessities include: 1) the patient should not live alone, 2) a domestic telephone is available, 3) the domicile has suitable washing and toilet facilities, 4) home visits by professionally qualified personnel can be arranged as necessary, and 5) the support of the family physician is obtained. This last is an important point as it will prevent a possibly hostile response to an unexpected emergency call, and the family physician can be an invaluable aid for the provision of safe home supervision.

Day case haemorrhoidectomy should never be offered to an isolated individual who is beyond immediate medical help.

Payment

If day case surgery is performed in a private facility, it is wise to make certain of payment, preferably at conclusion of the operation before the patient leaves for home. Dilatory or non-payment are a particular risk when the patient is confident about his cure and is at home.

Selection of Patients

Small non-prolapsing haemorrhoids do not need an operation. Large prolapsing haemorrhoids which are accompanied by many skin tags are inappropriate because the wounds are large and unsuitable for suturing; large open anal wounds cannot be properly dressed on an outpatient basis.

The ideal case is moderate-sized prolapsing haemorrhoids (Stage 2) which are too large for banding, but even Stage 3 haemorrhoids can be considered if no skin tags are present and skin bridges are easily preserved if an open operation is used.

Care must be taken to obtain all the relevant information regarding drug use and previous anaesthetic exposure. It is essential to learn of any allergic or other untoward reactions. Any history of substance abuse is a contraindication to day case surgery unless the period of abstinence is long (years).

Nervous or hysterical patients and older men with an enlarged prostate (i.e., liable to postoperative retention of urine) should not be offered day case haemorrhoidectomy.

Consent

Written consent for the procedure must be obtained. Particular care should be taken to make absolutely certain that the patient understands what he may expect during the postoperative period, and how the care of his needs will be provided. Patients must be furnished with a contact number that they can connect to on a 24-hour basis in the event of complications.

Preoperative Preparation

All patients should have their stools softened and their bowels regulated prior to surgery. It is an advantage if the patient arrives in the operating theatre with an empty rectum. This can be obtained by a same-day stimulatory suppository (Bisacodyl (Dulcolax) 10 mg) or a mini-enema (Fletcher's phosphate enema).

The patient is advised to avoid all food and drink for at least six hours prior to the operation and to arrive in the unit at least one hour before the time of surgery.

The Unit

This should be purpose-built and have medical (especially anaesthetic) and nursing staff trained for its requirements. The unit should be administered by competent managers who oversee every aspect of its functions, including the supply and servicing of equipment. Recovery trolleys and beds should be available on-site, and resuscitation equipment provided. Wall or ceiling supplies of oxygen and anaesthetic gases are valuable, and should be instantly serviceable in an emergency. Unconscious patients must be supervised and monitored by skilled staff.

If the unit is dedicated to proctological procedures (or has a large proportion of such cases), washing and toilet facilities must be sufficient to cater to the extra needs for such requirements. Because it is desirable for the patients to be accompanied by a relative or friend, some seating and catering opportunities should be provided for them.

Security of the unit is of prime importance. Medical records, on-site drugs and valuable equipment (which includes computers and video display units) must be adequately protected against unauthorised use and theft.

The view that day case haemorrhoidectomy can be performed occasionally in a minor surgery facility attached to a ward or an Outpatient Department must be condemned. Such practise does not fulfil the requirements for safe and expertly performed surgery.

Technical Aspects

The technique of haemorrhoidectomy does not need to be altered in any major way because it is being carried out as a day case. However, having stated this important general rule, certain modifications may be advantageous, as follows. 1) The closed (Ferguson) technique is preferable to the open (St. Marks) technique. 2) Haemostasis is of overriding importance, and extra time should be allowed for it to be achieved. 3) Anal sphincter tone should be preserved, consistent with anaesthetic requirements, which take precedence. Spinal and caudal anaesthesia both lower anal sphincter tone and may also promote postoperative retention of urine; whenever possible intravenous, regional bloc, or local infiltration anaesthesia are preferred, either alone or in combination with a light inhalation anaesthetic (see also Day case Anaesthesia). Normal anal sphincter tone is a protection against postoperative haemorrhage. 4) Anal dilatation as a prelude to dissection should be avoided whenever possible as it diminishes postoperative sphincter tone and promotes bleeding. 5) No intra-anal pack or dressing should be inserted at the end of the operation. They should be unnecessary if proper haemostasis has been achieved and their subsequent removal may cause difficulties; they also increase the incidence of postoperative retention of urine. 6) If the surgeon's technique does not include ligation of the haemorrhoid pedicle, this can be a possible safeguard against delayed secondary haemorrhage; some experts regard it as an unnecessary step, especially if dissection is carried out by diathermy or laser. 7) The operation should be unhurried and not be performed under time constraints.

Postoperative Care

Two requirements dominate postoperative care: one, the need for adequate pain relief and two, the need to restore normal defaecation as soon as possible.

Pain Relief

This is discussed also in the section on day case anaesthesia. Oral preparations, for obvious practical reasons, are the mainstay of pain relief after day case surgery. The patient should be advised to take the analgesic drugs by frequent small doses rather than by long-spaced large doses; also, the tablets should be taken before pain has reached its zenith. Useful preparations are diclofenac sodium (75–150 mg) and sublingual buprenorphine (200 mg every eight hours).

Topically applied local anaesthetic preparations are not recommended as they are usually ineffective (the wound is mainly within the anal canal) and have the risk of allergic side effects, which may be severe.

Metronidazole (400 mg BD) has been reported as reducing postoperative pain, and the author recommends its use for five days after surgery.

Frequent hot soaks provide substantial benefits, not only for relief of pain, but also to diminish other sources of anal discomfort, such as soiling and pruritus. Each bath can be followed by application of a bland cream to the anal verge; Nivea; E45; and zinc oxide cream are all suitable. In between soaks, the patient's clothing is protected by a pad of soft absorbent material (sanitary pad, gamgee or cotton wool) held in place by a T-bandage or elastic briefs.

While the patients are using analgesic drugs, especially strong ones, they must be warned that these can have side effects such as dizziness and drowsiness; these may increase risks of falls, with associated injuries, and the patients need to take precautions against them (e.g., by avoiding stairways or slippery floors), and, at first, may need assistance when getting in and out of bed or bath.

Re-establishing Defaecation

Most patients fear their initial defaecatory actions after any haemorrhoid operation, and day case procedures are no exception. Patients who are unusually nervous may benefit from a small dose of tranquilliser (e.g., Valium 2.0 mg twice daily) until defaecation has occurred; use of anxiolytics or tranquillisers can also reduce the need for analgesic drugs.

An early defaecation can be obtained by prescribing laxatives, and magnesium sulphate (5–10 gm in a tumblerful of water, twice daily) is an excellent preparation for this purpose, as it not only causes increased large bowel motor activity but also makes the stool soft or watery. If a closed haemorrhoidectomy has been performed (as it probably will have been), the prevention of hard stools is necessary to avoid breaking down the suture lines. Once defaecation has been established, a stool softener (e.g., Lactulose 15 ml twice daily) can be substituted for the laxative. Before the patients are discharged, they should be taking a normal diet with a bran or isphagula supplement, and be experiencing regular defaecation of normal stools. If postoperative defaecation is delayed for 72 hours, defaecation should be jump-started by an enema – ideally a mini-enema. If the patient presents unusual problems for establishing defaecation, admission to hospital is advised for a digital examination and possible resort to a rectal washout under anaesthesia. Short-term use of an anal dilator may also be necessary for some patients, but this is rare.

Provided early restoration of defaecation is achieved, early digital examination is not routinely required after day case haemorrhoidectomy, but should always be performed when the wounds have healed, prior to discharge.

Because care after day case surgery is given on an outpatient basis, the best way to make sure that it is both adequate and focussed is to provide a postoperative take-home packet containing all the medicines and dressings which will be needed for at least the first few days. Written instructions must be given for the use of all drugs provided. Analgesics should be prescribed in the form of individual doses, with a total provision that does not exceed a safe limit as patients are inclined to take more painkillers than they are advised, sometimes dangerously so.

The patients should be warned against two symptoms – bleeding and retention of urine. Slight bleeding can be expected, if not in all patients, then at least in a considerable number: they should know about this in advance, as this will prevent unnecessary alarm. Profuse bleeding is a potentially dangerous complication, and patients should contact the hospital immediately for re-admission. Retention of urine requires catheter relief, and this is done most appropriately in the hospital emergency room, but can also be done at home. On the first occasion, once the bladder has been emptied, the catheter is removed, and the patient can return home, provided no other problems are present; any further episodes of retention merit treatment by an indwelling catheter, for which the patient should be admitted and any further management carried out (e.g., by surgery for an enlarged prostate).

In addition to their pack containing all necessary drugs, dressings and documents, the patients should have in their possession a discharge operation note for their home carers, a 24-hour telephone number that they can use to contact the clinic for advice and emergency treatment, and the date they should return to the clinic. The first follow-up visit should be an early one, preferably within one or two days, and never longer than seven days if a haemorrhoidectomy has been performed. The final visit usually occurs between three and six weeks postoperatively, and depends upon the nature and circumstances of the individual operation, as well as the surgeon's choice. At the final visit, a digital examination is recommended but other investigations, such as proctoscopy and rectoscopy, are unnecessary if they have been carried out preoperatively.

Summary

The provision of safe and satisfactory day case surgery for haemorrhoids depends on four essentials, which are 1) dedicated units, 2) proper selection of patients, 3) excellent anaesthesia, and 4) good surgical technique. The results of the operations should not fall below those obtained by in-hospital treatment. A closed haemorrhoidectomy is preferred over an open technique. Anaesthetic considerations, discussed separately, are the ones that must be fully satisfied if the safety of day case haemorrhoidectomy is to be guaranteed. The main pressure for day surgery in the treatment of haemorrhoids is economic. The search for the cheapest provision of haemorrhoid surgery, of which day case haemorrhoidectomy is one, must not be allowed to diminish surgical standards. Postoperative care should be of high quality, with inbuilt provision for pain relief and bowel regulation. Day case surgery makes high demands not only on the surgeon's experience and technique, but also on his management and leadership skills. The provision of safe anaesthesia plays a more important part than surgery in preventing mortality. but also plays an essential role in preventing complications and reducing pain.

Day Case Anaesthesia for Haemorrhoidectomy

Day case surgery offers a number of advantages for both patients and healthcare providers. For the patient it means early return home, less chance of hospital-acquired infections, less chance of cancellation and a shorter waiting time. For healthcare providers, day surgery should increase efficiency and improve overall value for money. In England, most haemorrhoidectomy operations are still performed on an inpatient basis, patients staying an average of 3.2 days (Hospital Episode Statistics, 1999). This is despite the recommendation of the British Association of Day Surgery in 1999, that 50% of haemorrhoidectomies could be done with same-day discharge. Doctors and patients worry about postoperative pain and bowel function. These anxieties, together with the postoperative complications of bleeding and urinary retention, are what pose the main challenges to successful same-day discharge after haemorrhoidectomy.

Preoperative Selection and Preparation

Not all patients are suitable for day case anaesthesia. Success depends on careful patient selection and preparation. In assessing the patient for day case anaesthesia, both domestic and medical criteria are to be considered. In particular, patients undergoing haemorrhoidectomy need adequate social support.

They must have a responsible adult who will accompany them home and care for them over the following 24 hours. They must have access to a telephone and adequate bathroom facilities, and they should not live more than one hour's journey from the hospital. Medically, patients should be in good general health, with a reasonable exercise tolerance. They should be either ASA grades (American Society of Anesthesiologists, 1963) I or II, but stable ASA grade III patients may occasionally be considered. Patients with symptoms of bladder outlet obstruction will have a significant chance of developing urinary retention post haemorrhoidectomy and should be offered inpatient surgery. Day surgery patients should have no previous or family history of an adverse anaesthetic outcome, and they should have no major mobility problems. Obese patients pose special anaesthetic difficulties, especially if surgery is undertaken in lithotomy or in the prone jack-knife position. The Royal College of Surgeons recommends (RCS, 1992) that patients who have a body mass index (BMI) of over 30 are not suitable for day case surgery. However, these criteria were published some time ago, and with an impeccable anaesthetic technique, it is possible to care safely for patients who are obese. Many day case units now accept patients with BMIs of up to 35, so long as they are otherwise fit. Age as such is no bar to day surgery providing all the criteria outlined above are fulfilled. Detailed locally agreed guidelines for the selection process should be freely available and should be regularly reviewed.

Once the patient has been selected for same-day haemorrhoidectomy, they will require careful preparation. All patients undergoing general anaesthesia or regional block should be starved. Evidence suggests that patients should not eat for six hours before anaesthesia, but that it is safe to drink clear fluids for up to three hours before induction. It is important that haemorrhoidectomy patients do not become too dehydrated before surgery, as studies have shown that the use of peri-operative intravascular fluid is associated with postoperative urinary retention, and that this complication can be minimised by avoiding a drip (Hoff et al., 1994). Preoperative bowel preparation should also be considered. Various methods have been tried, including Lactulose two-to-four days preoperatively, sodium picosulphate with magnesium sulphate (Picolax) the day before surgery, and sodium citrate–sodium lauryl sulphoacetate–soritol (Microlax) enema on admission to the day unit. Lactulose softens the stool and has been shown to lessen postoperative defaecatory pain. Picolax has been used in the day case context, most commonly prior to colonoscopy. Patients find it difficult to cope with its effects at home, and it is associated with considerable dehydration. It is also important to consider other premedications at this time. These should be prescribed according to guidelines and may include preemptive analgesia and anti-emetics. Sedative premedication is rarely used in day surgery.

Providing adequate and accurate written and verbal information is very important to the success of day case surgery. This is particularly true for patients undergoing haemorrhoidectomy, who will be expected to take a lot of responsibility for their own welfare. Every effort should be made to ensure that both the patient and the home carer understand what to expect at each stage of treatment. If difficulties are experienced in communication, the patient should be looked after in hospital. Written patient information should contain a simple description of the operation, the risks and side effects accompanying the operation, clear descriptions of the preparation needed, a description of the aftercare, including a description of the various stages of recovery and how long recovery might take. Patients should be given a realistic idea of the amount of pain they could expect, but this should not be exaggerated and should be accompanied by reassuring instructions on how it can be controlled. Many bodies offer guidelines and assistance in developing effective patient information: the Patient Information Forum and The Plain English Campaign, to name but two. Information of varying quality is also available on the Internet.

Increasingly, preoperative assessment and preparation is being undertaken by nursing staff. With training and ready anaesthetic back up, nurses can perform this task extremely well. It is helpful for the assessment nurse to have a good understanding of the surgical procedure, so that the patients receive an authoritative and efficient service. By far the most time consuming part of assessment is the information giving, but allowing sufficient time to do this well helps to prevent problems on the day of surgery and after discharge.

Anaesthetic Technique

Several anaesthetic techniques have been described for haemorrhoidectomy and almost all of them have been used in day cases. Peri-anal surgery requires a relatively deep anaesthetic or, at least, profound analgesia. General anaesthesia combined with a local anaesthetic block is most commonly used. Any general anaesthetic technique should also provide a rapid smooth onset in the absence of sedative premedication, and rapid recovery with minimal side effects. If, however, insufficient time has elapsed for any local anaesthetic block to work, too-rapid emergence from anaesthesia will be a disadvantage. Propofol is the induction agent of choice for day case anaesthesia, partly for its good recovery characteristics, but mainly for its lack of emetic effect. Propofol is also the ideal induction agent for the smooth placement of a laryngeal mask. Any of the modern volatile agents are acceptable. The short-acting opioids Alfentanil and Fentanyl are both acceptable, as it is very unlikely that they will have a lasting effect on bowel function. Total intravenous anaesthesia is being increasingly used in day surgery. Remifentanil, a potent opioid, is rapidly metabolised by non-specific esterases in the body, and so allows profound analgesia during anaesthesia with minimal postoperative nausea and vomiting. As it quickly disappears from the body, patients are left with severe pain unless an effective block is present. Remifentanil also depresses the respiration such that patients often need respiratory assistance.

In an attempt to overcome many of the side effects of general anaesthesia, a variety of regional techniques have been described. With the widespread use of pencil-point, small-gauge needles, spinal anaesthesia can be used safely and successfully in the day case context. Spinal anaesthesia is associated with a high incidence of urinary retention after perianal surgery, so it is probably best reserved for those patients who have a positive indication for it: for example, those with difficult intubation, respiratory disease, or the risk of reflux. Kamphuis and others (1998) examined bladder function during spinal anaesthesia with lignocaine and bupivacaine, and found that spontaneous voiding did not occur until segmentary sensory analgesia had regressed to the third sacral segment and that this occurred much earlier in the patients receiving lignocaine. This study employed much larger doses of local anaesthetic, especially lignocaine, than those needed to achieve the saddle block required for haemorrhoidectomy. Although spinal lignocaine has a shorter duration of action than bupivacaine, there are some potential hazards associated with its use. Questions have been raised regarding the potential for neurotoxicity of single-dose 5% lignocaine. Pollock and others (1999) have shown a similar incidence of transient neurological symptoms using much lower concentrations of spinal lignocaine. Low-concentration subarachnoid lignocaine is hypobaric. Bodily and others (1992) assessed the characteristics of 0.5% lignocaine in day case patients having perirectal surgery in the jack-knife position, and found it to provide effective anaesthesia. While the patients were head down, the anaesthesia was confined to the lower dermatomes, but when patients were placed head up in recovery the sensory level of anaesthesia rose two-to-six dermatomes. This effect was observed for up to 60 minutes after injection. Perianal infiltration with local anaesthetic before incision prolongs postoperative analgesia after haemorrhoidectomy with lignocaine spinal anaesthesia (Morisaki et al., 1996).

There have been many papers describing the use of caudal analgesia for haemorrhoidectomy for inpatients using either local anaesthetic or opioids, but with variable results reported. Information is lacking for day cases. Caudal analgesia with local anaesthetic will interrupt sacral nerve transmission and the risk of urinary retention is likely to be similar to that for subarachnoid block. Caudal morphine slows bowel function.

Local anaesthetic infiltration alone has been used for haemorrhoidectomy. The injection is painful, both because the needle passes through the sensitive perianal skin, and because the local anaesthetic itself causes pain before it blocks. Nivatongs (1982) describes a less painful technique of local anaesthesia for ano-rectal surgery and Ho et al. (2000) have described how prior application of topical local anaesthetic (EMLA; Astra, Sodertalje, Sweden) (a eutectic mixture of lignocaine and prilocaine) reduces the pain of local infiltration.

Positioning

Although the prone jack-knife position may offer some surgical advantages, it has several anaesthetic disadvantages. These are especially relevant to day case patients. General anaesthesia is always started when the patient is supine, the patient then being turned prone, either from a trolley or directly on the operating table. Pronating an anaesthetized patient requires a level of anaesthesia that preserves autonomic function, and sufficient relaxation to allow gentle positioning and to avoid coughing. Patients who are prone must have a secure airway. These factors are achieved most reliably by intubation and ventilation. Patients undergoing perianal surgery in the lithotomy position do not normally require intubation. In addition, safely turning any patient prone requires at least five people, as well as the anaesthetist: two turners at the patient's side and one at the patient's feet, and two receivers. Great care in positioning is necessary as damage to the eyes, face, neck, brachial plexus, breasts, pelvis and genitalia have all been reported. All this adds to the complexity of the anaesthetic technique, to the time taken to perform the operation, and to the numbers of personnel needed in theatre. Venous air embolism, although uncommon, has been documented in prone patients, when the level of the incision is 10 cm or more above the heart. In the UK, the lithotomy position is preferred.

Analgesia

The biggest challenge to day case haemorrhoidectomy is the successful management of postoperative pain. Pain after haemorrhoidectomy fluctuates. It is worse immediately after surgery particularly with the first bowel action, and may then decrease around the third or fourth postoperative day. Pain that occurs while the patient is still in hospital can be controlled relatively easily using a combination of intra-operative local anaesthetic infiltration and systemic analgesics. Pain with defecation is lessened by the use of stool softeners before, and for up to two weeks after, surgery. Pain associated with anal sphincter spasm is reduced by avoiding anal canal dressings, and may be helped by chemical sympathectomy. (Carapeti et al. (1998) described the use of 0.2% glyceryltrinitrate ointment topically to the anal margin three times a day for two weeks.) Any analgesia prescribed should be taken regularly and not on a "demand" basis.

Non-steroidal anti-inflammatory drugs (NSAID) have had a long-established record in day case surgery. They act by inhibiting prostaglandin synthetase, leading to a decrease in the release of the pain mediators and inflammation in the tissues. They have a number of contraindications that should be sought before they are prescribed. Patients who are intolerant of NSAID may need planned hospital admission. The use of ketorolac injected into the anal sphincter at the time of surgery, followed by oral administration, has been described in day cases (O'Donovan et al., 1994). When this regime was compared to morphine, the analgesia achieved was similar, but patient satisfaction was higher as there were fewer opioid-related side effects. However, this is an unlicensed use of ketorolac, and there is no evidence that this mode of administration is superior to any other. It is now well established that NSAID act at central as well as peripheral sites. This favours systemic administration. Regular oral sodium diclofenac has been shown to be successful in controlling post-haemorrhoidectomy pain in day cases (Hunt et al., 1999). Regular paracetamol is very helpful as an adjunct to any NSAID prescribed, but is unlikely to be sufficient alone.

Opiates have also been used for post-haemorrhoidectomy pain. They are associated with increased postoperative nausea and vomiting, constipation, and urinary retention, and should not be routinely prescribed in this situation. Tramadol is an opioid-like analgesic with a mode of action that is not fully understood. It has weak affinity for μ receptors and yet is completely antagonized by naloxone. It enhances monoaminergic transmission, and is contraindicated in patients on monoamine oxidase inhibiters. It has the same analgesic potency as pethidine and can be administered orally, intravenously or intramuscularly. As it has less constipating effect and is less respiratory depressant than morphine, it may be more suitable than other opioids for patients who have undergone day case perianal surgery. It can cause nausea and dizziness and should therefore perhaps be reserved for treating breakthrough pain when regular NSAID have failed.

Metronidazole has been shown to reduce pain and analgesic consumption after haemorrhoidectomy, especially on the fifth, sixth and seventh postoperative day (Carapeti et al., 1998). It also results in the patient returning sooner to normal activity. The mechanism postulated for this is a reduction in bacterial colonization, secondary infection, inflammation and swelling. Carapeti and his team gave their patients 400 mg three times a day for seven days. Good general hygiene and regular warm bathing also helps to moderate the pain.

Postoperative Discharge and Follow Up

Patients undergoing perianal surgery may need several hours' hospitalisation before discharge, and are best operated on during a morning session. They are more comfortable if they are recovered supine rather than in a reclining chair. Precise discharge criteria vary between units, the most contentious factor being whether the patient should have passed urine or not. Patients who have emptied their bladder before surgery and are then fluid restricted may take several hours to pass urine. Hoff and others (1994) described 190 patients who underwent day case haemorrhoidectomy, following which the nursing staff were instructed not to inquire excessively about urination, nor were the patients required to urinate before leaving the hospital. Only one of these patients experienced urinary retention. All these patients had had general anaesthesia or sedation. Patients receiving a spinal or caudal are at much higher risk of urinary retention and should be required to void before discharge.

Patients who have returned home after haemorrhoidectomy must be offered as much support from the day case unit team as possible. Some of the research projects in this area attribute their success in part to home follow-up by research nurses for anything up to 10 days postoperatively. While this is currently beyond the capability of most day case units, the approach may well be needed, as more complex procedures are increasingly undertaken with same-day discharge. The minimum support the patient will need are access to round-the-clock telephone advice from an appropriately trained individual for the whole period of recovery, together with some district nurse visits in the early period. It is also helpful for the day case unit team to contact the patient on the day after surgery, to check that he or she continues to understand their medications, dressings and bathing. This simple phone call offers reassurance to the patient, pre-empts many problems and allows collection of audit data relating to minor morbidity that would not be otherwise available to the hospital team.

Day case haemorrhoidectomy is possible but requires attention to detail, a meticulous anaesthetic and surgical technique, and a carefully selected, well-informed patient who has adequate social support. Complications will occur, even in the best hands, and the patient must be capable of recognizing these, and of seeking and receiving early assistance. Successful outcome in day case surgery depends on recognizing those patients who need a planned hospital admission, just as much as it does on correct management of the day case patients themselves.

EDITORIAL COMMENT

The fact that day case surgery is possible does not make it desirable for all cases and in all circumstances. Anaesthesia must be of the highest standard possible, and the Editor tried to ensure that his anaesthetist had a special interest in this area.

In the Editor's opinion, a closed haemorrhoidectomy should be the preferred choice for day case surgery.

Day case haemorrhoidectomy places additional responsibilities on both surgeon and anaesthetist, and also for the provision of proper home-care staff and facilities. Unless these are properly provided for, and each patient is fully aware of, and supportive for, a day case operation, it is wiser for a surgeon not to become involved in day-case surgery for haemorrhoids. To an uncommitted observer, the main beneficiaries from this form of surgical treatment are hospital managers (reduced expenditure and shorter waiting lists) and healthcare providers (reduced costs for insurance companies and state treasuries).

References and Further Reading

American Society of Anesthesiologists (1963) New classification of physical status. Anesthesiology 24:111

Bodily MN, Carpenter RL, Owens BD (1992) Lidocaine 0.5% spinal anaesthesia: a hypobaric solution for short-stay perirectal surgery. Can J Anaesth 39(8):770–3

Carapeti EA, Kamm MA, McDonald PJ, Phillips RK (1998) Double-blind randomized controlled trial of effect of metronidazole on pain after day case haemorrhoidectomy. Lancet 17;351(9097):169–72

Ho KS, Eu KW, Heah SM, Seow-Choen F, Chan YW (2000) Randomized clinical trial of haemorrhoidectomy under a mixture of local anaesthesia versus general anaesthesia. Br J Surg 87:410–13

Hoff SD, Bailey HR, Butts DR, Max E, Smith KW, Zamora LF, Skakun GB (1994) Ambulatory surgical hemorrhoidectomy – a solution to postoperative urinary retention? Dis Colon Rectum 37(12):1242–4

Hospital Episode Statistics by the Department of Health. Year April 1998 to March 1999 for NHS patients.

Hunt L, Luck AJ, Rudkin G, Hewitt PJ (1999) Day case haemorrhoidectomy. Br J Surg 86(2):255–8

Kamphuis ET, Ionescu TI, Kuipers PW, de Gier J, van Venrooij GE, Boon TA (1998) Recovery of storage and emptying functions of the urinary bladder after spinal anesthesia with lidocaine and with bupivacaine in men. Anesthesiology 88(2):310–6

Morisaki H, Masuda J, Fukushima K, Iwao Y, Suzuki K, Matsushima M (1996) Wound infiltration with lidocaine prolongs

postoperative analgesia after haemorrhoidectomy with spinal anaesthesia. Can J Anaesth 43(9):914–8
Nivatvongs S (1982) An improved technique of local anesthesia for ano-rectal surgery. Dis Colon Rectum 25:259–60
O'Donovan S, Ferrara A, Larach S, Williamson P (1994) Intraoperative use of Toradol facilitates outpatient hemorrhoidectomy. Dis Colon Rectum 37(8):793–9
Pollock JE, Liu SS, Neal JM, Stephenson CA (1999) Dilution of spinal lidocaine does not alter the incidence of transient neurologic symptoms. Anesthesiology 90(2):445–50
Royal College of Surgeons of England (1992) Revised Guidelines for Day Case Surgery

Landmarks in the History of Haemorrhoids

Charles V. Mann

Date	Comments
c.2250 BC	Code of Hammurabi, King of Babylon. Description of anal symptoms (haemorrhoids).
1700 BC	Edwin Smith papyrus. Use of astringent lotions for anal symptoms (haemorrhoids?) described.
1552 BC	Eber papyrus. The most complete record of Egyptian medicine. Haemorrhoid remedies described.
460–375 BC	Writings of Hippocrates. Treatment of haemorrhoids by cautery and excision described.
Old Testament, Samuel 5:9	Philistines punished with "emerods".
Old Testament Samuel 5:12	After the Ark moved to Ekron, perpetrators smitten by "emerods".
25 BC–AD 50	Celsus describes ligature of piles with flax.
AD 130–200	Galen recommended conservative management of piles (laxatives, ointments, leeches) and regarded bleeding as therapeutic. Also described, however, use of a tight thread to induce sloughing of haemorrhoids.
Sometime between the fourth & sixth century AD	Susruta Samhita described use of treatment by clamp and cautery method.
10th century AD	El-Zahrawy described treatment by application of cautery irons.
10th–5th century AD	Treatment in Byzantine medical practise by twisting pile, application of ligature to its base, followed by amputation. A "modern" approach that lapsed for many centuries.

Date	Comments
1307–1370	John of Arderne published his treatise on the treatment of fistula and haemorrhoids, and the use of clysters (enemas).
1660–1734	Georg Ernst Stahl published a classic work on the treatment of haemorrhoids.
1835	Foundation of St. Marks Hospital, London by Frederick Salmon for the treatment of anal diseases, especially fistula in ano and haemorrhoids.
1849	J.G. Maisonneuve described treatment by forceful anal dilation. Subsequently, this treatment was revived by P.H. Lord.
1935	Development of the classical method of open dissection and ligature at St. Marks Hospital by E.T.C. Milligan and C. Naughton Morgan.
1955	Development of a closed method of haemorrhoidectomy by A.G. Parks, London.
1960	The closed surgical method of treatment established by J.A. Ferguson and colleagues at Grand Rapids, Missouri.
1963	Invention of the method of rubber band ligation of haemorrhoids as an office procedure by J. Barron (USA). Method widely adopted thereafter.
1970	New methods for physical destruction of haemorrhoids developed (cryotherapy infrared thermocoagulation, diathermy, laser). Some still used.
1975	Use of anal dilatation advocated by P.H. Lord. Was not widely adopted but of historical importance. Classical studies by W.H.F. Thomson into the nature of haemorrhoids, and their development from anal cushions, which are normal structures.
1990	Day-case surgery initiated in special centres.

Index

D

E

O

P

R

S